DATE DUE

NO 30 99	AP 26 '04		
	MAY 19 2004		
AP 29 '99	NO 29 04		
	MY 17 '05		
MY 24 '99	JE 7 05		
AP 27 00	MY 23 06		
DE 7 '00	MY 16 '07		
AP 19 01	DE 5 08		
	JY 10 09		
MY 24 01			
AP 25 02			
MY 16 '02			
AU 7 '02			
DE 02			
AP 21 '03			
NO 25 03			

Waterborne Disease

To Hilary, Anthony and Jonathan

Waterborne Disease
Epidemiology and Ecology

PAUL R. HUNTER
Public Health Laboratory Service, Chester, UK

JOHN WILEY & SONS

Chichester • New York • Weinheim • Brisbane • Singapore • Toronto

Copyright © 1997 by John Wiley & Sons Ltd,
Baffins Lane, Chichester,
PO19 1UD, England

243 779777
43 779777

customer service enquiries):
.co.uk.
on http://www.wiley.co.uk
or http://www.wiley.com

Commissioned in the UK on behalf of John Wiley & Sons, Ltd by Medi-Tech. Publications, Storrington, West Sussex RH20 4HH, UK

Other Wiley Editorial Offices

John Wiley & Sons, Inc., 605 Third Avenue,
New York, NY 10158-0012, USA

WILEY-VCH Verlag GmbH, Pappelallee 3,
D-69469 Weinheim, Germany

Jacaranda Wiley Ltd, 33 Park Road, Milton,
Queensland 4064, Australia

John Wiley & Sons (Asia) Pte Ltd, 2 Clementi Loop #02-01,
Jin Xing Distripark, Singapore 129809

John Wiley & Sons (Canada) Ltd, 22 Worcester Road,
Rexdale, Ontario M9W 1L1, Canada

Library of Congress Cataloging-in-Publication Data

Hunter, Paul R.
    Waterborne disease : epidemiology and ecology / Paul R. Hunter.
        p.   cm.
    Includes bibliographical references and index.
    ISBN 0-471-96646-0 (alk. paper)
    1. Waterborne infection–Epidemiology.   I. Title.
    RA642.W3H86   1997
    614.4'3–dc21   97–17109
                                                            CIP

British Library Cataloguing in Publication Data

A catalogue record for this book is available from the British Library

ISBN 0-471-96646-0

Typeset in 10/12pt Times from author's disks by Mayhew Typesetting, Rhayader, Powys
Printed and bound in Great Britain by Biddles Ltd, Guildford and King's Lynn

This book is printed on acid-free paper responsibly manufactured from sustainable forestation, for which at least two trees are planted for each one used for paper production.

Contents

Acknowledgements

There are quite a few people to whom I owe a debt of gratitude for their help in producing this book. I am especially grateful to Sue Horwood of Medi-Tech Publications for suggesting I write the book and encouraging John Wiley & Sons to publish it. Of the people at Wiley, I would most like to thank Phil Bishop, Geoff Reynolds and Alexa Dugan for answering my many questions.

I must also thank my colleagues at Chester Public Health Laboratory for their support, especially Maria Davies, Dorothy Williams and Christine Hill for filling in thousands of library request forms; also the library staff at Central Public Health Laboratory, London for all the photocopying of articles.

Finally, I would also like to thank my wife Hilary and my sons Anthony and Jonathan for putting up with me, especially as I was rushing to complete the book.

Introduction

The figures are enormous. In 1990 an estimated 5.3 billion people were living on this planet. That figure is set to rise to 6.2 billion in 2000 and 8.5 billion in 2025. However, that latter figure is open to considerable uncertainty and could be anything between 7.9 and 9.1 billion. All of these individuals will need a supply of safe water.

The prospects do not look good. Already 38% of countries report that more than half of their population does not have access to safe, adequate water supplies (Huttly 1990). Much of the projected increase in population will occur in Africa and South America, which already suffer from severe population pressure on their available water supplies. In these countries any improvement in supply is likely to be soon swamped by additional population pressures.

The worldwide incidence of waterborne disease can only be guessed at. It has been estimated that in 1989 there were some 1.362 billion episodes of diarrhoea in children under five worldwide (Huttly 1990). About 4.9 million of these children will have died as a result of these episodes of diarrhoea. Even if only a third of diarrhoea cases are waterborne, over 1.5 million children under five will have died in that year as a result of a waterborne diarrhoea. Figure I.1 shows the distribution of countries reporting inadequate supplies to their rural populations.

Even in otherwise affluent countries like the US and UK waterborne disease is not unknown. Outbreaks of waterborne disease still occur and there is evidence of sporadic disease linked to water risk factors. Morris and Levin (1995) estimated that, each year in the US, 560 000 (range 520 000–690 000) people suffer a moderate to severe waterborne infection and that 7 100 000 (range 400 000–27 000 000) suffer from a mild to moderate waterborne infection. They estimated an annual mortality of some 1200. These estimates were based on several assumptions that are open to significant debate.

OUTLINE OF THE BOOK

One of the problems in the investigation and management of waterborne disease is that a wide range of specialist knowledge is required by the outbreak team. Consequently, engineers and environmentalists, scientists, epidemiologists and doctors find themselves sitting round the same table. Not unexpectedly, this

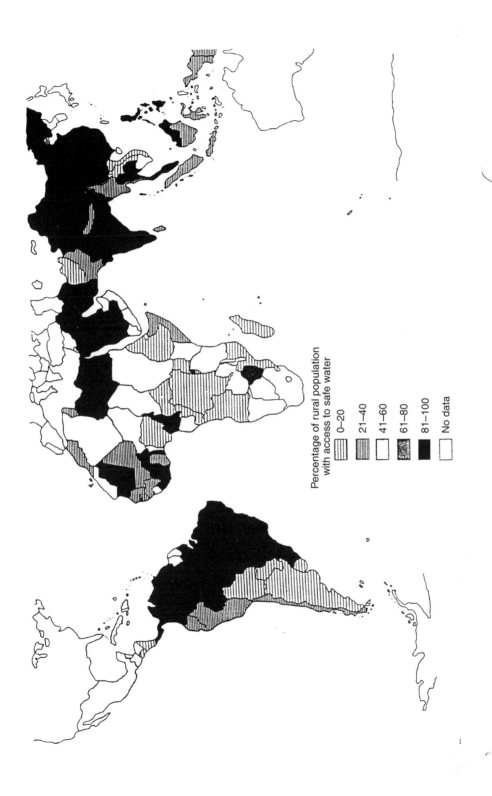

Percentage of rural population
with access to safe water

0–20
21–40
41–60
61–80
81–100
No data

causes difficulties in communication. Engineers and water scientists may not understand the epidemiological methods used by the medical personnel, who in turn may have only a hazy understanding of the engineering aspects of water treatment processes. Consequently, Chapters 1 and 2 aim to level the playing field by giving a basic introduction, firstly to epidemiological methods and then to water supply technology. Both chapters are intended to provide a basic vocabulary to aid understanding of subsequent chapters. It is hoped that the chapter on epidemiology will enable the reader to look more critically at the conclusions made by epidemiological studies.

Chapters 3 and 4 aim to provide some indication of the magnitude of the problem by reference to some national surveillance data and to prospective epidemiological studies.

Chapters 5–30 cover specific waterborne microbial diseases classified according to the genus of the infecting agent. As one proceeds through the book there is a general decline in the size of the pathogen or parasite under discussion. We start with the larger multicellular parasites, then discuss unicellular eukaryotic parasites, then bacteria and finally viruses.

Although the exact layout of each chapter varies slightly, I have tried to keep to a rough format. In most chapters I start with a thumbnail sketch of the biology of the organism, how it causes disease and the nature and severity of the illness that it causes. I also mention available treatments and diagnostic methods. A rather fuller description, with references, is given of the methods available for detecting the organism in water samples. The main sections of each chapter are the discussions of ecology and epidemiology. The sections on ecology discuss reports on the distribution and survival of each organism in the environment. Generally, I have restricted my discussion of this topic to work published between about 1986 and 1995. There has been a major change in the sensitivity of the technology available for detecting many pathogens in water samples over that time, so that the results of early studies are, in many cases, no longer valid. In the sections on epidemiology I have tried to give a fairly comprehensive survey of the English language literature from 1970 to 1995. Usually, I have discussed outbreak reports first, separating the discussion of drinking water outbreaks from that of recreational water outbreaks. Finally, I discuss prospective studies of sporadic disease. In these discussions, the main emphasis is given to understanding the mechanisms of transmission of the disease, how the outbreak teams arrived at the conclusions they did and what went wrong with the engineering that precipitated the outbreak.

The final three chapters are mainly concerned with the health effects of chemical pollution of drinking water. Because the epidemiological methods

---

Figure I.1 (*previous page*) Reported percentages of the rural population of various countries having access to safe water in 1988. Reproduced from Cairncross and Feachem (1993) *Environmental Health Engineering in the Tropics*, 2nd edn, by permission of John Wiley & Sons.

vary somewhat between the three areas, one chapter deals with water and cancer, one with water and pregnancy and the other with everything else. Within each chapter I have classified the discussion by chemical group.

INFORMATION SOURCES AND SEARCH STRATEGIES

To assess the value of any review, the reader needs to know how comprehensive and unbiased was the literature search. Information for this book was obtained from a mix of textbooks and MEDLINE searches.

General information in the first parts of Chapters 5–30 is derived largely from standard textbooks. Such information is rarely referenced in the text except where I have quoted the textbook writer. The four main texts that I used are *Principles and Practice of Infectious Diseases* (Mandell, Douglas and Bennett 1995), *Manson's Tropical Diseases* (Cook 1996), *Topley and Wilson's Principles of Bacteriology, Virology and Immunity*, Vol. 2 (Parker and Duerden 1990) and *Manual of Clinical Microbiology* (Murray *et al.* 1995). In my view, these four textbooks are the most comprehensive and well written in their fields of any English language book I have read. I also used *Infectious Disease* (Bannister, Begg and Gillespie 1996) and *Microbiological Methods* (Collins, Lyne and Grange 1995).

As a source in Chapters 31–33, I obtained chemical information from *Handbook of Poisoning* by Dreisbach and Robertson (1987) and *Guidelines for Drinking Water Quality*, Vol. 2 (World Health Organization 1984).

All other sources are referred to in the text or mentioned in the Further Reading sections. I have only really reviewed English language papers, largely because of their availability and because I knew I could understand the language of most of them. English language papers make up some 4500 of the 6500 papers identified under the epidemiology search.

For epidemiology searches I used DATASTAR, the online service, as text word searches, search title, abstract and descriptors. My search strategy used the text words '(WATER OR WATERS OR WATERBORNE OR SWIMMING) AND (EPIDEMIOLOGY OR OUTBREAK) AND HUMAN'. For papers on the isolation of pathogens and their ecology I used MEDLINE on CD-ROM and searched under each organism, limiting my search to papers on the isolation and detection subheading. For papers on chemical and radiological disease, I also searched the MEDLINE CD-ROM under adverse effects for WATER SUPPLY, WATER POLLUTION and WATER POLLUTANTS.

I am aware that not all possible papers were included. I offer my most sincere apologies to any person who feels slighted by my not referring to their work. I know that the first part of a book most scientists look at is the references, to see if they have been quoted. The other area of concern is whether the conclusions derived from reading each chapter could be biased by the selection of papers. This is certainly a possibility, because my search methods may not have detected epidemiological reports that included water as a possible risk factor, found it to be not significant and did not refer to that in the summary. This is likely to be more of a problem in the chapters on chemical disease and the reader should bear this in mind.

1   An Introduction to the Science and Art of Epidemiology

Epidemiology is the science and the study of the occurrence, distribution and control of disease in populations. Thus, the focus of study is groups of people rather than the individual. Epidemiology is the science that underpins most medical research. Unfortunately, any chapter on epidemiological methodology in a book of this size can do no more than scratch the surface of what is, to me, one of the more fascinating branches of medicine.

This chapter has three parts: (i) a brief discussion of risk and epidemiological proof, (ii) a basic introduction to the methodological tools of epidemiology and (iii) a model approach to the investigation of waterborne outbreaks.

RISK AND EPIDEMIOLOGICAL PROOF IN RELATION TO ENVIRONMENTAL CAUSATION OF DISEASE

Unfortunately, epidemiology does not offer simple absolute proofs of disease causation. At best we are left with the demonstration of statistically significant associations between environmental factors and disease. At the heart of these demonstrations is the concept of risk, and differences in risk between exposed and non-exposed populations.

Before progressing further we should define some epidemiological terms:

- Incidence: the number of new cases occurring in a certain population during a defined time period. If 1 in 20 people in an African village acquires schistosomiasis in a given year, the incidence rate would be 5% per year.
- Prevalence: the number of cases of a disease in a defined population at a particular point in time. If a medical team visits the village on a particular day and finds that 45 out of 100 people are excreting schistosome eggs the prevalence rate is 45%. More than a few authors on waterborne disease confuse incidence and prevalence.
- Absolute risk: the incidence of the disease. Unfortunately, the absolute risk of a disease in a population does not tell us much about the effect of a

Table 1.1 A comparison between cholera incidence rates in individuals drinking water from tube wells and other sources. Adapted from Levine *et al.* (1976a)

	Person-years	No. of cases	Annual incidence rate
Tubewell users	3725 (a)	53 (b)	1.42 (b×100/a)
Tubewell non-users	1545 (c)	13 (d)	0.84 (d×100/c)

Relative risk 1.7 (b×c)/(a×d)

Table 1.2 Consumption of a single brand of mineral water in a case-control study of an outbreak of hepatitis A. Adapted from Stroffolini *et al.* (1990)

Mineral water consumption	Cases	Controls
Yes	26 (a)	31 (b)
No	15 (c)	45 (d)

$$\text{Odds ratio} = \frac{\text{Odds of drinking water if ill}}{\text{Odds of drinking water if control}}$$

$$\text{Odds ratio} = \frac{a/c}{b/d} = ad/cb = 26 \times 45/(15 \times 31) = 2.5$$

particular environmental factor in the causation of disease. If an outbreak of hepatitis has been caused by drinking water and by shellfish, then knowing that the incidence in a town is 12% does not give any idea about the relative importance of the two factors. To estimate the importance of environmental factors we need to know the risk to exposed and non-exposed populations.

- Relative risk (RR): the ratio between the incidence of a disease in those members of a population exposed to a possible risk factor and the incidence in non-exposed individuals. Table 1.1 gives an example of how relative risk is calculated. Usually 95% confidence intervals are given.

- Odds ratio (OR): the ratio between the probability that someone with disease has experience of the potential environmental factor and the probability that someone without the disease has experience of the same factor (Table 1.2). In case-control studies relative risk cannot be calculated because cases and controls are not a random samples of the entire population. As with relative risk, the 95% confidence intervals are usually given.

- Statistical significance: this is presented in one of two ways. The most common way is to calculate the *p* value, an indication of the probability of the observed difference could have arisen by chance. In older studies particularly, *p* values were calculated using a non-parametric statistical test such as the chi-squared test. The result was usually deemed to be significant if $p < 0.05$. Increasingly, statistical significance is demonstrated by the 95% confidence interval of either the relative risk (RR) or the odds ratio (OR). As these ratios are usually calculated from samples of the study population, they are subject to random variations due to sampling. More frequently, epidemiologists use confidence intervals (CI): 95% confidence intervals represent the range within which the real relative risk or odds ratio should lie 95% of times. A result is deemed to be significant if the range of the 95% confidence intervals of the odds ratio or relative risk does not include 1.0.

In the mid-1960s Bradford-Hill (1965), one of the world's most eminent epidemiologists and medical statisticians, suggested nine epidemiological criteria to be used in assessing whether an environmental factor was associated with human disease:

1 Strength of association
2 Consistency
3 Specificity of association
4 Temporality
5 Biological gradient
6 Plausibility
7 Coherence
8 Experiment
9 Analogy

These will be discussed in turn, using the example of schistosomiasis. The chapter on schistosomiasis gives more detail about the relevant epidemiological studies.

Strength of association

The strength of association criterion relates to the statistical significance of disease, as measured by relative risk, odds ratios or probability rates between exposed and non-exposed populations.

Consistency

This refers to whether the same association between an environmental factor and a disease has been reported by several authors studying different populations. The association between water contact and schistosomiasis in tropical countries is not in doubt, as so many studies have reported this association over the years.

Specificity of association

This criterion relates to whether a particular type of exposure leads to a particular disease. This is usually a much more difficult criterion to satisfy. Many diseases other than schistosomiasis can be caught by swimming in tropical lakes.

Temporality

Exposure to the suspect agent must precede disease. It is clearly important to distinguish between illness caused by contact with an environmental agent and the possibility that patients suffering from the disease seek out contact with the agent. People clearly acquire their schistosomiasis from water contact rather than seek out water contact to relieve the symptoms of schistosomiasis.

Biological gradient

The criterion of biological gradient suggests that there should be a relationship between the amount and duration of exposure to an environmental agent and the severity of disease or the probability of developing disease. Investigation of the amount of water drunk each day in outbreaks of drinking water related disease is the classic example of such dose–response relationships. Several studies have shown such a link between the frequency of water contact and the amount of immersion and the likelihood of schistosomal infection.

Plausibility

The association of the disease with an environmental factor must be plausible, given existing knowledge about the biology or toxicology of the disease agent. A water link for schistosomiasis is clearly highly plausible given our knowledge of the life cycle of the schistosome.

Coherence

The data from the study should not conflict with what is known about the biology of the disease. For example, a study suggesting a link between schistosomiasis and aerosols from cooling towers would lack coherence.

Experiment

Can the link be supported by experimental studies such as randomized trial or by those studies that investigate the impact of changes aimed at reducing contact with the causative agent? Treating water bodies to reduce snail populations as a control measure for schistosomiasis and then observing the impact on the health of local children is an example of such experiments.

Analogy

Is there another disease in man or animals that can be used to draw conclusions about the possibility of contact? The evidence in favour of cercarial dermatitis being due to avian schistosomes in temperate climates is made stronger because of the known association with cercarial dermatitis associated with schistosomiasis.

TYPES OF EPIDEMIOLOGICAL STUDY USED IN THE INVESTIGATION OF WATERBORNE DISEASE

A variety of epidemiological studies have been used to investigate the relationship between water and disease. The advantages and disadvantages of these various studies are discussed in the following subsections.

Descriptive studies

As the name suggests, descriptive epidemiological studies set out to describe the pattern of disease in a community. Although descriptive studies rarely prove disease associations, they are an essential starting point in the investigation of any outbreak or possible waterborne disease. Such studies help to generate hypotheses for further study.

The data used in descriptive studies may be derived from routine surveillance data such as death reports, notifications of infectious disease, laboratory reports or case finding exercises. The critical areas of interest are the temporal, geographic and demographic distribution of disease. Thus, these studies will collect data on the date-of-onset, place of residence, travel history, age, sex and food history of cases. Analysis is usually restricted to summarizing and presenting these data in tabular and graphical form.

Because descriptive studies frequently rely on routinely collected data, such data is often incomplete. For example, cases may not be recorded if individuals with disease do not present themselves to a doctor. Even if a case is identified, important demographic data may not be available. In such cases epidemiological surveys may be done.

One frequently used variant of a descriptive study is the ecological study. In an ecological study, one attempts to draw conclusions on disease causation by correlating incidence or prevalence rates for several communities with possible factors, such as the proportion drinking well-water or the proportion unemployed. However, ecological studies are, at their heart, flawed (Hennekens and

Buring 1987). They are unable to link individual exposure to individual disease risk. They are also unable to control for many effects of potentially confounding factors. Finally, because ecological studies rely on average exposure levels, they may mask more complex relationships between exposure and disease. Because of these limitations, no reliable conclusion can be drawn from them either way. As will be seen in later chapters, most of the studies that have suggested a relationship between cancer and water supplies have been ecological studies and, as such, any conclusions drawn are open to considerable doubt.

Surveys

Epidemiological surveys are a special form of descriptive study. Surveys seek to describe the characteristics of individuals in the population, including their personal attributes, their experience of a particular disease and their exposure to putative causal agents. Surveys can be done in a variety of ways: by interviewing people in their homes or workplaces, by telephone and by postal questionnaire. Usually it is uneconomic, and unnecessary, to interview all individuals in a population. In this case only a proportion of the population – a sample – is interviewed.

Samples can be selected in several ways. The easiest sampling technique is the random sample. Here random number tables are used to choose individuals from a list of all such people in a population. Examples of such lists in the UK are electoral registers, telephone directories and family doctors' lists of patients. Sometimes, it can be very difficult and time consuming to select names randomly from a register. In this case, a more convenient method is to select names at regular intervals from the list, say every tenth name on the electoral register or the first name on every page of the telephone directory. This is called a systematic sample.

Random sampling is not appropriate when the study is concerned with only a section of the population, such as children, women or agricultural workers. In this case one would chose a stratified sample. For example, a random search of doctors' lists could be restricted to certain age groups. Studies of the prevalence of schistosomiasis could be limited to children in a town. If social class is known to be significant then the random selection of individuals could be followed until the correct number of individuals from each social class has been recruited.

If one were interested in the prevalence of a disease in a region it would be costly to select a truly random sample. A more economic sampling method in this situation is cluster sampling. Here several villages may be randomly chosen for more detailed study. Sampling all members of a random sample of households is another type of cluster sampling.

Whatever the sampling method employed, the major problem with surveys is one of bias, particularly selection bias. Selection bias may arise in one of three ways. The first is due to the identification of the population. For example, using telephone directories as a source of names would exclude people who have no phone. This could have a significant effect on studies of any disease that tends to affect the poor and homeless. The second source of selection bias is deviation from the selection rules. If a field worker is selecting individuals randomly from a community, the selection process may be biased if volunteers were accepted, rather than a truly random sample. The third way in which a survey could be biased is if many of the originally selected individuals could not be traced or would not cooperate. For example, in a survey of diarrhoeal disease those individuals who have been recently ill may be more likely to participate than those who have not been ill. Alternatively, if a high proportion of people with diarrhoea is admitted to hospital they may not be available for interview in the community.

Cohort studies

A cohort study is a study of a group of individuals for whom exposure data are known. Typically for prospective cohort studies, the group is followed over time to see if they develop illness or not. Cohort studies are said to have several distinct advantages. Because individuals are selected before illness develops, the study allows the investigation of the temporal relationship between exposure and illness. Furthermore, provided that the cases are not lost to follow-up, selection should not be biased by whether or not the individual will develop illness. Cohort studies are good at investigating the effect of several potential causes. Relative risk is used to compare the incidence of disease between those exposed and those not exposed to a potential causative agent.

A second type of cohort study is of a group defined by their exposure to a risk factor, for example in the investigation of an outbreak of diarrhoea after a swimming pool party. The cohort would be all those who attended the party. This is a retrospective cohort study.   .

Case-control studies

Case-control studies are retrospective studies of events that preceded the onset of disease in a group of individuals. They seek to test hypotheses by comparing the incidence of a preceding event in those with disease (cases) with that in a group of individuals who do not appear to have disease (controls). The key to success in case-control studies is the correct definition of cases and the selection of controls.

In order to know whether a particular individual should be included in a case-control study as a case, one needs a clear definition of what a case should be. This case definition may include clinical, epidemiological and microbiological or other laboratory features. Case definition is discussed in more detail below. In many waterborne outbreaks, it is likely that all individuals who satisfy the case definition can be included in the case-control study. However, provided sufficient numbers can be recruited, only a sample of cases may need to be interviewed. When only a sample of cases is included in the study the sampling techniques available and their pitfalls are similar to those described above under 'Surveys'. Frequently used cluster sampling methods include using only cases presenting to hospital or cases living in selected villages.

The crucial point in case-control studies is that controls should be a random sample of the population from which the cases were selected. This is not as easy as it sounds. Traditionally, case-control studies were done on matched pairs. Matched controls were chosen to be similar to cases on certain matching criteria, such as age, sex and location of residence. The weakness with matching controls is that any effect that the matching criteria may have on disease causation can not then be tested.

If cases were taken from a subgroup of a population then controls should also be selected from that same subgroup. For example, if cases are selected from those presenting to hospital with a disease, one may use patients presenting to hospital with an unrelated illness as controls. In the situation where cases are cluster sampled from certain villages, the controls should be selected from the same villages. If all cases occur in children, then controls should also be children. Other ways of identifying controls include using family doctor or health authority lists of patients, asking cases to nominate controls from their local area and selecting controls in a semi-random way from telephone directories. Each of these methods has its problems, as discussed above. In my experience, many cases are unwilling to name individual controls. If the number of cases is small, it is often necessary to interview more controls than cases to increase statistical sensitivity.

Because one can not extrapolate from the results of a case-control study to the incidence of disease in the general population, odds ratios rather than relative risks are calculated.

Case-control studies have the advantage of being relatively quick and inexpensive compared to other some other designs of epidemiological study. They can also be used to examine several hypotheses. However, statistical association in a case-control study does not necessarily imply causation. Care should be taken if very many hypotheses are tested. If twenty variables are tested in a case-control study and a p value of less than 0.05 is taken as indicating significance, then it is highly probable that at least one variable will achieve statistical significance. Furthermore, if the variables are not truly independent of one another, then confounding variables may appear significant. These are some of the reasons why newer statistical techniques such as logistic regression analysis are becoming the favoured tools for analysing the results of analytical epidemiological studies.

Intervention studies

Rarely do epidemiologists get the opportunity to conduct experiments into the causation of disease. In the field of waterborne disease, the situations where this may arise include: (i) monitoring the effects on health of putting a new water supply into an area previously without one, (ii) giving some households additional water treatment facilities and (iii) temporarily stopping water supply or issuing a boil water notice during the investigation of a waterborne outbreak. When such opportunities arise, they offer unparalleled opportunities for studying the relationship between water supply and health or disease.

AN APPROACH TO THE INVESTIGATION AND CONTROL OF WATERBORNE OUTBREAKS

The investigation of waterborne outbreaks, or any outbreak, should follow a logical process, which will be broadly similar in each case:

1 Preparation for the outbreak
2 Detection of an outbreak
3 Confirmation that an outbreak is occurring
4 Description of the outbreak
5 Generation of a hypothesis as to the cause of the outbreak
6 Implementation of initial control measure
7 Testing the validity of the hypothesis
8 Implementation of further control measures, if necessary
9 Learning the lessons for the future

These steps are not always followed in a strict order. Often, different stages of the process are carried out at the same time. For example, the description and confirmation steps can happen at the same time. Hopefully, however, the preparation step will precede the others. Figure 1.1 gives an outline flow diagram of the stages in the investigation of an outbreak.

Preparation for an outbreak

The investigation of waterborne outbreaks is a skilled and complex activity that requires the bringing together of individuals from a variety of organizations and professional backgrounds. It is too late to decide who should be involved in the investigation of an outbreak when it is already happening. All relevant organizations and authorities must have formal outbreak plans. These plans must make explicit who is to manage the outbreak, who should be members of the outbreak team and what is expected of them. These outbreak plans need to be approved by all organizations and authorities that are likely

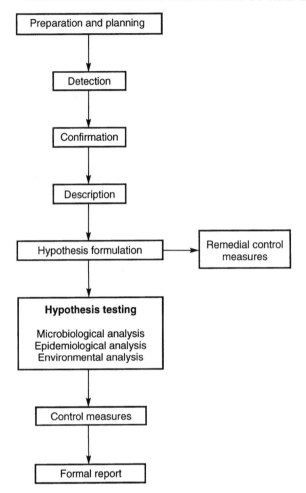

Figure 1.1 The stages in the investigation and control of a waterborne outbreak.

to be involved. It is not appropriate to have arguments over responsibilities in the full glare of publicity during an outbreak investigation.

Detection of an outbreak

The detection of an outbreak usually follows several steps. The first step is that individuals become ill and decide to visit their doctor or attend a hospital. The next step is that the doctor either makes a diagnosis or sends a specimen to a microbiology laboratory. The clinician may also decide to notify the relevant authority of the disease. Often the first person to identify an outbreak is the local medical microbiologist, who notices an increase in the laboratory diagnosis of certain diseases. The microbiologist may also notify the relevant public health authorities of the diagnosis of certain diseases or his suspicions of an outbreak. The public health department may be the first to identify a waterborne outbreak by seeing an increase in notifications by clinicians or microbiology laboratories.

This chain of events is not very efficient and it is likely that only a minority of waterborne outbreaks is ever diagnosed. Often people who are infected will not become ill or even if they do will not seek medical attention. Clinicians may not correctly diagnose the condition or, if they do, they may not take microbiological samples or ever notify the case. In my experience is it unlikely that a family or hospital doctor will ever see sufficient cases in an outbreak to realize that one is occurring. The microbiology laboratory may miss the diagnosis of individual patients by not performing the appropriate examinations. Many UK and US laboratories were still not examining faecal samples for cryptosporidiosis several years after the importance of this pathogen became clear. Even if the laboratory makes the correct diagnosis it may not report to the public health authorities or realize that this is part of an outbreak. Even if cases are notified to the public health authorities, outbreaks may be missed if the number of cases is small compared to the incidence of endemic disease in the community or if the outbreak is spread over more than one health authority area or country.

Rarely outbreaks may be identified because a water company is aware of some treatment failure or distribution failure and advises the public health authorities, who instigate prospective surveillance.

Outbreak confirmation

Before acting on the diagnosis of an outbreak it is important to consider whether the outbreak is real. Is the increase in cases an artefact as a result of increased testing or changes in reporting practices? Check that any micro-biological diagnoses are correct. Is the thing seen under the microscope really a *Cryptosporidium*? Have some family doctors suddenly realized that they have to notify a particular disease? Such confirmation should not take long but could save a lot of embarrassment. Once the outbreak is confirmed the outbreak team is called together.

Outbreak description

Outbreak description is the most important stage in the investigation of any waterborne outbreak (Palmer 1989). It should logically progress through several stages.

An explicit statement of the case definition is essential to know whether individual illnesses should be included in the outbreak. Case definitions may include a range of possible onset dates, clinical symptoms, geographical locations and microbiological results. Case definitions can be very broad or very narrow, to include either many possible cases or few. The broader the definition, the more cases will be identified, although many of these additional cases may not be related to the main outbreak. It is a matter of judgement how broad case definitions should be. A case definition does not have to be set in stone at this stage. It can and should change as new information becomes available.

Once a case definition has been agreed, case finding is the next step. For case definitions that include a microbiological diagnosis, the easiest way of identifying cases is to review microbiology laboratory results. A positive microbiological result will be very specific. However, relying on microbiological results will exclude those patients who have not had microbiology investigations taken. It is often necessary to encourage doctors to increase their sampling rate or to report all episodes of particular clinical syndromes. A frequent alternative is to develop more than one case definition, one of which includes microbiology data and one that relies exclusively on clinical features. These can be called confirmed cases and presumptive cases.

A basic set of data needs to be collected on every individual who satisfies the case definitions. As a minimum, this will include name, address, age, sex, date of onset, the results of microbiological examination and sufficient clinical information to prove that the individual satisfies the case definition. It is also usual to record place of work or schooling, a basic food or contact history and any travel history. This type of data may be collected by a trawling questionnaire, which asks a series of open questions covering activities during the period before the onset of illness. How far back the questioning should go depends on what is known about the incubation period of the particular disease under investigation.

The description of the outbreak then relies on the presentation of this early data, such as the epidemic curve, geographical mapping and age/sex distributions. The epidemic curve is probably the most useful descriptive technique in any outbreak investigation. It is simply a histogram showing the number of cases developing illness over time. Figure 1.2 shows some example epidemic curves. Geographical mapping represents cases by marking points representing home addresses on appropriate maps such as street plans. When waterborne disease is suspected the appropriate water supply zones may be superimposed on the map (Figure 1.3). Computer mapping packages are increasingly replacing the traditional 'pin in the map' technique.

Hypothesis formulation

Once the initial outbreak data have been collected and described, the outbreak control team has to decide what possible factors may be responsible for the

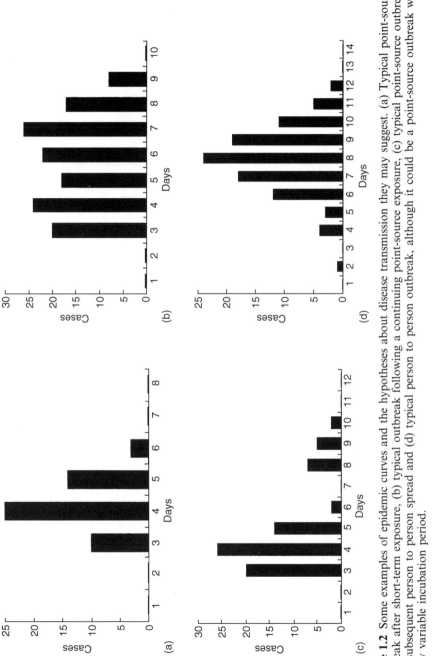

Figure 1.2 Some examples of epidemic curves and the hypotheses about disease transmission they may suggest. (a) Typical point-source outbreak after short-term exposure, (b) typical outbreak following a continuing point-source exposure, (c) typical point-source outbreak with subsequent person to person spread and (d) typical person to person outbreak, although it could be a point-source outbreak with widely variable incubation period.

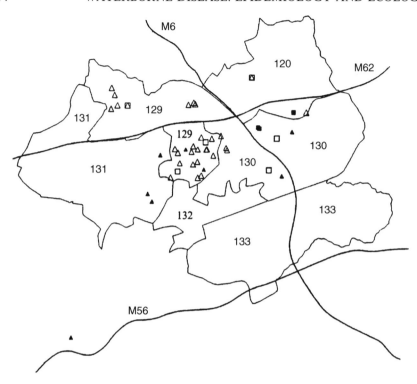

Figure 1.3 An example of the use of geographical mapping in the investigation of a waterborne outbreak. Reproduced from Bridgman *et al.* (1995) *Epidemiology and Infection* **115**: 559, by permission of Cambridge University Press.

outbreak. In the context of waterborne disease, it has to be decided whether a waterborne factor is part of the initial hypothesis. In deciding what hypotheses to test, the outbreak control team will rely on the initial descriptive epidemiology, initial environmental investigations, knowledge of the epidemiology or microbiology of the causative agent and their experience of previous outbreaks.

The epidemic curve will help to distinguish between an outbreak due to a single point source event, an outbreak due to continued problems and one due to person to person spread. Continued monitoring of the epidemic curve is also a good indicator as to whether control measures have been effective. The age and sex distribution is often helpful in suggesting possible hypotheses. Outbreaks of enteric disease spread by person to person transmission tend to affect younger children. However, high levels of immunity in the adult population can also skew the age distribution. Sex differences may reflect important occupational factors such as agricultural activities. The geographical distribution of cases, such as their restriction to certain water supply zones, is often one of the first indicators of a waterborne route of infection.

The early environmental investigations may also give important clues. Knowledge of water treatment failures in the days before an outbreak or early results of environmental microbiology will guide hypothesis generation.

Not to be underestimated, however, is the importance of experience in deciding what hypotheses to test. Nevertheless, always keep an open mind, as infectious disease epidemiology is usually able to surprise.

Remedial control measures

Once a mains drinking water has been implicated as a cause of an outbreak in the hypothesis generation phase of the investigation, the outbreak team has to decide whether any action should be taken at that stage to minimize any further hazard to the public. Essentially the measures available are to disconnect the mains supply, use water from another source or reservoir, issue advice to the public to boil water for drinking, or do nothing.

It is this stage of outbreak investigation that is the most difficult. Rarely has the team proven the source of the outbreak. Furthermore, it is often not known whether any contamination was a short-lived or continuing problem. Decisions taken can have far-reaching effects on the health of individuals. Even issuing boil water notices can have adverse health effects (Mayon-White and Frankenberg 1989). Needless to say, an innocent water company stands to lose money and reputation if it has to make major engineering changes and go public on a suggestion that is eventually disproved.

Hypothesis testing

Once one or more hypotheses have been generated, the outbreak team then has to attempt to prove them in a more rigorous fashion. There are usually three strands to this proof: microbiological, epidemiological and environmental. Microbiological proof rests, at best, on identifying the causative agent in the water supply or demonstrating microbiological evidence of treatment failure such as coliforms. Microbiological examination of patients and contacts is also essential in many outbreaks to identify new cases. The most common analytical epidemiological method is the case-control study. Environmental investigations can also provide important proof. These investigations include a search for possible breakdowns in standard procedures, such as evidence of chlorination failure. This will include a review of all recent records relating to the quality and safety of the relevant supply, along with a thorough inspection of the water source, treatment plant and distribution network. In borderline cases, investigators may have to develop some particular risk assessment of the system, looking at its design and operating principles. Such environmental evidence both supports the other evidence and suggests control measures. Both US and UK authorities have suggested protocols for determining the strength of evidence in favour of an outbreak being waterborne (Anon 1996; Kramer *et al.* 1996).

Control measures

Once a waterborne hypothesis has been confirmed, then one can have more confidence in the remedial measures already implemented. The water company can then institute more long-term control measures to prevent a recurrence of the problem in the future. This may mean a change in procedure or new engineering works such as the introduction of new filtering systems.

Formal report

In today's society, many different organizations and individuals will have an interest in the outcome of the investigation of an outbreak of waterborne disease. The water company and water regulators will need to know how the outbreak happened in order to reduce the risk of similar episodes happening in the future. The water regulator may be interested in knowing whether the failure was negligent if a prosecution is under consideration. Other water companies may want to put into effect the recommendations before the embarrassment of having an outbreak. Other public health teams may need to know the outcome of the investigations in case they also have a similar problem. Furthermore, local residents and the various enforcement authorities also need to know how the outbreak was handled and whether the control measures have been properly implemented, not least to decide whether to seek legal redress for any harm or loss suffered from the outbreak. It is for all these people that a formal report needs to be written and published.

In order for the wider public health community to learn any general lessons the appropriate national surveillance centre needs to know the outcome in order to record the nature and causes of the outbreak. Where more general lessons can be drawn, the essential aspects of the investigation should also be published in more widely read scientific journals, so that authors like me can include the outbreak in their own reviews of the literature.

FURTHER READING

Farmer R and Miller D (1991) *Lecture notes on Epidemiology and Public Health Medicine*, 3rd edn. Blackwell Scientific, Oxford.

Giesecke J (1994) *Modern Infectious Disease Epidemiology*. Edward Arnold, London.

Hennekens CH and Buring JE (1987) *Epidemiology in Medicine*. Little, Brown and Company, Boston, MA.

Riegelman RK (1981) *Studying a Study and Testing a Test, How to Read the Medical Literature*. Little, Brown and Company, Boston, MA.

2 Water Supply and Distribution

Perhaps the biggest improvement to public health in the western world came with the development of water supply treatment and distribution systems. This chapter aims to give an introduction to the general principles of water treatment for the novice. In many ways, it can only act as a glossary to some of the terms in common use. A more detailed, but still accessible, introduction is given by Gray (1994).

WATER SOURCES AND EXTRACTION

One of the most important geophysical process underpinning life on earth is the water cycle. The absolute amount of water on earth remains constant, but it is in constant flux from one state to another. Figure 2.1 shows a schematic diagram of this hydrogeological cycle, giving some idea of the vast, almost unbelievable, volumes of water involved. Most water for consumption comes from either surface water or groundwater sources.

Surface water is that freshwater present in streams, rivers, lakes and reservoirs. The quality of surface waters varies markedly from one place to another and in the same place over time as a result of various factors, such as geology and climate. All surface water originally fell as rain onto land, with the exception of that small proportion of rainfall which fell directly onto the water body itself. Much of this rainfall will then flow over the surface of the ground into a stream. This is runoff. Over impervious rocks most of the rainfall will run off into water courses in this way. As it runs off the ground it will pick up many organic and inorganic contaminants and it may become quite turbid. The water will also tend to be soft. In areas of chalk and limestone much of the rainfall percolates into the ground. Rivers in such areas often arise from springs or from seepage from the water table. Such water is usually clearer, but harder due to the presence of dissolved calcium salts. Extraction from surface waters is relatively easy. However, because of their greater risk of contamination, treatment is usually more complex and costly. Furthermore, because river flow relies on recent rainfall the security of supply may be problematic in drought years.

Groundwater is subsurface water in soils and rocks that are fully saturated. The volume of groundwater is vast, representing the world's largest volume of

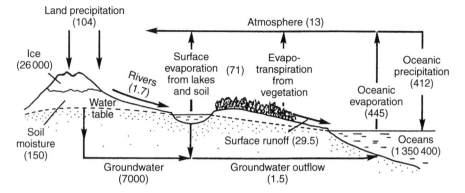

Figure 2.1 Hydrogeological cycle showing the volume of water stored (in 10^3 km^3) and the amount cycled annually. Reproduced from Gray (1994) by permission of the author.

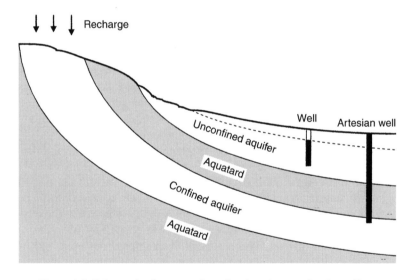

Figure 2.2 Schematic diagram of confined and unconfined aquifers.

liquid freshwater, some 7 000 000 km^3, approximately 95% of all freshwater other than that contained in ice sheets. Those geological formations that yield most water are known as aquifers. Typically, these form in porous rock or deposits overlying less permeable rocks, known as aquitards. Confined aquifers also have an aquitard overlying the water bearing rock (Figure 2.2). Unconfined aquifers have no such upper layer of rock. The upper surface of the aquifer is then known as the water table (the point at which the porewater pressure equals atmospheric pressure). All groundwater once fell as rain, known as recharge. The residence time is the time between water falling as rain and it leaving the aquifer. This can be very long, 300 years on average.

The quality and nature of groundwater depends on the geology of the aquifer, especially the nature of the rock, the residence time and the presence of local sources of pollution. For example, water from limestone aquifers is hard due to the presence of dissolved calcium. Young groundwaters may have higher organic content due to leaching from soils and atmospheric carbon dioxide. Older waters tend to be more mineralized. Groundwaters in lowland areas with substantial agricultural activity can have high nitrate contents. An increasing problem is the presence of polluting chemicals from human industrial activity.

Groundwater for consumption may come from natural springs where the water naturally issues from the ground or via an artificial borehole drilled into the ground. Usually the water will need to be pumped out of the well. Any borehole must be protected to prevent toxic or infective agents gaining access to the water from the surrounding land.

WATER TREATMENT

The role of water treatment is to render the water safe, palatable, clear, colourless and odourless, reasonably soft and non-corrosive (Gray 1994). Depending on its quality, raw water will have to undergo a series of physical and chemical treatments before it will be considered fit to go into the distribution system. The various processes that may be used in the treatment of a moderately polluted river are described briefly in the following subsections.

Pretreatment

1 Raw water is passed through one or more coarse screens to remove large solids such as plants or dead animals.
2 The water may spend time in a pretreatment storage reservoir. This improves quality by allowing much particulate matter to settle and exposing certain microorganisms to the lethal effect of sunlight. Sunlight will also reduce colour by bleaching, and some impurities that may adversely effect taste will be oxidized.
3 Before further treatment the water is usually passed through fine screens and/or microstrainers to remove fine solids and algae. When such solids build up on the microstrainers smaller microorganisms such as protozoan oocysts are also removed.
4 Pre-chlorination may be used when the raw water has high bacterial counts with low turbidity. A disadvantage of pre-chlorination is that large volumes of chlorine are often needed due to the very large chlorine demand of raw waters.

5 Aeration is needed when water is taken from the bottom of lakes or from underground aquifers. Waters with very low oxygen concentrations can adversely affect other treatment processes. Occasionally air is bubbled up through the water, although more usually the water is brought into contact with oxygen by a cascade or fountain system.

Coagulation and flocculation

After pretreatment small particles, less than 10 μm, remain suspended in the water body. These particles include microorganisms as well as various organic molecules and inorganic particulates. These will not sediment out by themselves. A chemical coagulant is, therefore, added to help precipitation of these particulates. Chemical coagulants include aluminium sulphate, aluminium hydroxide, ferrous sulphate and, increasingly, various synthetic organic polymers. Some very clear waters may not form a precipitate, even after the addition of coagulant. In such circumstances, coagulant aids may be added. Coagulant aids include various forms of clay, lime, activated silica and, more recently, synthetic water-soluble, high molecular weight polymers.

After the addition of the coagulant, the smaller particles come together to form flocs, which then settle out. To improve the efficiency of flocculation the water is gently mixed. Mixing is essential to good floc formation. After the addition of coagulant, floc formation will be almost instantaneous if the mixing is sufficiently violent. However, the flocs formed will still be relatively fine and will not sediment out efficiently. Thus, the initial mixing will be followed by more gentle stirring to allow the floc size to increase. A variety of technologies may be used for both the violent mixing and gentle stirring stages.

Clarification

Once floc formation is complete, flocs are removed by the processes of sedimentation followed by filtration. In the sedimentation tanks, water flows upward sufficiently slowly that the flocs settle to the bottom of the tank. Clarified water flows over the top of the tank towards the next treatment stage. The sludge formed during this stage is removed, either continuously or intermittently. Sludge is potentially hazardous due to the presence of pathogenic microorganisms and toxic materials. It must be disposed of safely.

Sedimentation alone becomes increasingly inefficient at removing particles below 100 μm. Filtration is designed to remove the remaining particulate matter. The most common forms of filter are based on layers of sand and gravel through which water passes under the influence of gravity. Rapid sand filters contain coarse (about 1 mm diameter) grains of sand. Slow sand filters use much finer grains of sand. Slow sand filters are more efficient at removing smaller particles, although water flow through the filter is about 50 times slower. In use, a layer of algae and bacteria builds up on the surface of slow sand filters, which assists in the removal of very small particles as well as nitrogen and phosphorus.

During use, retained particulates build up in the filters, which, if left, would cause the filter to fail. Filters need to be backwashed regularly to remove this material. Backwashing, as the name suggests, consists of forcing water back through the filter in the reverse direction. The backwash water is then run to waste or put back to the head of the treatment works. In sand filters, filter efficiency declines immediately after backwashing. Some outbreaks have been traced to the ineffective removal of this backwash water leading to a build up of oocysts in the plant.

Disinfection and other chemical treatments

After filtration it is normal to disinfect the water with chemical disinfectants. However, before the addition of disinfectant the pH of the water may be adjusted by adding alkalis such as lime, sodium carbonate or caustic soda if it is too low or adding acids if it is too high. Too acidic a pH can lead to corrosion of metal pipes and solder. As well as damaging the plumbing system, this can increase the concentrations of metals such as copper and lead in the water at the tap. If the water is too alkaline this can lead to salt deposition on the inner surfaces of the pipes.

The most common disinfectant is chlorine. Chlorine can be added as a gas, liquid or solid. Gaseous chlorine is stored in cylinders and injected into the water supply through a chlorinator. Once added to the water, the chlorine hydrolyses to form hypochlorous acid, which subsequently dissociates to produce hypochlorite:

$$Cl_2 + H_2O \rightleftharpoons HOCl + H^+ + Cl^- \rightleftharpoons 2H^+ + Cl^- + OCl^-$$

Chlorine gas   Hypochlorous acid   Hypochlorite ion

Chlorine added to treated water is very efficient at killing most microbial pathogens. Furthermore, if sufficient chlorine is added to the supply in the treatment works, bactericidal levels will remain in the water throughout the supply and prevent regrowth of bacteria in the distribution system.

One problem with the use of gaseous chlorine for water disinfection is the production of chlorination by-products in waters with a high organic content. Such chlorination by-products include trihalomethanes such as chloroform, 1,2-dicloroethane and carbon tetrachloride. These chlorination by-products have been implicated in the aetiology of bladder cancer (Craun 1988; Jolley, Brungs and Cummings 1985; Larsen 1989). Because of concerns about the potential adverse effects of chlorination by-products, some water treatment companies use a process of chloramination. Cloramines are formed by the reaction of ammonium and hypochlorous acids according to the following formulae:

$$NH_3 + HOCl \rightarrow NH_2Cl + H_2O$$
Monochloramine

$$NH_2Cl + HOCl \rightarrow NHCl_2 + H_2O$$
Dichloramine

$$NHCl_2 + HOCl \rightarrow NCl_3 + H_2O$$
Trichloramine

The exact proportion of each chloramine depends on the pH of the water.

The other main disinfectant in common use in commercial water treatment is ozone. Ozone is produced by passing dried air between two electrodes through which a high voltage alternating current is passed. It is a more expensive form of disinfection, largely due to the cost of electricity. It has the advantage over chlorination of having no apparent adverse health effects and also being effective against cryptosporidium oocysts. However, no disinfection residual passes into the mains supply and bacterial regrowth is a potential problem. In some systems small amounts of chlorine are still added to provide some protection against regrowth.

Other disinfection methods available include chlorine dioxide, ultraviolet irradiation and, in sunnier countries, exposure to solar radiation.

In addition to disinfection, other chemical treatments may be used. Most commonly this is water softening by the addition of lime or soda ash or by a resin-based ion-exchange system.

WATER DISTRIBUTION

After treatment, water is distributed to the eventual customer through a network of pumping stations, service reservoirs, water mains and service pipes.

Service reservoirs are the slack in the system, enabling the system to cope with marked variations in demand throughout the day. Usually the service reservoirs have a capacity equal to a little more than a single day's demand. They are constructed out of concrete, brick or steel and designed to be watertight in order to protect against the risk of contamination. In flat areas these service reservoirs will often be built in water towers to give added hydraulic pressure within the distribution system.

Trunk mains are the largest diameter main and are used for transporting large volumes of water over distance. They do not branch or have connections to service pipes. The distribution mains are designed to distribute water from a supply reservoir to the individual customers' premises. They range in diameter from 50 mm up to 500 mm and are made from a variety of materials, including iron, asbestos cement, unplasticized polyvinyl chloride (uPVC) and medium density polyethylene (MDPE). Service pipes are the final stage in water distribution, taking the water from the distribution main into the customer's home.

WATER SUPPLY IN DEVELOPING COUNTRIES

In some senses issues around water supplies in developing countries are no different to those same issues in the west. Indeed, for large systems there is likely to be little difference in much of the technology. Problems of water supply in many poorer areas include problems of funding water supply technology, poor maintenance of systems, poor volume and locality of supply, and pollution of supplies.

Where water is taken from rivers or streams it is often impossible to ensure safety without subsequent treatment, either by conventional water treatment including disinfection or by boiling. Where natural springs exist they can be protected by an appropriate construction to prevent pollution of the supply, either from faecal or toxic wastes above the spring or from individuals taking water from the spring.

The other source of water is from wells. There are several types of well construction suitable for small communities (Cairncross and Feachem 1993). Wells are either hand dug or tube wells. Hand-dug wells have the advantage of being dug by the community; they require little special equipment or technical knowledge. They also are wider than tube wells and so have a larger storage capacity. On the negative side they can be dangerous to dig, because there is a risk of the sides collapsing onto the diggers. Furthermore, because they are wider they are more liable to pollution.

There are four main methods of tube-well construction (Figure 2.3):

- The driven tube well, where a specially perforated tube is hammered into the ground. This can be sunk to about 10–15 metres.
- A bored tube well, which is sunk by hand with an auger, a type of giant corkscrew. This can be sunk down to about 25 metres.
- A jetted tube well, which is sunk into soft ground by water being pumped up or down a pipe. This type of well can be sunk up to about 80 metres.
- A borehole is drilled by a special drilling rig. Such boreholes can be sunk up to 100 metres. This depth is too great for hand pumps. Drilling rigs are also costly.

Open wells are subject to various forms of pollution (Cairncross and Feachem 1993). For example, wells can be contaminated by polluted ground-water if they are sited too close to latrines; surface water may carry pollution

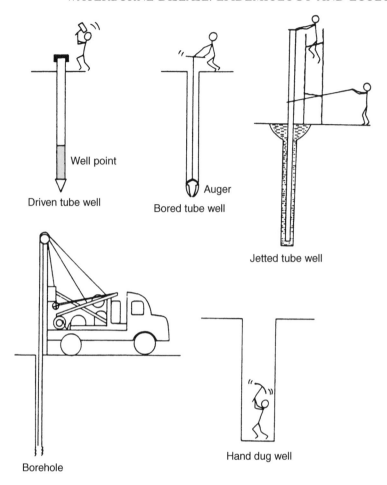

Figure 2.3 Examples of different tube well construction. Reproduced from Cairncross and Feachem (1993) *Environmental Health Engineering in the Tropics*, 2nd edn, by permission of John Wiley & Sons.

down the well (especially if cattle are allowed near the well); vessels used for drawing the water may be dirty; and rubbish may be thrown down the well. Indeed, as will be seen later in this book, some of these sources of pollution are not unknown in developed countries.

Dirty and polluted water can be further purified in the home. Boiling is the most effective method of rendering infected water safe. However, in areas where fuel is at a premium this may not be practicable. Boiling will not improve the appearance of visually dirty water. Such water can be strained through a clean cloth to remove larger solids and prevent guinea worm infection. Water filters can also be constructed out of clay pots, stones, sand and

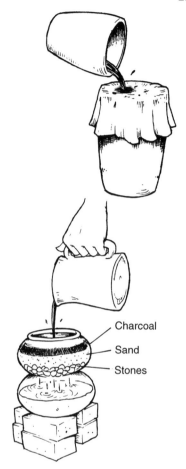

Figure 2.4 Example of a home-made device for filtering water for drinking. Redrawn from Fernando (1996); reproduced by permission of UNIFEM.

charcoal (Figure 2.4). Mintz, Reiff and Tauxe (1995) describe one approach to ensuring safe water in tropical countries by disinfecting water in the home and then storing it in narrow-mouthed, closed vessels to prevent subsequent contamination from dirty hands.

WATER SUPPLIES FOR THE TRAVELLER

Travellers, particularly those from relatively affluent countries, are at increased risk of waterborne disease compared to local residents. They have not had time to build up any effective immunity to many of the local pathogens. For the traveller, therefore, safe water is a priority. However, any water treatment technology must be sufficiently lightweight to carry easily. The safest approach is to boil any water intended for drinking or teeth brushing. Boiling kills all waterborne pathogens. It is good practice in many countries to boil up water just to place into bottles for future use. The second best option is bottled mineral water, provided it is a recognized brand with a tamper-proof top. It is not unknown for locals to earn a living from filling up used bottles. If in doubt, sparkling mineral water is much safer. Most 'home bottlers' do not have the technology to carbonate water, and carbonation is itself bacteriostatic. There are also a variety of filters on the market. These work by a mixture of filtration and disinfection. The quality is variable, so be sure you know which type you are buying. Chemical disinfection, either by chlorination or iodination, is effective against many pathogens when used in clear water. However, it is not 100% reliable and I would always use another method in preference to disinfection as the sole treatment.

FURTHER READING

Bitton G (1994) *Wastewater Microbiology*. John Wiley and Sons, New York.

Fernando V (1996) *Water Supply*. Intermediate Technology Publications, London.

Kerr C (ed.) (1989) *Community Water Development*. Intermediate Technology Publications, London.

Smethurst G (1988) *Basic Water Treatment*, 2nd edn. Thomas Telford, London.

3 Drinking Water and Waterborne Disease

In this chapter I attempt to identify how common is waterborne disease. Evidence on the incidence of waterborne disease comes from two sources. The first is national records of outbreaks and the second prospective epidemiological studies.

NATIONAL SURVEILLANCE OF WATERBORNE OUTBREAKS

United States of America

Probably the most comprehensive surveillance reports on waterborne disease are those relating to outbreaks in the United States. Since 1971 the Center for Disease Control (CDC) has been collating information on reported outbreaks of waterborne disease. To be included as an outbreak an incident has to involve two or more individuals with similar symptoms. Single, well-documented cases of chemical poisoning are also included. The CDC reports classify water sources as community water systems (which serve large or small communities with at least 15 service connections or 25 year-round residents), non-community systems (which serve institutions, industries, camps, parks, hotels or businesses that may be used by the general public) and individual systems (which supply one or a few residences or persons outside populated areas).

Craun (1992) published a review of reported outbreaks in the United States covering 70 years from 1920 to 1990. Table 3.1 gives the average number of outbreaks per year. From the table, it is clear that ascertained outbreaks from community systems declined steadily between 1920 to 1970 then increased dramatically again. This increase in outbreaks was related primarily to the start of CDC's interest in waterborne disease and so represents increased ascertainment rather than increased disease. The role of protozoal pathogens, such as *Giardia* and *Cryptosporidium*, in the aetiology of waterborne disease became clear during the 1970s and 1980s and so some outbreaks would have been identifiable for the first time during these two decades.

Table 3.1 Average number of waterborne outbreaks per year, USA, 1920–1990. Data from Craun (1992)

Time period	Community systems	Non-community systems	All water systems
1920–30	17.2	2.6	23.2
1931–40	12.8	8.1	30.6
1941–50	9.6	14.2	31.3
1951–60	4.1	3.9	11.1
1961–70	3.9	3.9	13.1
1971–80	12.3	16.1	32.6
1981–90	12.4	9.7	29.1
1920–90	8.9	7.1	20.2

Table 3.2 lists the diseases responsible for these outbreaks during the period 1920–1994. The most notable aspect of this table is the virtual disappearance of typhoid as a waterborne disease in the US during the 20th century. Unfortunately, the decline in typhoid has been matched by increases in chemical poisoning and the appearance of diseases such as giardiasis, crypto-sporidiosis and viral gastroenteritis. Gastroenteritis of unknown aetiology has been the most common diagnosis in waterborne outbreaks since 1941. As already indicated, the increase in reported outbreaks since 1971 probably represents the introduction of active surveillance of waterborne disease by CDC.

As well as recording outbreaks of waterborne disease, CDC has started indicating the engineering cause of the outbreak. The data for the period 1981–1990 are presented in Table 3.3. Groundwater was responsible for 77.3% of non-community outbreaks. This finding casts considerable doubt on the general belief that well-water and springwater are safe and require no further action. Inadequate disinfection of surface water was responsible for 28.2% of community outbreaks, and distribution difficulties were responsible for 24.2%.

United Kingdom

The regular publication of reports of waterborne disease in the UK only started in 1995 with the publication of the 1994 data. However, Galbraith and others (Galbraith 1994; Galbraith, Barrett and Stanwell-Smith 1987) have published what is probably the most comprehensive review of waterborne outbreaks outside of the US.

Table 3.4 shows the outbreaks associated with public water supplies identified by Galbraith (1994) for the years 1911–1986. Information for later years was obtained from other sources. During the years covered there were 57 outbreaks, almost half of which have occurred since 1980. Most of the first

Table 3.2 Aetiology of waterborne outbreaks, USA, 1920–1994. Adapted ˅ (1992) with additional data from Moore *et al.* (1993) and Kramer *et al.* (19˅,

Time period	Disease	Number of outbreaks	Number of cases
1920–40	Typhoid	372	
	Gastroenteritis	144	
	Shigellosis	10	
	Amoebiasis	2	
	Hepatitis	1	
	Chemical poisoning	1	
	Subtotal	530	206 000
1941–60	Gastroenteritis	265	
	Typhoid	94	
	Shigellosis	25	
	Hepatitis	23	
	Salmonellosis	4	
	Chemical poisoning	4	
	Paratyphoid	3	
	Amoebiasis	2	
	Tularaemia	2	
	Leptospirosis	1	
	Poliomyelitis	1	
	Subtotal	424	66 000
1961–70	Gastroenteritis	39	
	Hepatitis	30	
	Shigellosis	19	
	Typhoid	14	
	Salmonellosis	9	
	Chemical poisoning	9	
	Toxigenic *E. coli*	4	
	Giardiasis	3	
	Amoebiasis	3	
	Subtotal	130	46 000
1971–80	Gastroenteritis	181	
	Giardiasis	39	
	Chemical poisoning	38	
	Shigellosis	24	
	Hepatitis A	16	
	Viral gastroenteritis	12	
	Salmonellosis	8	
	Typhoid	4	
	Campylobacteriosis	3	
	Toxigenic *E. coli*	1	
	Subtotal	326	79 000

continued overleaf

Table 3.2 *(continued)*

Time period	Disease	Number of outbreaks	Number of cases
1981–90	Gastroenteritis	128	
	Giardiasis	71	
	Shigellosis	22	
	Chemical poisoning	18	
	Viral gastroenteritis	15	
	Hepatitis A	11	
	Campylobacteriosis	10	
	Salmonellosis	4	
	Cryptosporidiosis	2	
	Yersiniosis	2	
	Chronic gastroenteritis	2	
	E. coli O157:H7	1	
	Typhoid	1	
	Chlorine dermatitis	1	
	Cyclospora	1	
	Cholera	1	
	Amoebiasis	1	
	Subtotal	291	65 000
1991–94 (4 years)	Gastroenteritis	30	
	Giardiasis	9	
	Cryptosporidiosis	8	
	Shigellosis	5	
	Copper	4	
	Campylobacteriosis	3	
	Lead	3	
	Fluoride	3	
	Nitrate	3	
	Hepatitis A	2	
	Salmonellosis	1	
	Vibrio cholera non O1	1	
	Subtotal	72	423 000

half of the 20th century was characterized by a predominance of outbreaks due to typhoid, while the years since 1980 have been characterized by the rapid rise of cryptosporidium as a major waterborne pathogen. The decline of typhoid is undoubtedly real and reflects improved water treatment and the reduced prevalence of the disease in the general public. The rise of cryptosporidium probably is an artefact due to its relatively recent recognition as a cause of human disease. It is to be noted that despite the increase in reported outbreaks, the number of cases affected by such outbreaks has fallen.

Most waterborne outbreaks in England and Wales have affected public supplies. Table 3.5 lists known outbreaks from private supplies. Since 1941 there have been 20 such outbreaks. There has also been an increase in reported

Table 3.3 Causes of waterborne outbreaks, USA, 1981–1990. Date from Craun (1

Cause of outbreak	Community	Non-community	Other
Untreated groundwater	15 (12.1)	43 (44.3)	19 (27.1)
Inadequate disinfection of groundwater	17 (13.7)	32 (33.0)	
Ingestion of contaminated water while swimming			41 (58.6)
Inadequate disinfection of surface water	35 (28.2)	9 (9.3)	
Distribution deficiencies	30 (24.2)	3 (3.1)	3 (4.3)
Filtration deficiencies	16 (12.9)	1 (1.0)	
Unknown	7 (5.6)	3 (3.1)	1 (1.4)
Untreated surface water	2 (1.6)	4 (4.1)	3 (4.3)
Miscellaneous	2 (1.6)	2 (2.1)	3 (4.3)
Total	124	97	70

Table 3.4 Waterborne outbreaks associated with public water supplies in England and Wales, 1911–1995, number of outbreaks in 10-year periods. Adapted from Galbraith (1994) with additional data from Stanwell-Smith (1994) and Furtado et al. (1996)

Ten year period	Number of outbreaks		Number of cases[a] & (deaths)	Disease: *number of outbreaks*, cases & (deaths)
	Site of contamination			
	Source	Distribution		
1911–20	3	5	3630+ (28+)	Typhoid:[b] *6*, 359+, (28+) Paratyphoid: *1*, 71, (?) Dysentery: *1*, 1700, (?)
1921–30	5	3	2029+ (65+)	Typhoid: *4*, 459, (50) Paratyphoid: *1*, 31, (?) Dysentery: *1*, 1100, (12) Gastroenteritis: *2*, 439, (?3)
1931–40	6	0	7912+ (78+)	Typhoid: *3*, 686, (77+) Gastroenteritis: *3*, 7200+, (1)
1941–50	1	2	610 (0)	Typhoid: *1*, 22, (0) Dysentery: *2*, 588, (0)
1951–60	None identified			
1961–70	1	0	90 (0)	Paratyphoid: *1*, 90, (0)
1971–80	1	2	3222 (0)	Gastroenteritis: *2*, 3114, (0) Giardiasis: *1*, 60, (0)
1981–90	14	3	1925 (0)	Campylobacter: *3*, 629, (0) Cryptosporidiosis: *11*, 900+, (0) Gastroenteritis: *3*, 310, (0)
1991–95	11	0	1340+ (0)	Cryptosporidiosis: *11*, 1340+, (0)

[a] Case numbers are often estimates; + indicates a minimum estimate.
[b] One outbreak of typhoid was also associated with 1500 cases of gastroenteritis.

Table 3.5 Waterborne disease from private supplies, England and Wales, 1941–1995. Adapted from Galbraith, Barrett and Stanwell-Smith (1987), Stanwell-Smith (1994) and Furtado *et al.* (1996)

Ten year period	Number of outbreaks	Number of cases & (deaths)	Disease: *number of outbreaks*, cases & (deaths)
1941–50	4	47+ (5+)	Typhoid: *2*, 9+, (5) Paratyphoid: *1*, 1, (0) Amoebiasis: *1*, 17, (0)
1951–60	None detected		
1961–70	None detected		
1971–80	2	166 (0)	Paratyphoid: *1*, 6, (0) Gastroenteritis: *1*, 160, (0)
1981–90	5	962 (0)	Gastroenteritis: *1*, 138, (0) Campylobacter: *3*, 520, (0) Streptobacillary fever: *1*, 304, (0)
1991–95	9	299 (0)	Gastroenteritis: *1*, 56, (0) Campylobacter: *5*, 127, (0) Giardia: *1*, 31, (0) Cryptosporidiosis: *1*, 42, (0) Mixed campylobacter and cryptosporidiosis: *1*, 43, (0)

outbreaks associated with private supplies since 1980. The responsible pathogen has, unlike the situation in public supplies, been campylobacter, another 'new' pathogen.

The five chemical related incidents are listed in Table 3.6. The two copper poisonings were due to contamination at point of use. The other incidents will be discussed later in the book.

Benton *et al.* (1989) have done a similar review of waterborne disease in Scotland for the years 1945–1987. They identified 57 outbreaks, which affected 15 305 individuals. Of these 57 outbreaks, 18 (5252 cases) were associated with public supplies, 21 (9362 cases) were due to private supplies and 18 (418 cases) were water-associated. Water-associated outbreaks included cases where people had drunk from streams or inadequately plumbed vending machines. Surprisingly, the commonest incident was chemical poisoning (37% of outbreaks), although relatively few people were involved (0.71%). Viral gastroenteritis was responsible for only 5% of outbreaks, but 52.2% of cases, while shigellosis was responsible for 5% of outbreaks and 30.1% of cases. Gastroenteritis of unknown cause was responsible for 28 outbreaks, affecting 15.8% of cases.

Czech Soviet Republic

Šrámová and Kovácová (1984) identified 40 outbreaks of gastrointestinal disease associated with drinking water in the Czech Soviet Republic (CSR) during the four year period 1979–1982 (Table 3.7). The most notable aspect of

Table 3.6 Incidents of chemical contamination of water supplies in England and Wales

Year	Number affected (deaths)	Chemical	Comments
1950	6 (0)	Copper	Outbreaks associated with drinking
1956	5 (0)		tea made in copper geysers
1960	18 (1)		
1969	7 (1)	Arsenic	Back-siphonage from agricultural sprayer
1984	500+	Phenol	Industrial pollution of river
1988	?20 000	Aluminium	Accidental addition of aluminium to treated water

Table 3.7 Notified outbreaks of waterborne gastrointestinal infections in Czech Soviet Republic between 1979 and 1982. Adapted from Šrámová and Kovácová (1984)

Disease	Water supplies	Wells		
		Public	School	Private
Typhoid or paratyphoid				1 (15)
Other salmonella infections	2 (85)			
Shigellosis	6 (287)	10 (1450)	7 (1034)	2 (25)
Other bacterial infections		1 (25)	1 (80)	
Infections of unknown cause	3 (481)	6 (266)	1 (28)	
Total	11 (853)	17 (1741)	9 (1142)	3 (40)

[a] Number of outbreaks (number affected).

these reports is the predominance of shigellosis as a frequent cause of large waterborne outbreaks associated with drinking well-water. The cause of the other infections listed in the table is not clear from the paper.

Israel

Between the years 1976 and 1992 there were 130 documented outbreaks, affecting 23 743 individuals, of waterborne enteric disease in Israel (Tulchinsky *et al.* 1993). During the years since 1976 there has been a dramatic decline in the incidence of waterborne disease outbreaks, particularly after 1985 (Table 3.8). The authors of this review suggest that this decline is largely due to the introduction of mandatory chlorination, stimulated in part by a vigorous press interest in waterborne disease.

Scandinavian countries

Stenström (1994) has reviewed reported waterborne outbreaks of disease in Nordic countries (Sweden, Norway, Finland, Denmark and Iceland) for the

Table 3.8 Outbreaks of waterborne enteric disease in Israel, 1976–1992. Adapted from Tulchinsky *et al.* (1993)

	1976–80	1981–85	1986–90	1991–92
Non-community water				
Outbreaks	45	19	4	0
Cases	2465	577	207	0
Cases per outbreak	54	30	52	0
Community water				
Outbreaks	25	27	9	1
Cases	7619	10 880	1829	166
Cases per outbreak	305	409	203	166
Total				
Outbreaks	70	46	13	1
Cases	10 084	11 457	2036	166
Cases per outbreak	144	249	157	166

years 1975–1991. He identified 141 outbreaks, of which the majority (80) were in Sweden; 100 outbreaks were in community systems and 41 in private systems. The aetiological agent was identified in only 36% of outbreaks associated with community supplies and 46% with private supplies. Of the identified outbreaks, 46% were due to a bacterial cause, of which 12 were due to campylobacter, 43% were due to a viral pathogen, most commonly Norwalk, and 11% were due to a protozoan such as giardia or crypto-sporidium. Table 3.9 lists the causes of the outbreaks. Of the 100 community systems involved, 25% were without any disinfection.

PROSPECTIVE EPIDEMIOLOGICAL STUDIES

The analysis of reports of outbreaks of waterborne disease is essential to further our understanding of the prevalence and causes of waterborne disease. However, relying on such data suffers from significant weaknesses. In many countries, including many industrialized countries, there is no national monitoring and recording system even if outbreaks are identified. Even where good systems exist, many outbreaks go unrecognized and unreported. To gain a real understanding of the prevalence of such disease requires prospective epidemiological studies of populations with different degrees of exposure to the risk factor. These studies are rarely easy and usually require the inclusion of a large number of cases and controls.

One of the few prospective studies looking at the impact of the quality of mains drinking water on health to be conducted in the west was done in France in the years 1983 and 1984 (Ferley *et al.* 1986; Zmirou *et al.* 1987).

Table 3.9 Causes of waterborne outbreaks in Nordic countries between 1975 and 1991. Adapted from Stenström (1994)

Cause	Outbreaks (%)
Community systems	
Waste-water contamination of the raw water source in combination with deficiencies in disinfection	46
Cross-connection	20
Animal contamination	9
Regrowth in distribution system	5
Unknown	20
Private systems	
Waste-water contamination at source through infiltration	55
Back-suction of waste-water into source or reservoir	19
Cross-connection or growth in distribution system	18
Unknown and other causes	8

Table 3.10 Current European microbiological standards for drinking water

Indicator	Maximum permissible count (per 100 ml)
Coliforms	0
Faecal coliforms	0
Pseudomonas aeruginosa	0
Faecal streptococci	0

They conducted a prospective longitudinal study over 18 months in 52 French alpine villages. In all villages the mains water was untreated surface water. The two parts of the study were: (i) weekly microbiological monitoring of the drinking water and (ii) ascertainment of cases of gastroenteritis by physicians, pharmacists and primary school teachers. Waters that did not meet the EC standards (Table 3.10) were associated with an increased risk of gastroenteritis (RR 1.36, CI 1.24–1.49) in the village around the time of sampling. The authors further found that, of the microbiological counts, faecal streptococci were the most important indicators of risk and that faecal coliforms provided addition estimators of risk, but that total coliforms and total counts provided no additional information.

An experimental study to determine the relationship between apparently high quality drinking water and ill health was conducted in Montreal, Canada (Payment *et al.* 1991b). This study set out to determine the risk of human illness from normally treated and disinfected drinking water meeting current legislative standards. Half of the approximately 1200 participants drank tap-water while the others (controls) drank the same water after treatment by reverse osmosis. The study was repeated over two periods. Throughout the study, participants kept a health diary. During both time periods, the rate of highly credible gastrointestinal symptoms was significantly higher in the group drinking tap-water (0.99 versus 0.72, and 0.65 versus 0.48 gastrointestinal episodes per person per year). The implication of this study was that in the area of Montreal where the study was undertaken, about 30% of all cases of gastroenteritis were waterborne. No specific pathogen was identified to explain this result. An interesting aspect of this study was that many of the reverse osmosis filters became colonized with high bacterial counts. Gastrointestinal illnesses were higher in controls whose filtered water had higher bacterial counts.

At this point it is worth referring to the study by Laursen *et al.* (1994) from Denmark. This was a study of a population of about 2000 individuals supplied by water that had been contaminated by sewage as a result of backflow from a blocked sewer that contaminated a well. About 88% of respondents to a postal questionnaire (1455 individuals) reported gastroenteritis. Median duration of diarrhoea was 6 days. There was a very strong dose–response effect with water consumption ($p < 0.000\ 001$). However, no pathogen was isolated from stool samples. The authors estimated that 1658 work days were lost as a result of this incident, at a cost to the economy of 1 600 000 Danish kroner (£180 000) at 1991 prices. This is one of the few studies that have attempted to cost the economic impact of waterborne disease. The real cost would have been greater than this, because no account was taken of medical costs incurred.

In comparison to the relative paucity of research papers that have investigated the impact of water supply and water quality on health in the west, there have been numerous studies in the developing world. Sometimes it has been possible to investigate the changing incidence of potentially waterborne disease in a population over time and relate this to changing water quality. At other times it has been possible to observe the differing incidence of potentially waterborne disease in two communities with differing water qualities. Esrey *et al.* (1991) have reviewed 144 studies up to about 1990 that investigated the effect of water supply and sanitation on a community's health. Many of these studies were related to specific diseases such as schistosomiasis or dracunculiasis. For example, the authors reviewed 14 studies linking ascariasis to drinking water or sanitation; of these, 9 showed a positive effect while 5 did not.

A total of 84 studies looked at the impact of water supply or sanitation on the prevalence of diarrhoeal disease. Of these studies, 43 looked at the impact of water supply on health in isolation of any effect of changes in sanitation, but were unable to distinguish between improved water quality and quantity. A positive impact, with a median reduction in the incidence of diarrhoeal disease of 16%, was reported in 24 of these 43 studies. Only 22 of the 43 studies were deemed to be rigorous by Esrey *et al.* In those studies that demonstrated a positive effect, water was piped into or near the home. Those studies that identified no benefit were concerned with wells and standpipes.

Of 16 studies that looked at the effect of pure versus contaminated water supplies, 10 reported a positive benefit. The median reduction in morbidity was 17%. It was suggested that these studies indicate that improved water quality will have little impact on morbidity where there is widespread faecal contamination of the environment.

The biggest impact on diarrhoeal morbidity seems to come from increasing water quantity, independently of quality. Of 15 studies reviewed by Esrey *et al.* (1991), all but one found a reduction of morbidity (median 27%). This was especially marked in those families that took advantage of the increased availability of water. Diarrhoeal disease appears to be inversely proportional to the amount of water used in a family, even in the same environments. This latter finding is perhaps explained by six studies that reported the impact of hygiene interventions (i.e. providing soap and encouraging hand washing after defecation and before preparing food). All six studies found a reduction in morbidity, the median reduction being 33%.

The review by Esrey *et al.* (1991) was very comprehensive and should be essential reading for anyone interested in the impact of water and sanitation interventions in developing countries. I do not intend to discuss any research paper that was included in that review. I will, however, discuss several that have been published more recently.

Gross *et al.* (1989) investigated the impact of a new water supply, excreta disposal facilities and public removal of refuse on the health of two low-income communities in Brazil. Of 168 children surveyed, 70.8% carried one or more intestinal parasites of which the commonest was *Ascaris lumbricoides*. The presence of a piped water supply had no effect on the carriage rate of intestinal parasites. However, the prevalence of diarrhoea was lower in those receiving a piped water supply (26.1 days per child per year) than in those taking water from a neighbour's water hose (28.3) and in those taking water from a water tank (47.8) ($p < 0.001$).

A diarrhoeal disease surveillance study was conducted in five counties of Fujian province, southeast China (Chen *et al.* 1991). All of the people (20 488) living in five villages were studied for the 12 months from May 1986 to April 1987. A total of 14 168 episodes of diarrhoea were detected, giving an incidence rate of 729.9 episodes per 1000 people per year. Diarrhoea was more common in the younger age groups. During the study diarrhoeal pathogens were isolated from 7.13% of environmental samples, drinking water, dish water, food, flies and toilet areas. The incidence of diarrhoea was markedly affected by the source of drinking water: 575.0 episodes per 1000 persons per year in people drinking piped water, 845.5 in people drinking well-water and an astounding 4579.7 in people drinking river water ($p < 0.01$). Other significant factors included poor family sanitary conditions, overcrowding (<10 square metres per person) and low income.

A study in Cebu in the Philippines looked at the relationship between the microbiological quality of drinking water and the prevalence of diarrhoeal disease in 690 children under two years old (Moe *et al.* 1991). Faecal pollution as measured by microbiological indicator organisms was common. For example, 21% of 123 spring waters, 21% of 131 open dug wells, 14% of 52 wells with pumps, 6% of 751 boreholes and 60% of 5 non-municipal piped water supplies yielded greater than 1000 faecal coliforms per 100 ml. By contrast, only 5% of 138 municipal piped water samples yielded a count of >1000 faecal coliforms per 100 ml. The prevalence of diarrhoea ranged from 5.2 to 10.0% over the six subsequent two-month periods. In analysing the data for any effect of microbial indicators, the authors categorized indictor counts as high and low risk (<1000 and ≥1000 organisms per 100 ml). It appeared that there was little change in the prevalence of diarrhoea if indicator counts rose to 100 per 100 ml. The was a significant association between diarrhoea and ≥1000 *E. coli* per 100 ml (odds ratio (OR) 1.92, CI 1.27–2.91), enterococci (OR 1.94, CI 1.20–3.16) and faecal streptococci (OR 1.81, CI 1.10–3.00). The association with faecal coliforms was borderline significant (OR 1.49, CI 1.00–2.22). The probability of diarrhoea in a child during a 24-hour period was 0.09 in those exposed to <1000 *E. coli* and 0.15 in those exposed to ≥1000. The respective probabilities for enterococci were 0.09 and 0.16.

Mahalanabis *et al.* (1991) investigated possible risk factors for prolonged diarrhoea in Bangladeshi children for the years 1983–1985. The study was restricted to children under three years old who had attended the treatment centre of the International Centre for Diarrhoeal Disease Research. Cases were categorized as either long-term (more than 14 days) or short-term (less than 10 days) duration of diarrhoea. Those with intermediate duration of diarrhoea (10 to 14 days) were excluded from the study. Of 3690 children in the study 10.7% had diarrhoea lasting for more than 14 days. Children with prolonged illness were more likely to use unprotected surface water for drinking (OR 1.56, CI 1.18–2.06). Non-water risk factors included presenting with bloody diarrhoea or having mucoid stool, having vitamin A deficiency, a chest infection, being of low weight, having a high family income and not having been given an antibiotic before admission.

A case-control study of diarrhoeal illness was reported from Nicaragua (Gorter *et al.* 1991). Cases were 1229 children under five years with diarrhoea presenting to a health centre. Controls were children presenting with one of several non-water associated illnesses and matched for age-group and day of presentation. The authors found very little effect of type of water source (piped water supply versus protected well, unprotected well or surface water). There was, however, a significant ($p < 0.01$) increase in the rate of diarrhoea with distance from water supply. Those living more than 1250 m from their source had over three times the risk of diarrhoea compared to those with a supply in the home (adjusted OR 3.29, CI 1.13–9.61).

A study in seven rural villages in southern Thailand compared the incidence of diarrhoea in children using a piped water supply with that of those who did not (Chongsuvivatwong *et al.* 1994). All villages had a piped water supply, but this was not used by all families in a village. The cohorts consisted of 126 children under two years using piped water and 137 not using it. Each family was visited once a week to determine any diarrhoeal illness. Using the piped water supply was associated with a reduced incidence of diarrhoea (2.54% versus 3.52%, RR 0.74, CI 0.59–0.93). Unfortunately, the authors noted that during the study period fewer families were using the piped water supply due to distribution failures.

A very effective way of preventing the very young from acquiring potentially fatal waterborne disease is not to let them drink water. The only other readily available source of liquid is breast milk. Breast-feeding should have a major protective effect against waterborne disease. VanDerslice, Popkin and Briscoe (1994) reported a study that looked at the impact of breast-feeding, drinking water quality and sanitation on infant health in Cebu in the Philippines. Recruited into the study were 2555 pregnant women, of whom 2355 had singleton live births. Each mother was interviewed during pregnancy, soon after birth and every second month after that for two years. This study analysed data for just the first six months of age. As was expected in a multivariable model, full breast-feeding was found to be protective ($p < 0.05$); even small amounts of added water increased the risk of diarrhoea substantially. There was also a significant independently increased risk of illness with microbiologically poor water ($p < 0.05$) and poor standards of sanitation as indicated by the presence of excreta in the yard ($p < 0.01$), and with the absence of private excreta disposal facilities ($p < 0.01$). Further analyses suggested that the benefits of breast-feeding increased as standards of sanitation declined.

VanDerslice and Briscoe (1995) reported further on this study the following year. They found that in areas with poor environmental sanitation, improved drinking water would have little or no effect. However, in areas with good community sanitation, reducing faecal coliform counts by two orders of magnitude would reduce the incidence of diarrhoea by 40%, eliminating excreta from around the house by 30% and providing private excreta disposal by 42%.

The resistance of enteric bacteria to antimicrobial agents is even more of a problem in developing countries than in the west. Drug-resistant bacteria may themselves cause disease, making treatment more difficult and expensive. Even if the resistant bacteria are of low virulence, they may transmit antibiotic resistance to other, more virulent, bacteria. Shears *et al.* (1995) reported a study of the faecal carriage of multiply drug-resistant (resistant to three or more antibiotics) enteric bacteria in Bangladeshi children. They also cultured bacteria from village water sources. Most (81%) of the children carried multiply drug-resistant coliforms in the intestine. All of the tube wells examined had low coliform counts (<10 per 100 ml), but many (76%) of the storage pots in the home had high (>50 per 100 ml) counts. Of these, coliforms isolated from storage pots and all coliforms isolated from surface water drinking sources were multiply drug resistant.

Comments

The paper by VanDerslice and Briscoe (1995) is, in my view, one of the single most useful studies of the impact of water supply on diarrhoeal disease in developing countries. It summarizes and confirms many of the findings of previous studies in a single piece of research. My own rephrasing of the studies reviewed in this section is as follows:

1 The single most important intervention in reducing childhood diarrhoeal disease is education aimed at getting communities to take responsibility for improving the general sanitary standards in their area.
2 Education of women about the benefits of breast-feeding.
3 Provision of a water supply as close to people's homes as possible, whatever the quality.
4 Education of individuals, usually women, about the benefits of hand washing and making soap available.
5 Provision of excreta disposal facilities and sanitation.
6 Improving the quality of the water supply.

It is notable that in this list of priorities, education features most strongly, while improving water quality (the most expensive and difficult option) comes last. In the two studies from developed countries discussed at the start of this section (Payment et al. 1991b; Zmirou et al. 1987), it is doubtful whether any adverse water-associated health effect would have been seen at all, had not the studies been done in affluent communities with high standards of community hygiene and cleanliness. It is a sobering thought that so much apparently waterborne disease could be prevented by education, not requiring expensive civil engineering.

However, a study by Curtis et al. (1995) from Burkina Faso suggested that the relationship between the factors I have listed may be more complex than at first appears. They studied those factors that were associated with good hygiene practice when mothers disposed of their children's faeces. Those mothers who had access to a tap in their own yards reported using safe hygienic practices three times more commonly than those mothers taking water from wells outside the compound ($p < 0.05$). These reports were backed up by observation of faeces around the house. The authors suggested that this may be because the improved water supply was encouraging better hygienic practices or because women who spend a lot of time collecting water have less time available for hygiene. This impact of water supply was stronger than health education or family economic status.

WATERBORNE DISEASE IN REFUGEE CAMPS

One issue of increasing importance to water supplies and waterborne disease is the special problems of refugee camps. Supplying safe water to large numbers of people, many of whom are already debilitated from hunger, pre-existing disease and fear, is a colossal problem. Many of the fatalities in refugee camps are due to diseases that have the potential to be waterborne. I now review two papers that considered certain of the problems that were associated with major refugee camps.

During 1978 almost 200 000 refugees fled Burma into Bangladesh. These refugees were settled in 13 camps. Initially the camps were formed from locally available materials and had no latrines and no water supplies. Four clinics, which between them recorded 174 201 visits, were set up in the camps (Khan and Munshi 1983). Of these visits, 28% were for watery diarrhoea, 32% for dysentery and 40% for other illness. During the ten-month period from May 1978 to February 1979 there were 1306 deaths, an estimated mortality rate of 88.6 per 1000 per year. Fatality rates were highest in the young: 640 per 1000 per year for the under one-year-olds and 357 for the 1–4 year olds. Diarrhoeal disease was responsible for 11.8% of deaths. Coliform counts in locally available water from ditches, a shallow dug well and a pond were very high, over 17 000 per 100 ml.

An even bigger catastrophe was the Rwandan refugee crisis in 1994. Some 500 000–800 000 refugees entered the North Kivu region of Zaire in July of that year. During the first month that the camps were open, 48 347 deaths were recorded (Goma Epidemiology Group 1995). This number was probably an underestimate because it only included the counts of bodies that were collected by truck. The average crude mortality rate was between 19.5 and 31.2 per 10 000 per day. Unaccompanied children had an extremely high death rate, up to 120 per 10 000 per day. The first case of cholera was diagnosed on 20 July, and within six days there were over 6000 cases of diarrhoea occurring each day. Approximately 88% of all fatalities were associated with diarrhoea. Given the usual high rate of asymptomatic carriage of *Vibrio cholerae* O1, it was likely that most of the refugees had been infected. The rapid spread was thought to be due largely to the consumption of untreated lake water. Many of the refugees were located near to Lake Kivu. Indeed, it was not until three days after the peak of the epidemic that the relief operation was able to supply purified water, and then only 1 l per person per day (UNHCR recommendations are for a minimum of 15–20 l per person per day).

Discussion of other outbreaks in refugee camps will follow later in the book.

4 Illness Associated with Recreational Contact with Water

In this chapter we turn our attention to recreational water-associated disease. The epidemiology of this group of illness varies quite markedly depending on the type of water in which the affected individuals have immersed themselves. We will consider three classifications of water: surface waters, swimming pools and spa-pools/hot tubs. Surface waters include rivers, lakes and ocean waters, which are usually natural and unchlorinated. For all three categories we will first look at evidence from the US and UK national reporting of waterborne outbreaks. Prospective epidemiological studies will then be reviewed.

DISEASE ASSOCIATED WITH UNTREATED SURFACE WATERS

Outbreaks reported to national surveillance centres

During the ten years from 1985 to 1994, 55 outbreaks of disease affecting 3713 individuals associated with recreation water contact with surface waters were reported to the US Center for Disease Control (St Louis 1988; Levine, Stephenson and Craun 1990; Herwaldt et al. 1991; Moore et al. 1993; Kramer et al. 1996). Table 4.1 lists the number of outbreaks reported by causation. All but one of the outbreaks were related to inland waters and one was due to ocean water. In 24% of outbreaks a causative organism was not identified. Perhaps most surprising to the European audience is that 29% of outbreaks, affecting 1294 individuals, were due to shigellosis.

Until 1992 the UK Communicable Disease Surveillance Centre (CDSC) did not routinely collect and publish reports of waterborne disease. However, it would appear that recreational water outbreaks are uncommon in the UK. In their review of outbreaks between 1937 and 1986, Galbraith, Barrett and Stanwell-Smith (1987) found very few recreational water associated outbreak reports since typhoid in the 1950s. There were, however, 6 cases of primary amoebic meningoencephalitis and about 200 cases of leptospirosis. Since 1992 there has been only one outbreak associated with recreational contact with surface waters. This was an outbreak of viral gastroenteritis during 1994 affecting 7 of 11 canoeists who immersed themselves in river water.

Table 4.1 Outbreaks of disease associated with recreational contact with untreated surface waters reported to CDC during the ten years from 1985 to 1994 (St Louis 1988; Levine, Stephenson and Craun 1990; Herwaldt *et al.* 1991; Moore *et al.* 1993; Kramer *et al.* 1996)

Pathogen	Number of outbreaks	Number of cases
Shigellosis	16	1294
Acute gastroenteritis of unknown cause	13	1005
Adenovirus conjunctivitis	1	595
Cryptosporidium	1	418
E. coli O157: H7	2	187
Cercarial dermatitis	4	80
Giardiasis	4	65
Norwalk-like gastroenteritis	1	41
Leptospirosis	2	14
Amoebic meningoencephalitis	10	10
Aseptic meningitis	1	4

This marked difference between US and UK experience in part reflects different habits of the two nations' swimmers. Swimming in unchlorinated inland surface waters appears to be much more common in America than in the UK. In the UK the seaside is the preferred place to enjoy swimming out of doors.

Šrámová and Kovácová (1984) listed 20 outbreaks of intestinal disease reported in the Czech Soviet Republic during the four years from 1979 to 1982. All of these outbreaks were of shigellosis. Nine outbreaks affecting 494 people were after swimming in streams or rivers, eight (261 people) were from swimming in a 'natural outdoor bathing area' and three (62 people) from swimming in a swimming pool.

Evidence from prospective epidemiological studies

Cabelli *et al.* (1979) were the first to undertake adequate prospective epidemiological studies of the health effects of bathing. The early studies took place at the New York City beaches. There were cohort studies of all those who attended the beach on a particular weekend. They investigated two beaches; one was 'relatively unpolluted' and the other was 'barely acceptable'. Water samples were also taken and analysed for a variety of microbial indicators during times of maximum swimming activity. Individuals were assessed as swimming (exposure of the head to the water) or non-swimming. Details about subsequent illness were obtained by telephone interview 8–10 days later. Log mean faecal coliform counts were 565 per 100 ml at the barely acceptable beach and 28.4 at the relatively unpolluted beach. The gastrointestinal symptom rate for swimmers at the barely acceptable beach was significantly higher than in non-swimmers (4.2% versus 2.6%, $p = 0.005$). There were no statistically significant effects on other symptoms at either beach, and no effect on gastrointestinal symptoms at the relatively unpolluted beach.

Over the next few years Cabelli *et al.* (1982) repeated this study design at several US beaches. Over the several studies undertaken, the authors interviewed over 25 000 swimmers and non-swimmers. Excess attack rates of gastrointestinal symptoms and 'highly credible gastrointestinal symptoms (HCGI)' (vomiting or diarrhoea with fever) in swimmers were noted in most of the studies. No relationship between swimming and any other symptom was found. When the investigators calculated the correlation coefficients between attack rates of HCGI with counts of indicator organisms, the major association was with enterococci ($r = 0.96$); correlation coefficients of association with other organisms were much lower (e.g. *E. coli*, $r = 0.58$). This study confirmed an association of gastroenteritis and swimming in faecally polluted waters and showed that the best marker of risk was enterococcal counts.

The Cabelli study design was also used by Canadian workers to investigate the health effects of swimming at several Ontario beaches (Seyfried *et al.* 1985a). Over 6000 people were included in this study. A wide range of symptoms was associated with swimming in this study, including respiratory (2.84% versus 1.17%), gastrointestinal (1.53% versus 0.39%), eye (0.98% versus 0.61%), ear (0.69% versus 0.22%), skin (0.69% versus 0.22%) and allergies (0.69% versus 0.28%). Unfortunately, significance levels were not given, making interpretation of the results difficult. The authors then went onto compare illness with counts of indicator organisms (Seyfried *et al.* 1985b). The organisms associated with gastrointestinal symptoms were faecal streptococci, though this did not quite achieve significance ($p = 0.069$). Total staphylococci counts were associated with eye symptoms ($p = 0.002$) for people who had put their head under water.

A study, stimulated by anecdotal reports of illness among participants in a snorkel swimming event held annually in Bristol docks, compared illness rates between snorkelers and observers in the subsequent year's event (Philipp *et al.* 1985). This found that 27% of participants developed gastrointestinal symptoms within 48 hours of entering the water compared to only 2.4% of controls ($p < 0.001$). It was found that three water samples taken during the event all exceeded the mandatory EC limits for total and faecal coliforms.

A small case-control study in the English Lake District looked at people presenting to general practitioners with newly diagnosed diarrhoea or vomiting (Jessop, Horsley and Wood 1995). Controls were taken from the telephone directory or from temporary resident registrations at a local general practice. This study found no difference between cases or controls for the use of local lakes.

Dewailly, Poirer and Meyer (1986) took the opportunity of studying the health hazards of windsurfing during the 1984 Windsurfer Western Hemisphere Championship held on the St Lawrence river, Quebec. This was a cohort study, which included 79 competitors and 41 employees. Symptoms were recorded for

Table 4.2 EC microbiological standards for bathing waters

Parameters	Guide level	Mandatory level
Total coliforms/100 ml	500	10 000
Faecal coliforms/100 ml	100	2000
Faecal streptococci/100 ml	100	–
Salmonella/1 l	–	0
Enteroviruses: PFU/10 l	–	0

each of the nine days of the event. Significant excess cases of diarrhoea (RR 6.7, CI 1.1–41.7) and any symptom (RR 2.9, CI 1.3–6.6) were seen in competitors. Symptoms of skin infection, otitis and conjunctivitis were also elevated but not significantly so. The risk of 'water pollution related symptoms' increased with the number of falls the competitors reported ($p = 0.000\ 001$).

In a retrospective study, 5737 tourists in one of eight holiday camps were interviewed about their swimming in the River Ardech in France and about the presence of any symptoms (Ferley *et al.* 1989). Those who had been swimming were more likely to be symptomatic (RR 2.1, CI 1.8–2.4), have acute gastrointestinal disease (RR 2.4, CI 1.9–3.0), have objective acute gastrointestinal disease (vomiting and/or diarrhoea) (RR 2.3, CI 1.7–3.2) and have skin disease (RR 3.7, CI 2.4–5.7). Microbiological sampling of the river near the camps showed that of all the indicator organisms faecal streptococci were most strongly correlated with risk. The authors suggested that faecal streptococcal counts in water of 20 per 100 ml was the level at which statistically significant excess morbidity was seen in swimmers. This compares with the EC limit for bathing waters of 100 per 100 ml (Table 4.2).

Another Cabelli-type study was done at nine beaches in Hong Kong during the summers of 1986 and 1987 (Cheung *et al.* 1990). A total of 18 741 responses were included in the analysis, of which 14 464 were from people classed as swimmers. Significant excesses were noted in self-perceived gastrointestinal (RR 3.2), highly credible gastrointestinal (RR 5.0), ear (RR not calculable), eye (RR 3.9), skin (RR 2.4) and respiratory (RR 2.6) symptoms and with fever (RR 3.7). In this study *E. coli* counts were more highly correlated with disease than were faecal streptococci.

Calderon, Wood and Dufour (1991) set out to determine whether people were at risk of illness from swimming in water that was subject to animal but not human faecal contamination. They did a Cabelli-type study at a pond with no obvious source of external human contamination. Water quality criteria were within European and US standards. The study included data from 104 families. Swimmers experienced more gastroenteritis than non-swimmers (RR 8.7, $p < 0.001$). In descending order, the most significant factors associated with illness were the number of bathers in the pond (≥ 53 versus <53; $p = 0.011$) followed by counts of staphylococci (≥ 45 versus <45 per 100 ml; $p = 0.026$). Counts of faecal coliforms and *E. coli* were not associated.

Associations between illness and enterococcal counts ($\geq$20 versus <20 per 100 ml; p = 0.059) or rainfall (p = 0.089) did not quite achieve statistical significance. The authors concluded that, in this study, illness acquisition was from other bathers and that high faecal indicator counts where the source is animal, not human, do not predict disease. However, enterococcal counts were generally relatively low. The degree of faecal pollution from animal sources was, therefore minimal. As both rainfall and enterococcal counts were borderline significant, it is not clear whether the study was sufficiently powerful to confirm any association.

The first Cabelli-type study to be reported in a medical journal in the UK was of 2010 individuals on a beach in Ramsgate, Kent, undertaken during August 1990 (Balarajan *et al.* 1991). Bathers had significant increase in any gastrointestinal symptom (RR 1.47, CI 1.06–2.04) and diarrhoea (RR 1.88, CI 1.18–2.99) but not eye, ear, nose and throat, or respiratory symptoms. Divers and surfers also experienced an increase in eye (RR 2.65, CI 1.22–5.75) and respiratory symptoms (RR 2.85, CI 1.38–5.87).

A similar study, this time of 733 individuals, was reported from South Africa (Von Schirnding *et al.* 1992). This study looked at two beaches, one of which had high counts of faecal coliforms (median 76.5 per 100 ml) and enterococci (median 51.5 per 100 ml) and the other low counts (8.0 and 2.0 per 100 ml, respectively). The incidences of gastrointestinal, respiratory and skin symptoms were higher in the swimmers at the more polluted beach compared to non-swimmers and swimmers at the less polluted beach. These differences were not, however, statistically significant.

In another UK study, investigators followed up 939 children who attended a beach in northwest England (Alexander *et al.* 1992). Water samples regularly failed EC standards. The authors claimed that their study found very highly significant associations between entering the water and a variety of symptoms such as vomiting, diarrhoea, itchy skin, fever, lack of energy and loss of appetite. However, the statistical methodology that the authors used to support their conclusions was rather non-standard. They compared symptom rates before and after attending the beach in their two cohorts, one with water contact and the other without. They claimed significant effects of water contact if there was a significant increase in the swimmers cohort, but not in the non-swimmers cohort. This approach is, in my view, suspect, especially as the contact group was almost twice as large as the non-contact group. My own analysis of the results of this study does not support their claims with the exception of gastrointestinal symptoms.

Fewtrell *et al.* (1992) studied illness rates in white-water canoeists after attending events at two sites, one of which was a lowland water and the other an upland water. Both of these sites complied with EC bacteriological standards, although counts of faecal coliforms were higher in the lowland water. The lowland water failed EC standards for the isolation of enterovirus. The study included 146 canoeists at the lowland water site, 206 at the upland site and 173 non-canoeist controls. Compared to canoeists at the upland site, those at the lowland site experienced increased flu (RR 1.76, CI 1.31–2.37), respiratory (RR 1.51, CI 1.06–2.14), eye/ear (RR 3.53, CI 1.13–11.03), gastrointestinal (RR 2.97, CI 2.01–4.37) and skin (RR 2.02, CI 1.05–3.86) symptoms. Canoeists on the lowland water had significantly increased levels of flu, respiratory and gastrointestinal symptoms compared to non-exposed controls, while canoeists at the upland site only had a significant increased risk of respiratory symptoms. Among lowland white-water canoeists, 67% experienced some symptom compared with 42% of canoeists at the upland site and 33% of non-canoeist controls.

An Australian Cabelli-type study reported by Corbett *et al.* (1993) included 2839 individuals who had attended beaches in the Sydney area during the summer of 1989/90. (Geometric mean counts for faecal coliforms were 26.2 per 100 ml in the morning and 15.9 in the afternoon; mean counts of faecal streptococci were 16.4 and 11.5 per 100 ml in the morning and afternoon, respectively). They found that swimmers had excess cough (OR 1.9, CI 1.4–2.4) and ear symptoms (OR 3.6, CI 1.8–7.2), but not gastrointestinal symptoms (OR 1.5, CI 0.8–2.7). The presence of any symptom correlated better with coliform counts that with streptococcal counts. This negative result for gastroenteritis probably is more of an indication of the very clean microbiological state of the Sydney beaches.

Perhaps the most comprehensive and convincing studies into the relationship between bathing and ill health were conducted in the UK by Fleisher *et al.* (1993). The studies conducted at two beaches within the UK are among the very few experimental studies ever to have been done on human ill health and water contact. The authors conducted a randomized trial of bathing water contact at two beaches, both of which complied with European standards for bathing beaches. Participants were recruited before the study day. Before the trial, each participant was interviewed and given a medical examination. Those who completed the examination were then randomized into 271 bathers and 296 non-bathers. Non-bathers were given a packed lunch and had to spend three hours sitting on the beach in a roped-off area, where they were watched to ensure that they did not enter the water. Bathers were allowed into various 20 m-wide swim zones in which comprehensive microbiological examinations of the water quality were undertaken regularly. Therefore, the exact exposure to various water qualities was known. Participants were followed up 3, 7 and 28 days after the trial. Although the rates of subjective and objective gastrointestinal illness were raised in bathers at both beaches (17.5% versus 11.0% and 22.4% versus 14.4%), this was not statistically significant. However, when the results from bathers were classified on the faecal streptococcal counts, a very highly significant relationship was demonstrated. Attack rates of both subjective and objective gastroenteritis were higher than in non-bathing controls when the faecal streptococci counts rose above 20 per 100 ml and became significant above counts of 40 per 100 ml.

Of individuals exposed to counts greater than 80 per 100 ml, 41.2% suffered from subjective gastrointestinal symptoms. Interestingly, at one of the beaches the authors also found an association between gastrointestinal symptoms and the consumption of hamburgers.

The cumulative evidence from the outbreak reports and other epidemiological studies is clear: adverse health effects appear common in people who immerse themselves in surface waters for recreation. The link between gastrointestinal illness and recreational surface water contact is particularly clear. The evidence points squarely at faecal pollution (as measured by enterococcal counts) as the responsible factor for this excess. Furthermore, significant illness occurs after contact with faecally polluted waters, even when such waters satisfy current bathing water standards. Symptoms increase with increasing microbiological evidence of faecal pollution. However, most illness is mild and self-limiting. Very few people seem even to consult a doctor. A microbiological or clinical diagnosis is rarely made in prospective studies.

The evidence in favour of an association between water contact and ear, eye, respiratory and skin symptoms is less strong but still reasonably convincing. Interestingly, there is evidence that some of these illnesses may be common, even in water with low levels of faecal pollution, as in the Sydney study (Corbett *et al.* 1993) and the study by Calderon, Wood and Dufour (1991). These studies would suggest that such symptoms may be related to person to person spread in the water environment or be some direct effect of immersion itself.

Although much less frequent, more serious and potentially fatal disease is also a risk. For example, cases of amoebic meningoencephalitis, although rare, are usually fatal. The risk of such more severe disease cannot be identified from prospective studies, only from retrospective analysis of outbreaks and case reports.

Further evidence of adverse health affects comes from certain case-control studies of sporadic disease. For example Gallaher *et al.* (1989) reported that swimming in surface water increased the risk of cryptosporidiosis by 3.7 times. In a similar study, Dennis *et al.* (1993) found that swimming in a lake, pond, stream or river versus not swimming or swimming in a swimming pool or the ocean was associated with a 3.1 times increased risk of giardiasis. These and other disease-specific studies are discussed in more detail in subsequent chapters.

DISEASE ASSOCIATED WITH SWIMMING POOLS

Outbreaks reported to national surveillance centres

The US data for outbreaks associated with swimming pools is given in Table 4.3 (St Louis 1988; Levine, Stephenson and Craun 1990; Herwaldt *et al.* 1991;

Table 4.3 Outbreaks associated with swimming pools reported to the US CDC during the period 1985–1994 (St Louis 1988; Levine, Stephenson and Craun 1990; Herwaldt *et al.* 1991; Moore *et al.* 1993; Kramer *et al.* 1996)

Pathogen	Number of outbreaks	Number of cases
Cryptosporidiosis	7	801
Giardiasis	8	434
Pseudomonal dermatitis	4	127
Pseudomonal otitis and conjunctivitis	1	35
Chemical dermatitis	2	29
Enterovirus-like	1	26
Hepatitis A	1	20
Acute gastroenteritis of unknown cause	1	16
Shigellosis	1	10

Moore *et al.* 1993; Kramer *et al.* 1996). During that period 26 outbreaks affected 1498 people. Five of seven outbreaks of cryptosporidiosis occurred in the last two years covered by the reports, probably reflecting the relatively more recent interest in this disease by American laboratories compared to their European equivalents.

In their review of waterborne and water-associated outbreaks in the UK from 1937 to 1986, Galbraith, Barrett and Stanwell-Smith (1987) were unable fully to quantify the risks associated with immersion in treated water pools. However, they felt that skin infections due to *Pseudomonas aeruginosa* were probably common. They also suggested that there were probably about 100 cases of skin infection due to *Mycobacterium marinum* infections since the 1960s. Included in the paper was mention of an outbreak due to *Legionella*, which caused 26 cases of Legionnaires' disease and seven cases of Pontiac fever. The UK Public Health Laboratory Service (PHLS) has been collating waterborne outbreaks since 1992. In the years 1992 to 1995, there have been four outbreaks, affecting 52 individuals, reported to the PHLS from England and Wales (Furtado *et al.* 1996). All four outbreaks were due to cryptosporidiosis. After the review by Galbraith, Barrett and Stanwell-Smith (1987) but before the routine reporting by CDSC, I can find one further swimming pool outbreak in England. It was also of cryptosporidium and it affected 65 individuals in 1988 (Joce *et al.* 1991).

Evidence from prospective epidemiological studies

By contrast to the situation for raw waters, there have been relatively few prospective studies of bathers attending swimming pools. Gentles and Evans (1973) conducted an early study of foot infections in 10% of individuals attending a heated swimming pool over a one-week period. They examined 773 individuals and found an overall prevalence of tinea pedis of 8.5%. This was highest in male adults, 21.5%, 6.3% in boys, 3.3% in adult females and

0.9% in girls. *Trichophyton mentagrophytes* var. *interdigitale* was the commonest isolate (62.1%) followed by *T. rubrum* (13.6%) and *Epidermophyton rubrum* (10.6%). Very few adults had a verruca (1% of males and no females), while the prevalence was 4.2% in boys and 10.5% in girls. As this was apparently the first such survey, the authors were unable to say whether this prevalence was higher than one would expect to see in the general population.

Almost 20 years later Bolănos (1991) reported a further study of dermatophyte feet infections in swimmers. He studied a class of students on day one of a course of swimming lessons. The study was repeated one and a half months later after 12 lessons. He found a slight, but not statistically significant, increase in symptoms of tinea pedis from 12.0% to 15.2%. The number of asymptomatic carriers of dermatophytes increased from 1.2% to 7.0%. At the start *T. rubrum* was the most frequently isolated fungal pathogen, being responsible for 82% of isolations. At the end, *T. mentagrophytes* was the most frequent, at 70.6% of isolations. *T. mentagrophytes* was also isolated from 6 of 30 floor samples at the time of the second study.

Not all rashes associated with swimming pools are infectious. In the UK Rycroft and Penny (1983) reported a survey of swimming pools that showed 19 severe and 46 moderate rashes in three bromine-disinfected swimming pools compared to no severe and 6 moderate rashes in six chorine disinfected pools. Subsequently, Penny (1991) reported a survey of rashes after swimming in pools in Somerset. He advertised in local papers for anyone who believed that they suffered a rash after swimming in a pool to write to him. Most (43) of the rashes detected were from the two bromine pools in the survey. Only two rashes were diagnosed from 19 chlorinated pools. The incidence rate per number of annual swims per pool type was 1:865 000 for chlorinated pools and 1:715 for the bromine pools. It would appear that in 1990 the risk of skin rash after swimming in a bromine-disinfected pool was over a thousand times that of swimming in a chlorinated pool. The clinical features of the rashes identified were compatible with bromine-based dermatitis rather than any infection.

A Japanese study investigated the incidence of molluscum contagiosum (a viral skin disease) in 15 elementary schools and 9 kindergartens (Niizeki, Kano and Kondo 1984). Of 7472 children examined, 517 (6.9%) were found to be suffering from the infection. The prevalence in swimmers was higher than in non-swimmers (7.5% versus 3.6%).

A study from Israel investigated the relationship between otitis externa and swimming pool water quality (Simchen, Franklin and Shuval 1984). They studied 346 children from 11 kibbutzim. The overall infection rate was 29.5%. The available pools were classed as high contamination (a total bacterial count of ≥ 30 per ml, a coliform count of ≥ 100 per 100 ml and a faecal coliform count of ≥ 10 per 100 ml), low contamination (total bacterial count of <1 per ml, coliform count of <10 per 100 ml and a faecal coliform count of <1 per 100 ml) and medium contamination (i.e. all pools that did not fit into the high and low categories). Otitis externa was uniformly high (41.0%) in children who were divers, compared to only 24.7% in non-divers ($p = 0.02$). In non-divers there was a significant correlation between water quality and otitis externa (17.0% in low, 23.1% in medium and 35.7% in highly contaminated pools; $p = 0.03$). The remarkable finding in this study was the number of very heavily contaminated pools. Other studies of ear infection associated with swimming pools are discussed in the chapter on pseudomonas. It should be remembered that there are other, non-infectious, explanations for any increased risk of otitis externa in swimmers and divers. If divers go deep there may be significant pressure on the tympanic membrane, with resultant damage. Direct irritation of the eustachian tubes by chlorine, leading to obstruction and otitis media, may also be a factor.

The only study that I could find that looked at the general health effects of swimming in pools was done in Paris during 1990/91 (Momas *et al.* 1993). The authors followed up a cohort of 246 pupils, some of whom (210) reported bathing at least once, while the remainder (36) reported not swimming during the study period. Compared with non-bathers, bathers more frequently reported blotch (OR 5.03, CI 1.68–15.1), fatigue (OR 3.70, CI 1.08–12.7) and watery eye (OR not calculable, $p = 0.0215$). However, bathers were less likely to report verrucae (OR 0.36, CI 0.15–0.89). This last finding is not surprising because many non-bathers reported the presence of a verruca as the reason why they were excluded from swimming.

Although there are several reports of swimming pool associated disease, the risk must be kept in context. Swimming is a very popular sport that promotes fitness and good health. The small number of outbreaks reported are minute in comparison to the number of people who attend swimming pools. Learning to swim can also be life saving. The benefits of going to a swimming pool certainly outweigh the very small risk of infection for most people.

DISEASE ASSOCIATED WITH WHIRLPOOLS, SPA-POOLS AND HOT TUBS

Outbreaks reported to national surveillance centres

During the period 1985–1994 there were 53 outbreaks reported to CDC as being associated with spa-pools, whirlpools or hot tubs (St Louis 1988; Levine, Stephenson and Craun 1990; Herwaldt *et al.* 1991; Moore *et al.* 1993; Kramer *et al.* 1996). Of these outbreaks, 48, affecting 951 individuals, were of skin disease either definitely due to or compatible with *Pseudomonas aeruginosa*. The remaining five outbreaks were of Pontiac fever, which affected a total of 63 people. No comparable data is available from the UK, probably because the routine UK reporting systems tend to rely heavily on laboratory reports, which subsequently give a much higher importance to gastrointestinal illness.

5 Dracunculiasis (Guinea Worm Infestation)

Dracunculiasis is an infestation by the nematode worm *Dracunculus medinensis*. It is quite possible that dracunculiasis will be only the second major disease to be globally eradicated. Dracunculiasis was targeted for eradication by the World Health Organization during the International Drinking Water Supply and Sanitation Decade, 1981–1990. If current eradication efforts continue, success may happen during the first few years of the next millennium. If this does happen, then dracunculiasis will be an example of disease eradication undertaken largely through education and by the application of simple, low-technology measures.

LIFE CYCLE

As already mentioned *D. medinensis* is a nematode worm. *D. medinensis* has its adult stage in a human host and its larval stage in the freshwater crustaceans *Cyclops*. Humans become infected by drinking water that contains infected *Cyclops*. The larvae are released from the *Cyclops* into the stomach, from where they pass into the small intestine and penetrate the mucosa. They then migrate to the retroperitoneal space (the space behind the peritoneum and in front of the spinal column and lumbar muscles) where they mature and mate. About a year later the female worm, now up to 1 m long, migrates to the subcutaneous tissue of the legs. Here she penetrates the skin and extrudes her uterus through her head. Whenever the resultant ulcer is placed into water the guinea worm discharges her larvae. The larvae are then preyed upon by *Cyclops*. Once consumed by the crustaceans, the larvae become infective for humans in about 14 days. The life cycle is illustrated in Figure 5.1.

CLINICAL FEATURES

There are usually no symptoms of infection until the female worm reaches the skin surface and is ready to discharge her larvae. A stinging/burning sensation

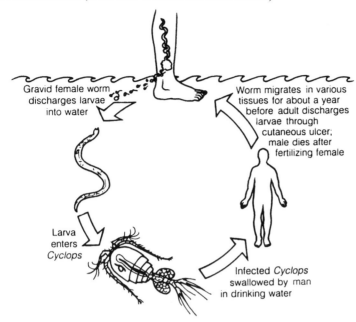

Figure 5.1 Life cycle of *Dracunculus medinensis*. Redrawn from Southgate (1996) in Cook GC (ed.) *Manson's Tropical Diseases*, 12th edn; reproduced by permission of WB Saunders.

heralds the appearance of a blister, which ruptures to form an ulcer when the site is placed in water. On examination of the ulcer, the worm's head may be seen protruding. This process takes place over just a few days. If the ulcer is placed in water, a milky fluid can be seen to be discharged. Occasionally there may be generalized symptoms of urticaria, nausea, vomiting and dyspnoea when the blister first appears. Once all the larvae have been discharged the worm dies and is reabsorbed or calcified. The ulcer usually heals with no scarring.

If the worm dies prematurely or breaks during an attempt to extract it, a large sterile abscess can develop. If this abscess becomes infected, the resulting cellulitis can affect nearby joints and tendons, causing significant disability. In endemic areas individuals can be affected by several such worms each year, restricting them to bed for up to a month at a time.

TREATMENT

The traditional method for removing a guinea worm is to attach the head to a matchstick and twist the stick a small amount each day until the worm has been removed. Specific chemotherapy with thiabendazole or metronidazole does not kill the worm but reduces the associated inflammation, allowing the worm to be removed more rapidly under local anaesthetic or even to extrude itself.

EPIDEMIOLOGY

All cases of dracunculiasis, almost by definition of its life cycle, are water-borne. Therefore, any study that investigates the epidemiology of dracunculiasis will look at the role of drinking water in its transmission. Especially since the implementation of the eradication strategy by WHO, there have been very many papers published describing the epidemiology of the disease in various tropical countries. I have concentrated on those studies that were particularly interested in the water connection, and have taken papers from the periods before and after dracunculiasis was targeted by the WHO.

In 1986 there were an estimated 3.5 million cases of dracunculiasis world-wide (Anon 1995). By 1990 623 000 cases were reported and this fell to only 165 000 in 18 countries by 1994. There is, however, some suggestion of gross under-reporting (Pilotto and Gorski 1992). The mid-1980s figure may have been closer to 10 million, although even this figure looks small compared to the estimated 48 million cases in 1947 (Stoll 1947). The original target year for eradication was 1996, but this will probably be delayed a year or two.

Belcher et al. (1975) studied the epidemiology of the disease in southern Ghana in 1973 after a health education aid reported the sudden appearance of the disease in his area. The investigators conducted a series of detailed interviews with adults in the area. In the survey, 32 out of 159 villages had cases. All affected villages relied on ponds for their water supply during the dry season, with the highest incidence occurring in those villages with access to only one pond. In affected villages the attack rate ranged from 3% to 28%. Villages near perennial rivers were not affected. In two villages with a long history of infection, two groups of people, railway workers and prisoners, had always been free of the disease. Both of these groups had water supplied by tanker. Guinea worm infection was uncommon in children, with the highest incidence in adults between the ages of 15 and 29. Untreated, 60% of sufferers had five or more weeks of disability, although with treatment this was reduced to less than 20%. Given the predominantly agricultural employment of the affected individuals, this disability posed a severe threat to their families' livelihood.

In a study of 17 rural villages in western Nigeria over five years from 1971 to 1975, the incidence of dracunculiasis was 13.5% of a population of 8200 (Kale 1977). Infection rates in males and females were similar. The predominant occupation among adult males was farming. The average duration of disability in an affected individual was 100 days. Of the 17 villages, 11 depended exclusively on waterholes and ponds, most of which became dry in the dry season, 5 had wells, of which 4 were badly constructed and poorly maintained, and 1 had access to a flowing stream. Although the incidence ranged between villages from 2.2% to 58.5%, the author did not attempt to link the different attack rates with the village water supply.

Johnson and Joshi (1982) studied the epidemiology of dracunculiasis in Rajasthan, India. The overall infection rate was 6.0%, 7.5% in males and 4.1% in females ($p < 0.001$). In the 11 affected villages, the attack rate ranged from 0.1% to 13.4%. Among people using pondwater, the attack rate was 6.4% and only 0.1% in those using well-water ($p < 0.0001$).

Watts (1986) studied human behaviour patterns likely to increase the transmission of infection in Nigeria between 1979 and 1984. The area under study had an extremely high prevalence of disease, 55%, with one village at 78%. This study was particularly important in that it identified many specific behavioural factors at which control strategies could be targeted. The study also reinforced the central importance of women in the control of dracunculiasis, as with other waterborne diseases. Collecting water is a major burden for women in tropical countries, especially in the dry season, when they may have to walk several kilometres each day. It is not surprising that women will use a nearer source of water if one is available. Watts showed that if they are aware that some waters are polluted, women will walk further to get safe water. Protection of surface water sources from wading water collectors was rarely done. Boiling water was impracticable in people's homes because of the extra burden that would place on women to collect firewood. At the time of the study few women were aware of the benefits of filtering drinking water through a fine cotton sieve. Population mobility is an increasingly important factor in the transmission of dracunculiasis. The local movement of women to collect water is one such factor, and wider movements associated with religious festivals or migrant workers increase the geographical distribution of the disease.

A survey of dracunculiasis in northwestern Uganda was done in 1994 to provide epidemiological base data in a water programme target area (Henderson, Fontaine and Kyeyune 1988). Among 2014 people in 221 households surveyed, 389 (19.3%) reported a guinea worm in the previous year. In this study, the incidence of dracunculiasis was bimodal, with a peak in August, the wet season, and a peak in February, the dry season. Compared to those who used boreholes for their drinking water, the attack rate was higher in people who drank from ponds, reservoirs and valley tanks in the dry season (4.9% versus 24.6%, RR 5.01, $p < 0.01$). In the wet season, the attack rate in borehole water users was only 0.9%, compared with 24.9% (RR 25.9, $p < 0.01$) in those using ponds, reservoirs and valley tanks, 12.1% (RR 12.5, $p < 0.01$) in those using all sources in water courses and 4.7% (RR 4.9, $p < 0.05$) in those using other unsafe sources.

Mazmum, a small town of 17 313 inhabitants in central Sudan, experienced a sudden increase in the number of cases of dracunculiasis in 1990 (Abdel-

Hameed *et al.* 1993). A review of the hospital records showed that 73 cases were recorded in 1990, 131 in 1991 and 643 in 1992. A house survey was also conducted in the town to assess the incidence (23.4%) between November 1991 and November 1992. The incidence of disease was higher in households that obtained their drinking water from Soba natural pool (28.6% versus 18.0%, $p < 0.005$). From a survey of schools it was clear that the incidence of the disease was lower in primary school (13.5% versus 26.2%, $p < 0.0005$) and secondary school children (6.6% versus 33.3%, $p < 0.0001$) than in similarly aged children who were not in school. In a survey of water sources, all water samples revealed *Cyclops* spp. The density of these copepods was higher in the natural pool.

6 Schistosomiasis

Schistosomiasis is a group of diseases caused by infection with trematode flatworms. More than 200 million people in 73 countries are affected. It is a disease that is on the increase. Most disease is caused by five main species, which differ in their pathology and geographical distribution. These five species are: *Schistosoma haematobium, S. mansoni, S. japonicum, S. intercalatum* and *S. mekongi*.

LIFE CYCLE

With the exception of *S. mekongi*, whose definitive host is the dog, the definitive host of all species causing schistosomiasis is man. Eggs are passed in the urine or faeces. When they come into contact with freshwater, the eggs hatch, releasing the first larval stage, a miracidium, which then penetrates the body of its intermediate host, a specific freshwater snail. Within the snail the miracidia multiply asexually to form numerous sporocysts, which, after a period of four to six weeks, are released from the snail as free-swimming cercariae. These cercariae have at most 72 hours to penetrate the skin of their new mammalian host, man. During penetration these cercariae lose their tails and become schistosomula, which then migrate to the lungs or liver where they mature and mate over about six weeks. Once mature, the adult worms migrate through the venous system to their main resting place. For *S. haematobium* this is the veins of the bladder; for the other species it is the mesenteric vein. The adult worms survive for about 5–10 years, although sometimes for much longer. The life cycle is demonstrated in Figure 6.1.

CLINICAL FEATURES

The clinical features of schistosomiasis are many and varied depending on the infecting species, the stage of infection and the worm load. There are two forms of acute disease: schistosome dermatitis and Katayama fever.

Schistosome dermatitis (swimmer's itch) is due to penetration of the free-swimming cercariae through the skin. It is an itchy papular skin rash, which occurs within about 24 hours of penetration. The eruption is probably allergic

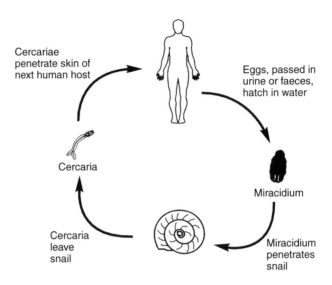

Cercariae
penetrate skin of
next human host

Eggs, passed in
urine or faeces,
hatch in water

Cercaria

Miracidium

Cercaria
leave
snail

Miracidium
penetrates
snail

Figure 6.1 Life cycle of *Schistosoma* spp.

in nature. The most severe forms of swimmer's itch are due to schistosomes whose primary hosts are not man and which are present in all five continents.

Katayama fever occurs about four to six weeks after infection, usually due to *S. japonicum* or *S. mansoni* and rarely to *S. haematobium*. There is an acute onset of fever, headache and cough. There is also enlargement of the liver, spleen and lymph nodes. Examination of the blood film shows eosinophilia. Occasionally Katayama fever results in death.

The nature of the chronic disease associated with schistosomiasis depends on the primary organ affected. *S. haematobium* tends to reside in the veins of the genitourinary system, so causing bladder and kidney disease. The remaining species tend to reside in the mesenteric veins draining the intestines, and so cause intestinal and hepatic disease. Schistosomiasis can also affect other organs from time to time such as the heart, lungs and nervous system.

Urinary schistosomiasis, especially when the infestation is light, is frequently asymptomatic. Painless haematuria is usually the first sign. Terminal haematuria, passing small amounts of blood at the very end of micturition is characteristic. More serious disease is due to damage of the bladder and kidneys as a result of obstruction to the flow of urine. Severe contraction of the bladder can occur, with fibrosis and calcification. This causes frequency, made worse by the increased risk of urinary tract infections. There is an increased risk of bladder cancer. Urinary outflow obstruction can lead to hydronephrosis, nephrotic syndrome and even renal failure.

Intestinal schistosomiasis can also be asymptomatic in light infections. Patients may complain of fatigue, abdominal pain and diarrhoea, which can be bloody. Anaemia is common due to the blood loss. There is polyp and ulcer formation, which can occasionally cause bowel obstruction. Perforation of the bowel is rare.

Hepatic schistosomiasis can occur when there is a heavy infestation. This usually presents as a symptomless hepatomegaly, with or without enlargement of the spleen. In advanced cases portal hypertension may develop, with massive enlargement of the spleen and the appearance of oesophageal varices, which can bleed repeatedly. Liver function is frequently normal.

DIAGNOSIS

All patients will give a history of residence or travel in an endemic area. A definitive diagnosis will only be made by finding the eggs in faeces, urine or a biopsy specimen. Eosinophilia seen on examination of the blood film is also a strong pointer.

Urine for microscopic examination is best collected between 10 a.m. and 2 p.m. Urine should be filtered to concentrate the eggs. Faeces should also be concentrated before microscopy. Biopsy specimens of the rectum or bladder walls should be compressed between glass slides before low-power microscopic examination. Microscopic examination also enables speciation of the schistosome as the eggs have their characteristic morphology.

An enzyme-linked immunosorbent assay (ELISA) test is available, although it is of limited use in residents of endemic areas. The ELISA test is, however, useful in early disease in travellers returning from an endemic area. It is also a useful way to reassure the worried well.

TREATMENT

Treatment of this disease has been revolutionized in recent years with the introduction of the broad-spectrum oral antihelmintic praziquantel. It is effective against all pathogenic schistosomes. Other drugs are available but with a more limited spectrum. Metrifonate is effective against *S. haematobium* and oxamniquine is effective against *S. mansoni*. In advanced and ectopic disease, surgery may be indicated after antihelmintic therapy.

ECOLOGY

As will be obvious from a knowledge of the life cycle of *Schistosoma* spp., the ecology of the disease outside of man will follow that of its specific snail species. Most of the snail hosts for the human schistosomes require freshwater. The snails also require calcium for their shells, so that an alkaline, rather than acidic, water is preferable. The waters need to be warm, over 20 °C and less than 39 °C. Heavily shaded waters are not suitable for snails because the plants on which they feed grow best in good light. Still or only slowly flowing waters encourage snail populations, as do muddy waters that contain many nutrients.

EPIDEMIOLOGY

The literature on schistosomiasis is vast and, because all infections are acquired from contact with water, all papers that discuss its epidemiology have as an element its waterborne nature. Consequently, it was not possible to give a comprehensive review of the subject in a single chapter. I have, there-fore, had to take a rather subjective choice of articles to discuss. Nevertheless, I have tried to concentrate on those studies that have set out to determine patterns of water exposure that are related to infection rather than those that have merely described the prevalence of infection in various populations.

Studies of the effect of domestic water supply provision

Jordan *et al.* (1978) reported the effect of providing a piped water supply to some villages in St Lucia and not others. The effect of the installation on the prevalence of schistosomiasis in children under ten years old was dramatic. Before and during installation of the piped supply the prevalence ranged from 22.7% to 30.6%. After installation it fell to 12.9% or less. Similar declines in prevalence were noted in all age groups. In villages not provided with a piped water supply the prevalence of infection remained high. Studies of the infec-tion of snails mirrored the findings in humans. The authors expressed disappointment that the disease did not decline further in the experimental area but noted that many children from the experimental area visited the control area to attend school.

In order to identify high risk factors for *S. haematobium* infection among schoolchildren, Savioli *et al.* (1989) analysed urine samples from about 25 000 children on two separate occasions. This study was done on Pemba Island, northeast of Zanzibar. In the first study, in November 1986, haematuria was found in 13 290 (54.3) of 24 462 children examined. Gross haematuria was present in 15.8%. All children with haematuria were then given a single dose of 40 mg of praziquantel. Six months later 26.0% had haematuria, of whom only 2.4% had gross haematuria. Those towns that had the most irregular piped water supply had the highest prevalence of haematuria before and after treatment.

The effect of water demand on the prevalence of schistosomiasis and other parasitic infections was studied among the Gumau people of Bauchi State, Nigeria (Akogun 1990). There was a significant positive correlation between 'water demand index' (the number of individuals per well in a town) and infection with *S. haematobium* ($r = 0.95$, $p < 0.01$) and *S. mansoni* ($r = 0.95$, $p < 0.01$). There was also a positive association with infection by *Taenia* spp. ($r = 0.70$, $p < 0.05$) but not other parasitic infections. The study also identified a significant negative correlation between distance from the nearest river and infection with *S. haematobium* ($r = -0.94$, $p < 0.01$) and *S. mansoni* ($r = -0.88$, $p < 0.01$). The author did not try to disentangle the correlation between water demand index and distance from river. Fewer wells are probably dug if surface water is readily available.

Studies of the effect of human behaviour

A study of a small village of 200 people in Ghana investigated the relationship between human behaviour and degree of infection with *S. haematobium* (Dalton and Pole 1978). The village concerned was situated on the shores of Lake Volta. Trained observers were employed to record the villagers' activities on the lake. Quantitative urine microscopy was then done. Multiple regression analysis revealed that the most important factors affecting egg counts in urine were the duration of domestic contact with the lake and the frequency of entering canoes. Some years later, Barbour (1985) reanalysed the results from this study and suggested that all the variation in schistosomiasis could be explained by age and sex differences.

Cheesmond and Fenwick (1981) reported a study of human excretion behaviour in Gezira, Sudan. From the top of a Land Rover they watched local people in the act of excretion. After observing an act of excretion the investigators visited the site to determine whether the individual had defecated or urinated. It was noted that several individuals washed themselves or bathed naked in the water near to where they had defecated. Where defecation could have contaminated a water body, snails were collected for examination. Snails from six of ten such sites contained schistosomes compared to only five of twenty sampled from sites not known to have been faecally contaminated.

A study of *S. haematobium* infection in 269 male children, aged 6–17, was done in El Ayaisha village, Upper Egypt, from 1978 to 1980 (Kloos *et al.* 1990). In March 1979, children in the study were treated with metrifonate. In July and October 1979 and March 1980, all water sites were observed and water activities recorded for children in the study. This included recording the type of activity involved and the degree and duration of exposure to the water. The authors calculated an index of exposure based on total body minutes (TBM). Thus, if 50% of the body was submerged for two minutes, this would give a TBM value of 1. The prevalence of egg excretion varied from 39% to 88%. Geometric mean egg counts increased between October 1978 and March 1979 when treatment was given. Counts were then lower in October 1979, but increased once more in March 1980. Overall frequency and TBM were only correlated with egg counts in the 9–11-year-old group. When analysis took into account the results of a water survey of cercarial counts at various sites in the area, there was a significant correlation between exposure to six of seven positive sites and urine egg counts. This study highlights the importance of combining ecological with epidemiological data in assessing the risk of various water-exposure behaviours.

Lima e Costa *et al.* (1991) studied the effect of sociodemographic factors and water contact patterns on the prevalence of *S. mansoni* infection in 506 individuals in a Brazilian village. The prevalence of infection was 37.5%. Significant sociodemographic factors included age, sex, colour and quality of the house. Those reporting water contact had increased risk of infection. Individuals reporting contacts less than once per week (OR 3.0, CI 1.3–6.6) had a smaller excess risk than those reporting contacts at least weekly (OR 4.3, CI 2.6–7.0). In a multivariate model that included age, those reasons for water contact that were independently associated with increased risk of *S. mansoni* infection were agricultural activities (OR 3.16, 1.69–5.92), fishing (OR 2.14, CI 1.50–3.05) and swimming or bathing (OR 1.97, CI 1.25–3.10).

A similar study in the town of Santo Antonio de Jesus, also in Brazil, studied children between the ages of 12 years 8 months and 14 years 11 months (Barreto 1991). This study correlated mean egg counts in faeces with a variety of factors. Significant associations were found with distance of relationship to head of household (for example, child servants had much higher counts than children or grandchildren of the head of the house) (OR 7.2, CI 3.6–14.7), being born in a rural area (OR 1.8, CI 1.4–2.3) and number of years living in a rural area ($p < 0.001$). The were also significant associations with poverty, as measured by family income ($p < 0.025$), and lack of education ($p < 0.025$). Compared to those who had flush latrines with sewage disposal, those with pit latrines (OR 1.9, CI 1.3–2.4) and no latrines (OR 1.8, CI 1.3–2.4) had increased risk, as did those who took their water from open bodies of water (OR 3.4, CI 2.0–6.1) or had piped water with no wastewater disposal (OR 1.6, CI 1.2–2.0). Increased egg counts were seen in those who had sporadic (OR 1.9, CI 1.5–2.6) or frequent (OR 4.5, CI 3.2–6.5) water contact. Fishing and playing in water or swimming in the past month were also associated. Areas of high human infection mirrored the pattern of snail infection.

Chandiwana, Woolhouse and Bradley (1991) studied the reinfection rates of approximately 500 people in rural Zimbabwe after treatment with praziquantel. In the initial survey 40.1% of 429 individuals were infected by *S. haematobium*. Heavy infections, which were largely confined to children under 16 years, were seen in 11.0% overall. Of 102 initial positives who were treated, 13 were reinfected after 14 weeks. Reinfection was found to correlate with water exposure index but not with number of exposures or duration of exposure. This water exposure index took account of area of skin exposed, duration of exposure and infectivity of the site as measured by survey of water snails. In a subsequent paper the authors reported that males and children were more likely to have contact with a variety of sites, which, they argued, could explain their increased rate of infection in the initial survey (Chandiwana and Woolhouse 1991).

The potentially debilitating effects of acute schistosomiasis were demonstrated by an outbreak of Katayama fever that affected three scuba divers who had been diving in a dam in the eastern Transvaal Lowveld (Evans, Martin and Ginsburg 1991). Two of the three were only in the water for about 25 minutes, the third for about 40 minutes. One diver who had a history of repeated water contacts had only a relatively mild illness. The other two were more severely affected. These latter two patients had not been previously exposed. Despite repeated treatments, it took 30–36 months for them to recover fully.

The epidemiology of *S. intercalatum* was studied in a village in southeast Gabon for a year from July 1989 (Martin-Preval *et al.* 1992). *S. intercalatum* has a distribution limited to central Africa. Stool samples were obtained from 354 residents of the village and 101 (28.5%) were positive. Egg excretion reached a peak of 65.2% among females aged 10–14 years and 60.0% among 15–19 year old males. A survey of two rivers found the intermediate snail host in one river but not the other. Water contact patterns of a subset of the population were then estimated by interview and direct observation. There was a highly significant association with average duration of water contact per week and egg excretion (0.89 $\pm$ 0.56 hours per week for egg excreters compared with 0.36 $\pm$ 0.45 hours per week for non-excreters; $t = 8.4$, $p <$ 10^{-9}). The effect of water contact was independent of age.

A Chinese study done in 1989 looked at factors affecting reinfection after treatment with praziquantel (Zhaowu *et al.* 1993). In March 1988 the prevalence of schistosomiasis in the study areas ranged from 13.0% to 49.7%. The 781 people who were positive were treated with a single oral dose of praziquantel. In March the following year, 740 of the 781 people were re-examined and 179 (24.2%) were positive once more. Reinfection was associated with the frequency of water contact, the type of water contact (fishing was associated with higher reinfection rates than either playing or herding animals), and the proximity of residence to a snail-infected water.

Marcal *et al.* (1993) used a 1:1 matched case-control design to study risk factors for *S. mansoni* in Pedro de Toledo, Sao Paulo State, Brazil during 1987, in which 96 case-control pairs were evaluated. In the univariate analysis, any water contact (OR 3.00, CI 1.19–7.56), water contact during fording (OR 3.20, CI 1.17–8.73), daily water contact (OR 8.00, CI 1.00–63.96), degree of water contact (OR 2.46, CI 1.29–4.69) and 'bad hygiene' (OR 3.00, CI 1.19–7.56) were linked to risk of schistosomal infection. In a multivariate analysis the three remaining variables were swimming, playing and fishing (OR 2.46, CI 1.21–4.98), fording (3.39, CI 1.11–10.36) and bad hygiene. The authors suggested that these results indicated recreational contact as a significant risk factor and that alternative recreational activities should be provided as part of a prevention campaign.

A 14-year schistosomiasis control programme in Peri-Peri, Brazil, succeeded in reducing the prevalence of schistosomiasis from 43.5% to 4.4% (Coura-Filho *et al.* 1994). In 1988 the programme was stopped, and three years later the prevalence had risen to 19.6%. Surveys of a rural and an urban population were done at that time to investigate possible risk factors for disease. The prevalence of the disease was higher in the rural area (28.4%) compared to the urban area (16.0%) ($p = 0.004$). Multivariate analyses were done separately for each area. In the rural area, living less than 10 m from a water source (OR 2.82, CI 1.24–6.44) and having an agricultural occupation (OR 3.25, CI 1.20–8.83) were associated with infection. Significant water use associated with infection included any water contact (OR 2.79, CI 1.19–6.85), daily fishing (OR 2.57, CI 1.10–56.03) and weekly (OR 6.13, CI 1.58–24.35) or daily (OR 6.87, CI 2.56–18.70) domestic agricultural activities. In the urban area, living less than 10 m from a water source (OR 2.94, CI 1.52–5.57), the absence of drinking water in the home (OR 5.87, CI 1.75–19.71), absence of a sewer (OR 3.84, CI 1.84–10.18) and living in a poor quality home (OR 9.21, CI 4.60–18.66) were associated with infection. Unexpectedly low family income appeared to be protective of infection (OR 0.23, CI 0.12–0.44). Significant water contact included any water contact (OR 3.08, CI 1.59–5.94), swimming weekly (OR 2.26, CI 1.18–4.33), fishing weekly (OR 3.01, CI 1.10–8.12) and daily domestic agricultural activities (OR 4.30, CI 1.06–14.44).

Ndamba *et al.* (1994) surveyed 2552 children aged between 5 and 15 years in Harare, Zimbabwe. They found that 13.7% were infected by *S. haematobium* and 6.7% by *S. mansoni*. It was noted that the suburbs with the highest incidence of infection were the ones without municipal swimming pools. Many of the boys in these areas went swimming in a dam just outside the city boundary.

The first cases of schistosomiasis in Kumba, southwestern Cameroon, were reported in the mid-1980s. Sama and Ratard (1994) conducted a house-to-house survey in high-incidence areas of the town. This included 171 households with a total of 1025 residents. The investigators noted that although clean drinking fountains were available, many residents still used the river for bathing and recreational activity. In a multiple logistic regression analysis, age, ethnic group, water contact and knowledge about schistosomiasis were associated with the risk of infection. The 10–19 age group had the highest risk, as did the Nigerian ethnic group. Risk increased with degree of water contact. Interestingly, the incidence of disease was higher in those people who knew most about schistosomiasis, although this was thought to be because of previous treatment.

A study of Zimbabwean athletes found an increased prevalence of schistosomiasis in triathletes (80%) compared to runners (38%) ($p < 0.05$) (Jeans and Schwellnus 1994). The swimming part of the triathletic events have recently been moved from chlorinated to freshwater, although the race organisers have taken measures to try to reduce the risk of schistosomiasis by spraying molluscicide over race areas. At the start of the season positive athletes were treated; retesting at the end of the season suggested a seasonal incidence of 64%.

Etard, Audibert and Dabo (1995) studied reinfection with *S. haematobium* after treatment with praziquantel in Mali between 1989 and 1991. Once again, this study showed increased risk with exposure to water.

Taylor *et al.* (1995) reported a sero-epidemiological survey for Norwalk virus, hepatitis A and schistosoma among canoeists in South Africa. They compared the seropositivity rates for each of these pathogens in canoeists and non-canoeists. Seropositivity to schistosomiasis was significantly raised among the canoeists (49.7% versus 6.8%, OR 13.6, CI 7.54–25.12).

In an Egyptian study 210 fishermen were compared with the same number of farmers from two villages (El-Hawey *et al.* 1995). The prevalence of *S. mansoni* was greater in fishermen (57.1%) than in farmers (45.7%) ($p < 0.01$), as was a history of swimming or bathing.

Studies of the effect of water resources and their management

Abdel-Wahab *et al.* (1979) studied the prevalence of schistosomiasis in an Egyptian village that had previously been the area of a study in 1935. In the earlier study *S. haematobium* had affected 74% of the population and *S. mansoni* only 3.2%. By 1979 *S. mansoni* had become more common, affecting 73%, and *S. haematobium* had declined to only 2.2%. The increase in *S. mansoni* was worrying because this schistosome is more likely to cause serious liver disease. The authors noted a recent change in the distribution of the snail vectors that favoured *S. mansoni*, which they suggested was due to the building of the Aswan High Dam. This would have affected river ecology.

A large study of 34 434 people from 225 villages in Mali looked at the effect of water management and irrigation schemes on the prevalence of schistosomiasis (Brinkmann, Korte and Schmidt-Ehry, 1988). The prevalence of schistosomiasis was six times higher in areas with artificial irrigation than in savannah villages and three times higher than in villages with natural water courses. Furthermore, high intensity infections were much more common in irrigated areas.

Schistosomiasis in travellers

In January 1982, five cases of Katayama syndrome were identified out of 11 individuals who had returned to the US and Sweden after rafting on the Omo River in Ethiopia (Philpot *et al.* 1982). One additional person was found to be an asymptomatic carrier. No differences in water exposure patterns were found between infected and non-infected individuals.

During 1992, two US Peace Corps volunteers were evacuated home because of infection of the central nervous system by *S. haematobium* (Wolfe *et al.* 1993). Both cases had been snorkelling at Cape Maclear, Lake Malawi. The infection left one of the cases, a woman, with incontinence of urine that requires periodic self-catheterization. Subsequent investigations were undertaken in Malawi. Infected vector snails were found in areas adjacent to the resort areas. A serological survey of 917 expatriates in Malawi found detectable schistosomal antibody in 302 (33%). Furthermore, this level of positivity was present among 427 people whose only ever recreational water exposure was at Lake Malawi.

Visser, Polderman and Stuiver (1995) reported another outbreak among travellers returning to the Netherlands after visiting Mali, west Africa. Of 30 travellers in two groups, 29 had swum in freshwater pools in the Dogon area. After presentation of the index case, the group was followed up for a period of 12 months; 28 of the 29 (97%) became infected, of whom 10 developed cercarial dermatitis and 15 Katayama fever. Eggs of *S. mansoni*, *S. intercalatum* and/or *S. haematobium* were found in faeces or urine samples. In four cases all three species were identified.

Schistosome dermatitis

Schistosome dermatitis (swimmer's itch) is not restricted to tropical countries. Many outbreaks of the disease have been reported from western countries. A small outbreak of itchy eruptions affecting more than 10 people occurred during August 1976 on the shores of Lake Michigan north of Chicago (Kirschenbaum 1979). Histological examination of one case, six days after onset, revealed only non-specific changes. Although no cercariae or infected snails were found, it was noted that ducks had been seen in the area for some weeks.

In August 1981, 16 people were affected by itching within an hour and a half of swimming in a Californian river. Examination of snails taken from the site found them to be emitting cercariae (Humphry *et al.* 1982).

During July 1987 more than 65 people developed an itchy rash accompanied by fever, nausea and vomiting after attending a water sports park in Suffolk, UK (Eastcott 1988). Histological examinations of two skin biopsies were consistent with cercarial dermatitis. Snails from the lake were emitting cercariae. These cercariae caused a rash when applied to the author's arm.

In the summers of 1985 and 1986, a total of 118 people presented with dermatitis, consistent with cercarial dermatitis, after swimming in one of four reservoirs in central Bohemia, Czechoslovakia (Kolarova *et al.* 1989). Surveys of the reservoirs found many infected snails. The outbreaks were controlled by the chemical and mechanical control of the snail populations.

On 19 October 1991, 37 students aged 13–16 years and their teacher visited a state park in Delaware (Wiley *et al.* 1992). They had spent between 1.2 and

6 hours wading in a shell fishing area. Of 37 persons who had contact with seawater, 30 (81%) developed itching or a macular rash within 2 hours of exposure and itching papular lesions after 12 hours. Cases occurred in only 5 (45.5%) of 11 individuals who had worn long pants compared with 25 (96%) of 26 who had worn shorts (RR 0.5, CI 0.3–0.9). On 7 November, mud-flat snails (*Nassarius obsoletus*) were collected from the same site. *Microbilharzia variglandis* were seen in a dish containing two snails and in two of 300 crushed snails.

An outbreak of cercarial dermatitis was also reported from Thailand in November 1988 (Kullavanijaya and Wongwaisayawan 1983). The outbreak affected 58 farmers after planting rice after a period of flooding. The itching had developed within about 15 minutes of entering the water. Snails from the area were captured and monitored. After about 16 days numerous cercariae of *S. spindale* were seen.

COMMENTS

The transmission of schistosomiasis depends on the contamination of freshwater with human (or animal in the case of *S. mekongi*) faeces containing infected eggs, the presence in the water of the appropriate species of snail and subsequent human contact with that water. Prevention of the disease is aimed at each of these three stages:

1 Reducing contamination of freshwater by treating infected individuals, educating people about the hazards of defecation into water sources and provision of latrines.
2 Reducing the snail population by using chemical moluscicides, or using biological control and covering irrigation channels.
3 Reducing contact with infected waters by educating people about the risks, siting villages away from particularly infected waters, providing piped water and providing safe water environments for bathing.

Schistosomiasis is a preventable disease and is potentially eradicable, provided that the will is there and sufficient resources are made available.

7 Giardiasis

Giardiasis is due to infection by the flagellate protozoan parasite *Giardia lamblia*, now called *G. duodenalis*. It is a common disease throughout the world, although outbreaks of waterborne disease appear more common in North America than in Europe.

LIFE CYCLE

G. lamblia exists in two forms. The trophozoites, which measure 12–18 μm, possess a concave sucking disc on the anterior end, while the posterior end tapers and terminates into two flagella. These trophozoites are normally found adherent to the mucous membranes of the upper small intestines. It is this form that is responsible for causing disease by damaging the mucous membrane. As the trophozoite is passed along the intestines it may form itself into an oval cyst, 9–12 μm long. These cysts are passed in the faeces and are the infective form. Once ingested by a new host the cyst passes through the stomach into the duodenum, where it produces two daughter trophozoites, which then colonize the small bowel. The consumption of as few as 10–25 cysts can cause infection.

CLINICAL FEATURES

The incubation period is usually about one to two weeks, although it can be as long as several months. The severity of any clinical illness varies considerably and only about a quarter of people will become symptomatic. In symptomatic patients the predominant feature is the acute onset of diarrhoea, which is often explosive, abdominal cramps, bloating and flatulence. There is no blood or pus in the stool, which is often pale and at times almost white in colour. Malaise is common and sulphuric belching is quite characteristic. Untreated, the acute illness usually lasts for at least 10 days and often for much longer – 4–12 weeks. Indeed, untreated, it can sometimes last for as long as 3–4 years. During this illness patients often lose considerable weight. Malabsorption can develop in about 10% of cases, and in children it is a cause of failure to thrive.

DIAGNOSIS

Diagnosis is usually made by light microscopic examination of a wet preparation of the patient's faeces. Identification of the characteristic cysts is diagnostic. Duodenal aspiration or biopsy of the small intestine is also used in the diagnosis of difficult cases. A variation of this is to get the patient to swallow a small weight to which is attached a fine thread, the other end of which is taped to the patient's cheek for a few hours. Once the weight is pulled out, the characteristic trophozoites can be seen attached to the thread. Serological ELISA tests are also available for detecting antibody in serum or antigen in stool.

TREATMENT

As with all diarrhoeas, fluid replacement is the most important aspect of treatment, although specific antimicrobial agents certainly have a role. The two drugs that seem to be most effective are metronidazole and tinidazole. Mepacrine is used as an alternative when the imidazole drugs are contra-indicated or have failed.

ENVIRONMENTAL DETECTION

Detection of giardial cysts in waters requires the filtration of large volumes of water (10 litres upwards). Cysts are recovered from these filters, by destruction of the filter followed by resuspension by washing. After further concentration by centrifugation, the deposit is examined microscopically. To assist detection the deposit is stained by iodine or monoclonal antibody (HMSO 1989). Recent developments in isolation and detection methods include:

- use of a cDNA probe rather than immunofluorescence, after disruption of the cysts with glass beads (Abbaszadegan, Gerba and Rose 1991),
- an antibody-magnetite method where anti-giardial antibodies are placed on magnetic beads, enabling capture and subsequent concentration of cysts in a magnetic field (Bifulco and Schaefer 1993),
- a method using flocculation concentration followed by flow cytometry with fluorescence activated cell sorting (Vesey et al. 1994).

ECOLOGY

Giardia spp. affect a wide range of animals, including amphibians, birds and mammals. While the infectivity of many of these animal strains for humans is not clear, the evidence from several outbreaks discussed below does indicate that infection in beavers, and possibly in small rodents such as muskrats, is a source of human infection.

Giardial cysts can be identified quite frequently in surface water supplies. LeChevallier, Norton and Lee (1991a) reported finding cysts in 81% of raw surface water samples from fourteen American states and one Canadian province, at counts ranging from 0.04 to 66 cysts per litre (geometric mean 2.77). There was high correlation with both faecal and total coliform counts and turbidity. On average, surface waters from urban areas contained ten times more giardial cysts than waters from protected watersheds, suggesting human sewage as the main source of environmental contamination. These authors were also able to demonstrate that 17% of filtered drinking water samples in these areas were also positive (range 0.29–64 cysts per 100 litres) (LeChevallier, Norton and Lee 1991b). However, in a Canadian study 32% of water samples from remote pristine sources where human faecal contamination is extremely unlikely, as well as 21% of animal faeces from these areas, were positive (Roach et al. 1993). They also found cysts in 17% of drinking water samples from one city, and in raw sewage.

Although giardial cysts are inactivated by both chlorine and ozone, they are relatively more resistant to chemical disinfection than many waterborne pathogens (Lin 1985; Finch et al. 1993). Consequently, disinfection alone cannot be relied on as the only control measure, especially if dosing and contact times cannot be guaranteed.

EPIDEMIOLOGY

Giardiasis is a common disease throughout the world, affecting all age groups, although the highest incidence is in children. It is a common cause of traveller's diarrhoea. Endemic disease is often spread directly from one person to another, especially in children or in poor hygienic circumstances. Person to person spread associated with anal intercourse in homosexuals has also been described. Waterborne outbreaks are particularly common and foodborne outbreaks appear to be becoming more common.

Outbreaks associated with drinking water

Brady and Wolfe (1974) describe the investigation into the cause of a 44-year-old woman's illness. She had been particularly ill with giardiasis, having up to 20 bowel movements per day for a month. Although she lived in the city she frequently visited her parents' farm. The water supply for the farm was from a brick underground cistern, which collected rain-water. Examination of water from this cistern revealed numerous trophozoites. Of ten individuals living in the area of the farm, five were positive for giardial cysts.

Of 54 campers on a two-week trip into the mountains of Utah in September 1974, 34 developed diarrhoea (Barbour, Nichols and Fukushima 1976). Of 28 symptomatic campers, 22 (79%) were stool positive for *Giardia*, as were four (29%) of 14 asymptomatic campers. Because of the small number of people not affected, epidemiological study was unable to identify any risk factor other than *not* drinking untreated water before the trip. Presumably this was because those who drank such water regularly had developed immunity. The authors also took this opportunity to examine faecal samples from another 25 campers, both before and after their trip. While none had positive stools before the trip, six (24%) were positive after the trip.

Laboratory-confirmed giardiasis occurred in 350 residents of Rome, a city in central New York State, between November 1974 and June 1975 (Shaw *et al.* 1977). Using a case definition of diarrhoeal illness lasting five or more days, there was a community attack rate of 10.6%. In a case-control study the only risk factors were drinking from the city system as opposed to drinking from a private water supply ($p = 0.038$) and drinking one or more glasses of unboiled water per day ($p = 0.0015$). The water supply was chlorinated, but neither filtered nor subject to sedimentation. Raw water was filtered through sand and the backwash water from this filter coagulated and the sediment examined. Although no cysts were seen, two of ten pathogen-free beagle puppies developed giardiasis after consuming the deposit. It was noted that human settlements in the watershed area could have been the source of contaminating human waste.

After receiving reports of diarrhoeal disease in Americans returning from the Island of Madeira in October 1976, the US Center for Disease Control undertook a postage survey of returnees (Lopez *et al.* 1978). Of 859 who responded, 39% had experienced diarrhoea and 33% a diarrhoeal illness compatible with giardiasis (i.e. diarrhoea lasting more than one week or less than a week with abdominal distension). Giardial cysts were seen in 47% of stools examined. The most significant factor for giardiasis was drinking local tap-water in Madeira ($p < 0.001$). Eating raw vegetables and local ice-cream were also significant ($p < 0.05$), although these were probably either confounding variables or due to contamination from tap-water. A follow-up survey the following year revealed no increase in disease.

In March 1976, 128 persons developed laboratory-confirmed giardiasis in Camas, Washington (Dykes *et al.* 1980). The water supply to Camas came from two sources: a set of seven deep wells and two mountain streams. Water tracer experiments were conducted to identify the distribution of these two sources through the city. Although a case-control study did not identify water consumption as a risk factor, it was noted that those districts with 70% or greater surface water had attack rates of 4.7%, while the rate in areas receiving less than 70% had 0% attack rate. Giardial cysts were identified in the raw water intake from the surface water and also from some filtered and chlorinated water from storage reservoirs. The passage of cysts through the filtration system was blamed on inadequate flocculation, coagulation and sedimentation as well as deterioration of the filters. Three beavers trapped below the water intake had giardia in their stools.

An outbreak was identified in Berlin, New Hampshire during April and May 1977 (Lopez *et al.* 1980). During this period 213 cases of giardial infection were identified by stool examination. Giardiasis was significantly more common in Berlin than in nearby towns that had a groundwater supply. Although the rate of illness was higher in residents who drank the local water (5.8%) compared to those who did not (3.1%) this was not significant. As part of the case-control survey, 74 residents were randomly chosen to give a faecal sample. Of these 74, 34 (46%) were positive for giardial cysts. It was estimated that of people infected with giardia in Berlin city, only 24% developed clinical symptoms. Cysts were found in both raw and treated water. Examination of the water treatment system showed that about 50 000 gallons of unfiltered water was leaking past the filter each day due to faulty joints in the filter.

During the summer of 1980 an outbreak of gastroenteritis affected an estimated 780 people in Red Lodge, Montana (Weniger *et al.* 1983). This number was estimated from a telephone survey of residents, which found an attack rate of 33% in urban residents and 15% in rural residents ($p = 0.000\ 45$). Stool samples from 24 (51%) of 47 symptomatic individuals were shown to contain giardial cysts, as did 3 (13%) of asymptomatic individuals. The illness in rural residents was associated with the frequency of visiting the town each month. This survey did not identify a significant association of illness with consumption of water among city residents. At the time of the outbreak, the water supply to Red Lodge was unfiltered, marginally chlorinated surface water from an unprotected watershed. Cysts were not identified in water samples. However, it was noted that the epidemic curve of the outbreak showed a bimodal pattern. Each peak was preceded by about 10 days by marked increases in the turbidity of the water at the water intake. This increase in turbidity corresponded to increased runoff because of heavy rains.

Vogt *et al.* (1984) reported the investigation of an outbreak in a small Vermont community in December 1981. Although *G. lamblia* was identified from only four cases the authors undertook a serological study of the at-risk population. People who drank the town water had a significantly higher immunofluorescent antibody titre to *G. lamblia* trophozoites than those who were not water drinkers. The water supply was an unprotected, unfiltered and unchlorinated spring.

An outbreak of waterborne giardiasis in November at Aspen, Colorado, affected about 20 of 110 people interviewed living in one area (Istre *et al.* 1984). The epidemiological study found a striking dose–response relationship with drinking town water ($p < 0.01$) and living in the neighbourhood for less than two years ($p < 0.01$). Furthermore, the attack rate did not vary with water consumption in those people who had lived in the area for more than two years. These data suggest that individuals living in the affected area for any length of time were becoming immune to giardiasis, probably as a result of previous waterborne outbreaks. Both raw and filtered water samples showed large numbers of giardial cysts. Defects in the water system included inadequate chlorination, lack of chemical coagulation pretreatment and damage to the filter.

There were 324 laboratory-confirmed cases of giardiasis affecting people in Reno, Nevada, during 1982 (Navin *et al.* 1985). The peak of the outbreak was in October and November. There was a significant association with drinking town water but not untreated stream water. The water supply was treated by chemical coagulation, flocculation, sedimentation and chlorination but not filtration. Giardial cysts were found in raw water and in a captured beaver. This beaver had built its lodge in a pipe leading to the reservoir. The outbreak terminated when chlorine concentrations were increased and the infected beaver removed.

The first UK waterborne outbreak of giardiasis occurred in the Bristol area in the summer of 1985 (Jephcott, Begg and Baker 1986). In all, 108 cases were detected. In a case-control study there were highly significant associations with the amount of water drunk at home and at work. Because of the geographical distribution of cases – all lived in an area supplied by a single water main – it was felt that the source of contamination must be in the distribution system, although the exact problem was not identified. Faecal samples from this outbreak were also examined by antigen capture enzyme immunoassay (EIA) (Green *et al.* 1990). The EIA was compared with microscopy after formal ether concentration. Of 136 faeces from people who had illness, 66 were positive and 61 were negative by both methods. Three were negative by EIA but positive by microscopy and six were positive by EIA but negative by microscopy. The authors concluded that EIA was more sensitive, and that it had time advantages over microscopy. An additional seven stools from asymptomatic people were found to be EIA positive. All seven lived in the same area.

An outbreak of giardiasis in Sweden in 1982 was of interest because there appeared to be an association with an outbreak of another but unknown pathogen (Neringer, Andersson and Eitrem 1987). This outbreak affected a small village of just 600 inhabitants in the southeast of the country. On 16 October, tree roots penetrating the village sewer caused an obstruction and backflow. This flooded the water treatment plant and the cellars of local houses. The sewage flooded into the waterworks through a previously unknown connection. Within 24 hours of this incident an outbreak of gastroenteritis affected about 557 people. The attack rate for residents was 76%. Another 103 people who visited the village over the incident period also reported gastroenteritis. No pathogen was isolated from water samples or from the stools of affected patients. This initial outbreak was over within seven days of the pollution incident. A few weeks after this outbreak it became clear that some individuals had not recovered from the acute illness or had developed diarrhoea a second time. Giardial cysts were identified in stool samples from 31 (60%) of 52 people who still had diarrhoea, and 25 (28%) of 88 people who had been ill but had recovered. Cysts were not seen in stool samples from any of 27 villagers who had not been ill. Cysts were not detected in any water samples one month after the pollution incident.

Over a three-month period from November 1985 to January 1986, 703 cases of giardiasis were reported in Pittsfield, Massachusetts (Kent *et al.* 1988). A variety of telephone questionnaires were administered to cases and to random controls. The water supply to this community was chlorinated but not filtered. It came through three different reservoirs. Epidemiological analysis showed that cases were more likely to drink more than two glasses of water per day (OR 9.2, CI 4.2–19.9) and be aged over 20 years (OR 3.3, CI 1.7–6.2). The attack rate also depended on the water source. For those living in the zone fed from reservoir A, the attack rate was 0.72%, from reservoir B it was 0.61%, from reservoir C 3% and from mixed sources 1.24%. The outbreak started about one week after reservoir C was brought back into operation after a period of three years. Giardial cysts were found in all three reservoirs, although at higher counts in reservoir C, suggesting that this was the initial contamination point. Inspection of reservoir C found graffiti in a controlled area and evidence of beaver activity. One beaver captured near reservoir C was stool positive. The outbreak was controlled by the issuing of a boil water notice and by taking reservoir C out of operation.

Between April and June 1986 an outbreak of giardiasis affected residents of a trailer park in rural Vermont (Birkhead *et al.* 1989). All 122 residents of the park completed an epidemiological questionnaire. Of these, 37 (30%) fitted the case definition of giardia positive stools or diarrhoea lasting over five days. The risk of disease increased with increasing water consumption, from 0% in those not drinking water to 42% in those drinking more than three glasses of water per day ($p = 0.001$). Drinking water from the park was chlorinated but unfiltered surface water. However, it was noted that chlorination contact times were probably inadequate at times of peak demand. Giardial cysts were present in the water. It was noted that the outbreak was preceded by the destruction of a beaver dam upstream, which led to the release of a large volume of water into the stream. Blood samples were taken from 24 residents and 20 non-resident controls. Of the 24 residents, 9 met the case definition. Levels of anti-giardial IgG and IgA, but not IgM, were significantly elevated in residents compared to non-residents. Among the residents IgA, but not IgG or IgM, was elevated. IgA levels were also raised in residents who drank tap-water, whether or not they had the illness.

An unusual outbreak affected just four people in a block of flats in Scotland in late June 1990 (Ramsay and Marsh 1990). The flats were supplied with cold water from four tanks in the roof. Inspection of these tanks showed that one tank had been deliberately contaminated with human faeces. Giardial cysts were also found in this tank.

A total of 362 cases of laboratory-confirmed giardiasis affected residents of Penticton, British Columbia from June to August 1986 (Moorehead *et al.* 1990). A case-control study of 77 cases did not find any significant association between illness and age, sex, water consumption or geographical location. A random telephone survey of 112 households found 14 cases, an attack rate of 12.5%. Extrapolating to the total population of 25 000, this would suggest that 3125 cases had occurred, hence the laboratory ascertainment rate was little more that 10%. A survey of physician records suggested that about 1500 people attended with the disease. The city was supplied from three sources: a creek, a lake and a well. The creek water was very turbid at the time due to the spring runoff. Although no giardia cysts were isolated from water, four of seven beavers trapped in the creek were stool positive. Two muskrats trapped from the lake were also positive. The creek was felt to be the main risk and it was closed. The outbreak subsequently declined. The authors noted that as the town was a tourist resort there was reluctance to issue a boil water notice. However, because of increasing demand for water during the tourist season, water extraction from the creek started again though from a higher level. After sanitary work was conducted around the original creek extraction point, it was reintroduced the following year, to be followed by recurrence of the giardial outbreak.

Hopkins and Juranek (1991) reported an outbreak among university students and staff on a geology field course in Colorado in June 1983. The authors investigated two groups. Disease was higher in the first group. Stool specimens were positive from 31 of 42 members of the first group, compared to none of 36 in the second group. Forty members of the first group drank untreated stream water compared to only five of the second group. Furthermore, within the first group the risk of stool positivity was strongly related to the amount of untreated water consumed ($p < 0.000\ 001$).

One of the largest European outbreaks of waterborne giardiasis affected more that 3000 individuals over Christmas 1986 at a ski resort in Sweden (Ljungstrom and Castor 1992). Of these, 1400 people were diagnosed microscopically. The cause of the outbreak was an overflow of sewage into the drinking water system. Serum samples were taken from 352 people who were exposed to the water at that time and 428 healthy, non-exposed individuals. These serum samples were analysed for IgG and IgA by indirect immunofluorescence. Of the non-exposed group, 10% had either IgG or IgA, or both antibodies. Of the exposed group, 41% had anti-giardial antibodies. Specific IgG was present in 60% and IgA in 28% of those who had giardia present in their stool, whether or not they were symptomatic. In those who were stool negative the equivalent percentages were 20% and 4%. IgG was present in 44% of those with diarrhoea and 27% of those without. The corresponding figures for IgA were 16% and 18%. The authors also noted that more sera were positive (66% versus 49%) if collection was delayed for three weeks after onset of illness. This study emphasized the point that in outbreaks of giardiasis, rather more individuals are infected than are identified either by symptoms or stool microscopy. This would explain the difficulty in getting statistically significant results in case-control studies of outbreaks.

Isaac-Renton *et al.* (1993) were the first people to investigate an outbreak of waterborne giardiasis by propagating the organism and then typing it. The outbreak occurred in Creston, a town of 4200 inhabitants in British Columbia. Over an eight-week period, 124 laboratory-confirmed cases were identified. Although no analytical epidemiology was done, the questionnaire of cases found drinking water to be the only common factor. A beaver upstream of the water intake was found to be excreting large numbers of cysts. The drinking water was found to be positive on several occasions up until the infected beaver was removed but not after. Non-outbreak strains from elsewhere in British Columbia and strains isolated from beavers distant from the water intake were also typed. The isolates were examined by both isoenzyme electrophoresis and pulsed-field gel electrophoresis (PFGE). Of eight different types found, the outbreak strains, strains from the water supply and the implicated beaver were all of the same type. Non-outbreak human and beaver strains were heterogeneous. This outbreak gives the best evidence yet that beavers are a source of waterborne outbreaks of giardiasis in humans. This outbreak was, in fact, the second to affect this town (Isaac-Renton *et al.* 1994). A previous waterborne outbreak of giardiasis had occurred five years earlier. Those residents who had been infected during the first outbreak were significantly less likely to be infected during the second (4% versus 68%, *p* < 0.001). This finding suggests that immunity to giardiasis probably lasts for at least five years.

Of the 19 outbreaks reviewed here, a suspect cause was identified in 18. Of these 18 outbreaks, 14 were due to the consumption of unfiltered or inadequately filtered surface water, and 6 of these 14 outbreaks were associated with contamination from animal faeces. The remaining four outbreaks were probably due to post-treatment contamination by sewage or human faeces.

Outbreaks associated with recreational water contact

In contrast to the large number of outbreaks of waterborne giardiasis resulting from drinking water published in peer-reviewed journals, there have been relatively few recreational water outbreaks reported.

Following the notification of giardiasis in a child who participated in a infant and toddler swim class, 70 other child participants were screened and 61% were stool positive (Harter *et al.* 1984). The swim class took place at a motel in Washington State. Also, 39% of 53 mothers and 28% of 21 fathers were positive for giardia. No non-swimming siblings were positive. From the pool records it was noted that high turbidity and low chlorine levels were an occasional problem. It was also noted that faecal accidents often occurred in this group of very young children.

Nine cases of diarrhoea fulfilling the case definition for giardiasis were identified in people who had been swimming at a pool in New Jersey during one day in September 1985 (Porter *et al.* 1988). Of these nine cases, eight were stool positive. It was found that a handicapped child had had a faecal accident on the day when all cases had been swimming. This child, as well as eight others in his group of twenty, were stool positive. Unfortunately, chlorine levels were not tested on the implicated day, but a sample the following day showed no chlorine because a gas cylinder was empty.

After reports of cases of giardiasis among guests who had stayed at a hotel in Manitoba, 107 people were interviewed (Greensmith *et al.* 1988). Of these 107, 59 (55%) met the case definition. Of 35 stool examinations, 30 were positive for giardial cysts. In a case-control study the most significant association was with using the water slide on one of three days, 21 March (p = 0.031), 22 March (p = 0.001) and 23 March (p = 0.007). Cases were also more likely to have used the slide on more than one occasion (p = 0.001). Swallowing pool water (p = 0.001) and drinking hotel water (p = 0.006) were also significant. The pool water was filtered and brominated. It was unclear how the slide became contaminated, although it was found to be possible for a faecal accident in the toddlers' pool to contaminate the slide pool. The speed at which people entered the slide pool would have predisposed to the injection of pool water.

Epidemiological studies of endemic disease

A state-wide survey of Colorado laboratories during 1973 found that 691 (3%) of 22 743 stool samples were positive for giardia (Wright *et al.* 1977); 256 cases were eventually included in a telephone questionnaire. Controls were selected randomly from the telephone directory. Cases were more likely to have visited the Colorado mountains (69% versus 47%, p < 0.001), camped out overnight (38% versus 18%, p < 0.01) and drunk raw mountain water (50% versus 17%, p < 0.001). Thus, almost one-third of cases may have resulted from drinking mountain stream water.

Esrey *et al.* (1989) investigated the relationship between the presence of giardial infection in pre-school children and drinking water source, use of water and latrines in rural Lesotho, South Africa. Stool samples and socio-economic data were collected from 267 children in 21 villages. Of these 267 children, 63 (23.6%) were stool positive for giardial cysts. Using less than 8 l of water per head per day was strongly associated with giardiasis (OR 2.42, CI 1.12–5.23) but not the source of water or the use of a latrine. Also associated with giardiasis were being aged over 24 months (OR 6.79, CI 2.41–19.09) and having a mother aged less than 20 years (OR 5.18, CI 1.48–18.09). Possessing agricultural tools was found to be protective (OR 0.70, CI 0.51–0.96). This study suggested that in this population personal hygiene and maternal experience were more important (i.e. person to person transmission) than water source in the transmission of giardia.

Birkhead and Vogt (1989) reported a study of 1211 cases of laboratory-confirmed cases of giardiasis, not linked to outbreaks, that occurred in Vermont between 1983 and 1986. Each case was interviewed by a public health nurse. No controls were interviewed. Using state census data, the authors estimated that residents with non-municipal water systems had an increased risk of disease of about 30% (RR 1.3, CI 1.0–1.7). Furthermore, the type of water supply affected the risk of giardiasis. Compared to municipal filtered surface waters, all other water sources had an increased risk. The risks for the other types of water were municipal non-filtered surface waters (RR 1.9, CI 1.1–3.3), municipal well-waters (RR 1.8, CI 0.9–3.4) and private waters (OR 1.3, CI 1.3–3.6). Person to person transmission in the under-five age group was suggested by the finding of increased risk in those attending day-care (RR 1.5, CI 1.0–2.3).

A study from New Zealand reported the rates of endemic giardial disease in Dunedin (Fraser and Cooke 1991). The city took its water from two different supplies. While most water was filtered by mechanical micro-strainers, one part of the city received water that had been treated by coagulation/flocculation and direct dual media filtration. This latter process would be expected to be much more efficient at removing cysts. The incidence of disease in the less efficiently treated water was more than three times higher (0.99 versus 3.29 per 10 000 person-years, RR 3.3, 90% CI 1.1–10.1, $p = 0.04$). A small case-control study undertaken at the same time also found an increased risk with the micro-strained water (OR 1.8, 90% CI 0.5–6.5) although this was not significant, possibly due to the small number of cases.

A case-control study of giardiasis in a Vancouver population of 1.4 million served by a non-filtered but chlorinated supply found no association with drinking water (Mathias, Riben and Osei 1992). The only risk factors identified were a child under 6 in the family (OR 2.2, CI 1.3–3.5), travel abroad (OR 2.3, CI 1.3–3.9) and travel elsewhere within British Columbia (OR 3.2, CI 1.7–6.2). It is tempting to speculate about whether the travel-associated cases were waterborne. That this speculation is indeed possible is suggested by a further case-control study elsewhere in British Columbia (Isaac-Renton and Philon 1992). This study, of 228 case-control pairs, found that drinking water was the most important risk factor for laboratory-confirmed giardiasis. People who drank non-chlorinated and unfiltered surface water were at a greatly increased risk compared to those who drank well-water (OR 12.0, CI 5.9–24.7). The risk between people who drank chlorinated and unchlorinated, unfiltered surface water was little different. Those who travelled to 'third world' countries and drank the local water were also at increased risk compared to those who travelled and did not (OR 6.3, CI 1.1–35.8). Furthermore, those travelling to Mexico, Pakistan or India were at increased risk compared to those travelling to other 'third world' countries

(OR 7.7, CI 1.6–37.0). Drinking local tap-water or engaging in recreational water activities was also a risk factor in those who travelled to rural areas of British Columbia (OR 2.2, CI 1.1–4.4).

In a study of endemic giardiasis in the Canterbury area of New Zealand from October 1990 to June 1991, 100 questionnaires were sent to laboratory-confirmed cases (Mitchell, Graham and Brieseman 1993). Eventually 51 case-control pairs were included in the analysis. Contact with sewage (OR 10.6, CI 1.31–85.12) and travel abroad (no controls travelled abroad, making calculation of OR impossible) were the most significant risk factors. Handling raw meat (OR 0.2, CI 0.07–0.89) and eating raw food (OR 0.4, CI 0.15–0.90) appeared to be protective, presumably due to increased immunity from previous exposure. Drinking non-Christchurch water was more likely in cases, though this did not achieve statistical significance (OR 2.9, CI 0.92–9.25).

A study of 273 cases and 375 matched controls during 1984 and 1985 was reported from New Hampshire in New England (Dennis et al. 1993). This found the following significant risk factors: drinking water from shallow wells compared to municipal supplies or artesian wells (OR 2.3, CI 0.4–14.1), drinking untreated surface water (OR 4.5, CI 2.0–9.8), personal contact with a known case (OR 2.4, CI 1.1–5.3), contact with a person in day care (OR 1.9, CI 1.1–3.8) and swimming in a lake, pond, stream or river versus not swimming or swimming in a swimming pool or the ocean (OR 3.1, CI 1.5–6.4).

Gray, Gunnell and Peters (1994) reported a case-control study undertaken from July 1992 to May 1993 in the counties of Somerset and Avon in southwest England. The analysis included 74 cases and 108 matched controls. Unadjusted risk factors were swimming (OR 3.0, CI 1.4–6.2), drinking potentially contaminated water (OR 5.7, CI 1.6–19.8), travel to developing countries (2.9–173.1) and 'type of travel', i.e. camping, caravaning or using holiday chalets (OR 6.9, CI 1.5–32.1).

As part of a larger study of risk factors for diarrhoeal disease in infants and young children in Egypt, specific risk factors for giardiasis were also analysed (Mahmud et al. 1995). A total of 152 infants were recruited at birth and followed for one year. Factors associated with an increased risk were: living in a house without a latrine (RR 2.63, CI 1.4–4.9), having a mud floor in the sleeping rooms (RR 1.79, CI 1.03–3.0) and household exposure to more than 10 chickens (RR 2.5, CI 1.13–5.56). Decreased risk was associated with having a mother educated to more than primary school level (RR 0.28, CI 0.09–0.85), storing household drinking water in metallic, rather than clay, containers (RR 0.33, CI 0.11–0.98) and male gender (RR 0.52. CI 0.3–0.89). The authors suggested that metallic containers for drinking water are less likely to be associated with giardiasis because water in them gets warmer, leading to reduced viability of cysts.

8 Cryptosporidiosis

Cryptosporidium is a coccidial protozoan parasite that was first described in the first decade of the twentieth century. However, it was not until the 1980s that its role in causing human disease was really recognized. It is now recognized to be a common cause of diarrhoea throughout the world. About 20 species are now known, of which *C. parvum* is pathogenic for humans. Until recently, it appeared that Cryptosporidium was more of a European than an American problem. This was undoubtedly because of the earlier interest shown in the pathogen in UK clinical laboratories compared to most American ones.

LIFE CYCLE

Infection can occur with as few as 30 oocysts (DuPont *et al.* 1995). Initially, the oocyst is ingested and passes through the stomach, where excystation occurs with the release of four motile sporozoites. These sporozoites then attach to the epithelial cell wall, where they are taken into superficial parasitophorous vacuoles. Here, a sporozoite matures into a trophozoite, which then divides, forming a meront, which eventually releases merozoites. Merozoites infect other epithelial cells, perpetuating the infection. Eventually, some merozoites form microgametes and macrogametes. The microgametes then fertilize the macrogametes, which become zygotes. These zygotes mature into an oocyst. The oocyst is the infective stage and is passed in the faeces. It is surrounded by a protective wall to ensure its survival in the environment. The whole life cycle of Cryptosporidium can be completed within a single host (Figures 8.1 and 8.2).

CLINICAL FEATURES

The incubation period is normally about 7–10 days (range 4–28 days).

The main clinical feature is diarrhoea which varies considerably in its severity from one case to another and in the same patient from one day to another. The stool may be watery and offensive and contain mucus or slime

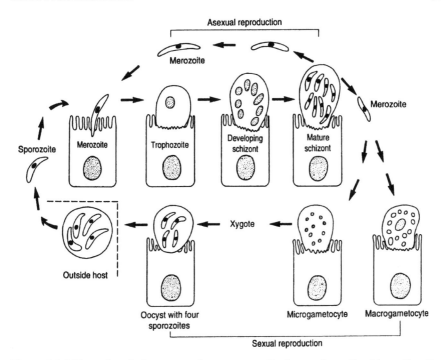

Figure 8.1 Life cycle of *Cryptosporidium parvum*. Redrawn from Farthing, Cevallos and Kelly (1996) in Cook GC (ed.) *Manson's Tropical Diseases*, 12th edn; reproduced by permission of WB Saunders.

but rarely pus or blood cells. Patients may also complain of mild abdominal pain and a few also have a mild fever. Symptoms usually last from 2 to 26 days, although illness has persisted for several weeks even in otherwise healthy individuals.

In immunocompromised individuals such as those suffering with AIDS, the disease is much more severe and more persistent. Illness can last for several months or until death. Severe diarrhoea is associated with marked weight loss. Malaise and fever are also more common. Non-gastrointestinal illness, such as cholecystitis, hepatitis and respiratory disease, may also occur in such individuals.

DIAGNOSIS

Diagnosis usually rests on microscopic demonstration of cysts in faeces of a case. To aid identification specimens are usually stained either by a modified acid-fast procedure or a fluorescent stain such as auramine. Specific monoclonal antibodies are also available for staining specimens prior to

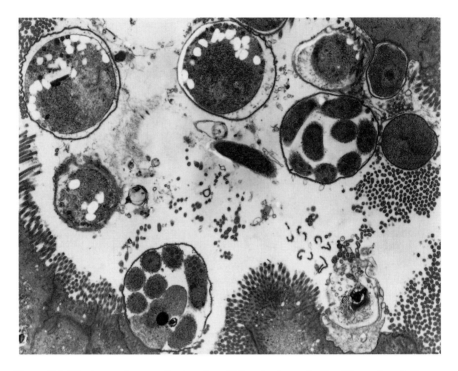

Figure 8.2 Electron micrograph showing different stages in the life cycle of *Cryptosporidium parvum*. Provided by Dr A Curry.

examination. Serological tests are available, though they are not used frequently for routine diagnosis.

TREATMENT

There is no specific curative therapy for cryptosporidiosis. Management of the illness is supportive where necessary.

ENVIRONMENTAL DETECTION

Detection in water samples usually requires the filtration of large volumes of water (up to 100 l or more). The filter matrix is then destroyed and the cysts resuspended by washing the filter elements. The resulting suspension is further concentrated by centrifugation before being examined microscopically after labelling with a fluorescent monoclonal antibody (HMSO 1989). Unfortunately, this method is laborious and recovery of oocysts is poor, especially at the final centrifugation stage (LeChevallier *et al.* 1995). Recent advances in methods for the detection of oocysts in water samples include:

- a membrane filtration method where the membrane was subsequently dissolved rather than cut up and washed (Aldom and Chagla 1995). This is said to increase recovery of cysts by 70.5%.
- detection of oocysts by the polymerase chain reaction (PCR), which was found to be only as sensitive as immunofluorescence (Johnson *et al.* 1995).
- the use of flow cytometry has made the detection of oocysts in water samples considerably easier and has also permitted the sampling of smaller samples of water (Vesey *et al.* 1994). It is more sensitive, faster and easier to perform than conventional methods (Vesey *et al.* 1993).

ECOLOGY

Cryptosporidium spp. infect a wide range of animals, including mammals (especially cattle), birds and reptiles. Oocysts have also been detected in surface water, groundwater and in treated water samples, both associated with outbreaks and as incidental findings. The source of environmental contamination can be both human sewage and animals.

Musial *et al.* (1987) were able to identify oocysts in treated sewage effluents with a turbidity of 4.8 nephelometric turbidity units (NTU). Given an estimated efficiency of detection of only 9%, the authors calculated that counts in the two samples were 5 and 17 oocysts per litre. Ongerth and Stibbs (1987) reported that each of 11 samples from 6 rivers in western USA were positive at counts ranging from 2 to 112 oocysts per litre. In the largest study of various waters throughout western United States, Rose (1988) found oocysts in 75% of reservoirs and lakes, 77% of streams and rivers, and 91% of both treated and raw sewage samples. The geometric mean counts were 0.94, 0.91, 17 and 28.4 oocysts per litre respectively. Another study of river water samples, this time mainly in eastern USA, found oocysts in 87% (LeChevallier, Norton and Lee 1991a).

In the Yukon, Canada, drinking water is treated only by chlorination. Roach *et al.* (1993) reported on the detection of cryptosporidial oocysts in various water samples. Cryptosporidial oocysts were not detected in pristine water samples. However, *Cryptosporidium* sp., at counts of up to 74 per litre, was identified in raw sewage samples and also in treated sewage.

In the UK, all of ten sites on three rivers yielded positive samples (National Cryptosporidium Survey Group 1992). The percentage positivity of sites ranged from 0.9% to 57% and counts were as high as 4.0 per litre. Worryingly, as groundwaters are often not filtered, *Cryptosporidium* sp. was identified in up to 6.8% of samples of one of two groundwaters surveyed at counts up to 0.922 per litre.

Oocysts have also been regularly isolated from potable water. Rose (1988) found oocysts in 50% of four non-filtered drinking waters (mean count 0.006 oocysts per litre) and 20% of filtered drinking waters (mean count 0.001 oocysts per litre) in western US. Roach *et al.* (1993) reported the detection of cryptosporidial oocysts in 5% of drinking water samples from one of two cities in the Yukon, Canada.

Newman *et al.* (1993) reported a survey of animal stool and environmental samples from an urban slum in Fortaleza, Brazil. Of 64 animal stools examined during the dry season, 4 (6.3%) were oocyst positive. During the rainy season 9 (14.3%) of 63 were positive. Dog faeces were the most frequently positive. Two of eight water samples were positive in the dry season and two of ten positive in the rainy season. Positive samples were from city tap-water and three closed wells.

Oocysts are able to survive for several months in water kept at 4 °C, but at higher temperatures viability declines (Barer and Wright 1990; Smith and Rose 1990).

EPIDEMIOLOGY

Outbreaks associated with drinking water

The first recorded waterborne outbreak of cryptosporidiosis occurred in Texas during 1984 (D'Antonio *et al.* 1985). A telephone survey of 100 households identified an attack rate of diarrhoeal disease of 34%. This survey identified two peaks of illness, in May and in July. The first peak was probably due to Norwalk virus, because symptoms were compatible with this pathogen and six sera tested from that time showed rising titres to Norwalk. However, of 79 stools examined during July, 47 were positive for *Cryptosporidium* oocysts. In the second outbreak, being absent from the community between 1 and 11 July, especially 2 July, was protective. There was a linear relationship between diarrhoea in July and total daily intake of tap-water ($p = 0.002$). The water supply for this community was chlorinated but unfiltered artesian well-water. Microbiological analysis of the unchlorinated well-water showed it to contain faecal coliforms. Dye added to the community's sewage appeared in the well-water, indicating cross-contamination.

An outbreak of gastroenteritis affected an estimated 13 000 people out of 64 900 living in western Georgia, USA, between 12 January and 7 February 1987 (Hayes *et al.* 1989). *Cryptosporidium* oocysts were detected in the stools of 58 out of 147 patients examined. The estimated size of the outbreak was made by extrapolating the results of a telephone survey of residents within the water supply zone. This same survey found an increased incidence of disease among residents exposed to the public supply compared to those not exposed (RI 3.1, CI 2.4–3.9). Oocysts were detected in treated water on several occasions during January and February. The public water system took its water from a small river. This water was treated by the addition of alum, lime and chlorine, rapid mixing, mechanical flocculation, sedimentation and rapid sand filtration. Environmental examinations revealed a previously unsuspected sewage overflow, which was draining into the river above the treatment works. Defects in the treatment plant included: the mechanical flocculators had been removed, awaiting new ones; the efficiency of the filtration was impaired due to poor control of water flow; and the filters were sometimes restarted without being first backwashed. It was noted that when such filters had been restarted without backwashing the turbidity from that filter was often higher than normal for a few hours.

An outbreak of cryptosporidiosis affected two towns on the coast of Ayrshire during April 1988 (Smith *et al.* 1989). By the end of April, 27 stool positive cases had been identified. However, telephone discussions with general practitioners in the area indicated that 'many hundreds' of people were affected. Although epidemiological studies were inconclusive as to the source of the outbreak, all cases lived within the area supplied by a single water treatment works. It was noted that drinking water microbiology failed testing on two occasions during the last week of March. From 27 environmental samples of various types, two final waters, one raw water, one back-flush water, two sludge samples, a soil sample and a grass sample were positive for oocysts. For the water samples oocyst counts ranged from 0.13 to 1000 per litre. An old fire-clay pipe was discovered that, after heavy rainfall, drained surface water from fields into a tank holding treated water for distribution. Scouring among calves in the area had been reported to the Veterinary Investigation Centre and although cattle had not been grazed on the fields drained by the suspect pipe, cattle slurry had been spread on them.

During May and June 1986, there was a marked increase in laboratory diagnoses of cryptosporidiosis in the Sheffield (UK) area (Rush, Chapman and Ineson 1990). There was a significant association between confirmed cryptosporidiosis and drinking water supplied from two suspect reservoirs (p < 0.001). All 14 surface water samples from these reservoirs were positive, as were the intestinal contents of 14 out of 18 brown trout. Two treated water samples were negative, although relatively small samples were analysed. It was noted that most samples from cattle in the area were oocyst positive. Although the water treatment system was not described, it was noted that heavy rainfall preceded the outbreak.

Probably the biggest recorded European outbreak of cryptosporidiosis occurred in Swindon and Oxfordshire, UK, during January and February 1989 (Richardson *et al.* 1991). During the outbreak 516 stool positive cases of diarrhoea were identified. No case-control study was done. However, all cases' home addresses were mapped. Most cases were in areas supplied by one of two water treatment works. During the latter part of February and early March, 34% of water samples taken from customers' taps in this area were found to contain oocysts in the range 0.002–24 per litre. The larger of the two suspect treatment works extracted its water from the River Thames. Treatment was by storage, screening, flocculation, rapid sand filtration and chlorination. It was not established how the water came to be contaminated. However, one possibility was that oocysts built up in the sand filters by the process of backwashing and reusing the backwash water to such an extent that breakthrough occurred.

An outbreak during December 1990 and January 1991 affected the Isle of Thanet, UK (Joseph et al. 1991), in which 47 stool positive cases were identified. A case-control study included 29 of these cases and 80 controls. The consumption of more than one cup of unboiled water per day was significantly associated with illness (OR 8.7, p = 0.002), as was drinking water outside of the home (OR 5.2, p= 0 .01). Drinking bottled water was protective (OR 0.1, p = 0.034). There was also a significant dose–response curve to drinking water (p < 0.001). No water sample was positive for oocysts. The implicated treatment works only operated on an occasional basis. Water treatment was by flocculation with aluminium sulphate coagulant, flotation and filtration. Turbidity readings from this treatment works showed an increase from <1 to 2 NTU for a few days towards the end of November. This increase in turbidity corresponded to an increase in river flow after heavy rains.

Probably the largest waterborne outbreak ever reported occurred in Milwaukee in the spring of 1993 (MacKenzie et al. 1994). In the area supplied by the Milwaukee Water Works (MWW), 739 cases of laboratory-confirmed cryptosporidiosis were reported. To gain an idea of the real incidence of the disease, a telephone survey was done. This showed that 30% of people in the survey had experienced a compatible illness during the weeks of the outbreak. Extrapolating this information to the rest of the population and subtracting the expected background incidence of diarrhoea suggested that 403 000 people were affected. Thus, for every stool positive case identified there were at least 500 people affected. Attack rates varied according to water zone. Compared to people living outside the area supplied by MWW, the risk was highest for residents of the southern area (OR 3.6, CI 3.0–4.3). This compares with the increased risks in the MWW middle (OR 2.4, CI 1.8–3.3) and northern (OR 18, CI 1.39–2.3) regions. Furthermore, of those living outside the area affected but working outside the home, the risk of infection was higher if they worked in the southern region (OR 2.6, CI 1.6–4.2). Oocysts were found to be present in concentrations of 13.2 and 6.7 per 100 litres in ice made from MWW water. Water was extracted from Lake Michigan. Both MWW plants treated water by the addition of chlorine and polyaluminium chloride coagulant, rapid mixing, mechanical flocculation, sedimentation and rapid sand filtration. The filters were cleaned by backwashing the water, which was reused. Although no specific failure was identified, it was noted that unusually high turbidity readings were recorded at the start of the outbreak.

During January and February 1991 an outbreak of cryptosporidiosis affected 44 people in south London (Maguire et al. 1995). Data from 15 cases and 81 controls were included in a case-control study. All of the cases and 70% of the controls lived in the area supplied by a single water provider (OR undefined, $p = 0.018$). Among residents in the area supplied by the suspect water company, drinking more than a glass of water per day was associated with illness (OR 4.77, CI 1.1–28.5). Oocysts were not identified in any water sample. The water supply to this area was slow sand filtered and dual filtered. No obvious defect or operating problem was identified in the treatment works.

An outbreak affected 125 cases in Bradford, England, in November and December 1992 (Atherton, Newman and Casemore 1995). In an analysis of 35 case-laboratory control pairs, drinking water from the suspect supply was associated with an increased risk (OR 13.5, CI 3.8–51.7). Residence within the supply area and increasing water consumption were also highly associated. A small study of 20 cases and neighbourhood controls also found an association with drinking tap-water (OR 4.6, CI 0.8–28.5). *Cryptosporidium* oocysts were detected in the supply system early in the outbreak. It was noted that following heavy rainfall, turbidity of the treated water had increased. No other abnormality was found.

Between November 1992 and February 1993, an outbreak of cryptosporidiosis affected 47 cases in Warrington, northwest England (Bridgman *et al.* 1995). Most people affected were residents of a single water supply zone. Two case-control studies were done, one using neighbourhood controls and the other laboratory controls. In the neighbourhood control model drinking unboiled water from the affected zone was associated with illness ($p = 0.003$). Furthermore, the risk of illness increased with increasing consumption of this tap-water ($p = 0.0008$). In the study with laboratory controls, both drinking unboiled tap-water and residence in the affected zone were significant associations. No oocysts were identified in any water sample. The water supply to the affected zone was an unfiltered borehole supply. Environmental investigations revealed several possible mechanisms for contamination: cattle had been grazing in a field close to one of the boreholes; there had been very heavy rains just before the start of the outbreak; and there was staining evidence of water ingress into this same borehole. It was also noted that there had been a small but unusual increase in turbidity in water samples from this borehole during early November.

From 1 April to 31 May 1993, 64 stool positive cases were identified in the southwest of England (Morgan *et al.* 1995). Of 40 primary cases, 35 lived within the area supplied by one of two water companies that served the town. The risk of infection was much greater to people living in the affected area than in the area supplied by the other company (OR 15.1, CI 7.1–32.2). When data was analysed from a case-control study of people living in the affected area, there was a significant dose–response relationship with water consumption ($p = 0.03$). Oocysts were detected in 4 of 70 water samples, although at very low concentrations. The water supply to the affected area was from three boreholes and a well. No defects were identified.

Of the eleven outbreaks described here, three were associated with unfiltered well-water and four followed unusually high rainfalls. Five of the outbreak reports also mentioned increases in water turbidity, usually still within prescribed limits, before the outbreak developed. Turbidity remains one of the easiest and most useful routine water quality indicators.

Outbreaks associated with recreational water contact

Probably the first outbreak of cryptosporidiosis to be linked to a swimming pool occurred during July and August 1988 (Sorvillo et al. 1992). Of 60 people who were members of five different swimming groups using the same pool in Los Angeles, 44 (73%) developed gastroenteritis. Cases continued to occur for four weeks. Oocysts were identified in five of eight stool samples examined. The attack rate increased with the numbers of hours exposure to the pool, from 39% for 1–3 hours to 89% for more than 6 hours exposure ($p < 0.001$). Inspection of the pool revealed that one of the filters was inoperative.

The second such outbreak, by a matter of only a few weeks, affected residents of Doncaster, northern England (Joce et al. 1991). The local hospital laboratory identified 67 cases spread fairly evenly between 1 August and 31 October. Epidemiological analysis found a significant association between illness and head immersion at a particular swimming pool, using both laboratory-based controls (OR 14.4, CI 1.46–673.41) and neighbourhood controls (OR 6.2, CI 1.41–31.36). A questionnaire was administered to children through local schools, of which 139 were returned. Thirty-one children were reported to have gastroenteritis, although none of them had submitted stool samples. This study also found a significant association between illness and swimming at the implicated pool (OR 2.88, CI 1.06–8.00). Samples from the learner pool contained oocysts at a concentration of 50 per litre. In the months before the outbreak pool managers had noticed a smell in the changing rooms and had found difficulties in controlling the levels of free chlorine. Initial inspection revealed no other problems, although when the learner pool was drained about 30 cm of liquid sewage appeared in the deep end. A foul drain had apparently become blocked and sewage backflowed into the pool.

Another swimming pool outbreak was reported from Vancouver, British Columbia (Bell et al. 1993). Using the case definition of 'gastrointestinal symptoms of abdominal cramps with watery diarrhoea or vomiting lasting four days or more in November or December 1990', 89 cases were identified of whom 20 were stool positive. In a small study of 23 matched case-control pairs, cases were more likely to have swum in the children's pool (OR 4.5, CI 0.97–20.83) although this did not achieve statistical significance. Subsequent analysis of unmatched 66 cases and 23 controls found a much greater association (OR 12.8, CI 3.68–46.77). The pool water was sand filtered. Examination of the pool records revealed an increase in the number of defecations into the pool during November and December from the usual one or two per month to one or two per week.

During an outbreak of cryptosporidiosis in Oregon from June to October 1992, 9 of 18 cases in early studies reported swimming at a local wave pool compared to none of the controls (McAnulty, Fleming and Gonzalez 1994). Altogether, 55 stool positive cases were identified, of whom 37 were the first to be affected in their house. The suspect pool was filtered by rapid sand filtration.

At the same time as the massive outbreak of cryptosporidium in Milwaukee described above, there was a smaller outbreak among guests of a resort hotel some 70 miles from the city (MacKenzie, Kazmierczak and Davis 1995). A case search exercise among people who had been guests at the hotel between 11 and 18 April 1993 revealed 51 who satisfied the case definition, 22 of whom were laboratory- confirmed cases and the remainder probable cases. Swimming in the resort hotel's pool was significantly associated with illness (OR 9.8, CI 3.4–29.7), as was using the whirlpool (OR 3.7, CI 1.5–9.3) and the consumption of ice from ice making machines (OR 2.3, CI 1.01–5.2). When stratified for swimming in the pool, use of the whirlpool was found to be not significant. When analysis was restricted to confirmed cases, the association with ice also disappeared (OR 1.1 CI 0.4–3.3). No defect in the pool structure or maintenance was found. The authors concluded that the most probable explanation for the outbreak was a faecal accident within the pool. They noted that cryptosporidial diarrhoea is watery, which would make it more difficult for the pool operator to detect such an accident.

Epidemiological studies of endemic disease

During August 1986, Gallaher *et al.* (1989) did a case-control study of laboratory-confirmed cases of cryptosporidiosis in New Mexico, in which 24 stool positive cases and 46 matched controls were studied. Significant risk factors included drinking untreated surface water (OR ∞, CI 2.44–∞), swimming in surface water (OR 3.7, CI 1.02–13.5) and attending a day care centre where other children were ill (OR 13.1, CI 2.58–66.4). Altogether, 8 of the 24 cases were exposed to surface water and 8 attended day schools.

A telephone-based case-control study of 51 matched case-control pairs was reported from Adelaide, Australia (Weinstein *et al.* 1993). Drinking only rainwater was found to be protective ($p < 0.001$). Drinking only bottled spring water did not quite achieve statistical significance as a risk factor ($p = 0.063$). It was noted that most bottled spring waters sold in Adelaide come from relatively shallow aquifers in areas of moderately intensive agricultural land use. There was also the possibility that some bottling operators were diluting spring water with mains water.

To test the effectiveness of filtration to reduce the risk of cryptosporidiosis, a study in Los Angeles compared the prevalence of cryptosporidiosis among persons with AIDS living in areas that consistently had filtered water with those that did not (Sorvillo *et al.* 1994). During the four years, 1983–1986, in which area A had unfiltered water the prevalence of cryptosporidiosis was lower than that in Area B, which consistently received filtered water (OR 0.75, CI 0.49–1.16). During the four years after the introduction of water filtration to Area B, the prevalence declined from 4.2% to 3.4%. However, a similar decline was also seen in the area that had always received filtered water. It does not appear that water supply was a significant factor for cryptosporidiosis in Los Angeles.

In a study of 1000 elementary school children in Jordan, oocysts were detected in 4% of faecal samples (Nimri and Batchoun 1994). It was noted that the prevalence was higher (5%) in villages where drinking water was from wells than in Embed City (3.3%) where it was a main supply ($p < 0.05$). However, contact with animals could also explain the difference.

9 Cyclospora

Cyclospora are the most recent in the list of 'new' waterborne diseases to have been described. Indeed, it is only since about 1990 that the organism's role in human disease has even been identified, and then it was erroneously though to be a cyanobacterium. To avoid over-repetitive disclaimers, I will refer to *Cyclospora*, even if the original article referred to the organism by another name. The tentative name is *Cyclospora cayetanensis* and it is known to be a coccidial protozoan parasite. There is still much that is unknown about the biology and ecology of this pathogen.

LIFE CYCLE

The life cycle remains to be described.

CLINICAL FEATURES

The incubation period appears to be between one and seven days. Symptoms are similar to those of cryptosporidiosis, namely diarrhoea, abdominal pain, nausea, vomiting and anorexia. Flatulence and bloating are also features. The diarrhoea is characteristically prolonged, lasting from one to eight weeks. Weight loss can be profound in cases of prolonged illness.

DIAGNOSIS

The diagnosis is made by microscopic demonstration of the oocysts in stool samples after staining, as for cryptosporidium. The oocysts look remarkably like those of cryptosporidium, other than that they are rather larger, about 10 μm in diameter.

TREATMENT

No specific treatment is available.

ECOLOGY

Other than what is described below under 'Epidemiology', little is known about the ecology of *Cyclospora*.

EPIDEMIOLOGY

Most reports of human infection with *Cyclospora* spp. have been in residents of developing countries or in travellers returning from such countries. Indeed, the first report of illness was in travellers returning from Haiti and Mexico (Soave *et al.* 1986). Further reports seemed to indicated that the infection was a disease associated with travellers with AIDS (Hart *et al.* 1990; Long *et al.* 1990).

The first outbreak of disease linked to *Cyclospora* occurred in Nepal between June and November 1989 (Shlim *et al.* 1991). The organism was seen in the stools of 55 people who presented with prolonged diarrhoea. Of the 55 people, 52 were foreign residents and 3 were tourists. None had any other illness. Rather more residents than tourists were affected than generally seen in the clinic ($p < 0.001$). This initial study was unable to identify a probable source for the infection. The following year, 85 cases were detected between May and October. *Cyclospora* were only detected in one sample (the head of a lettuce from which a patient had eaten) out of several samples of water, raw vegetables and cow manure (Cohen *et al.* 1991).

A case-control study of *Cyclospora* disease in Nepal was eventually done in 1992 (Hoge *et al.* 1993). This study was of foreign residents and tourists. *Cyclospora* were identified in the faeces of 108 (11%) of 964 patients with gastroenteritis compared to only one (1%) of 96 asymptomatic individuals. Of the 108 symptomatic cases, 93 completed a questionnaire, as did 96 controls. Cases were more likely to have drunk untreated water (OR 3.98, CI 1.29–13.14) or local milk that was not boiled before consumption (OR 6.17, CI 1.22–42.17) in the week before symptoms. However, only 28% of cases reported either water or milk consumption so other modes of transmission may still be present.

Wurtz *et al.* (1993) described nine cases of *Cyclospora* infection. One case, a 35-year-old man, developed illness four days after he had cleaned out a saltwater aquarium by oral siphoning. A six-year-old boy also became ill the day after swimming in Lake Michigan.

In June 1994 an outbreak of *Cyclospora* infection affected British soldiers in a small military detachment in Nepal (Rabold *et al.* 1994). *Cyclospora* organisms were detected in the concentrate of a 2 litre water sample taken from the water storage tank. The water had been filtered, but not sufficiently to remove *Cyclospora*-sized particles, and chlorinated. The routine boiling of water in the camp was implemented.

10 Naegleria

Naegleria fowleri are free-living amoeboflagellates that normally live in warm waters and survive by feeding off bacteria. The first case of human infection was described as causing a disseminated fatal infection. Normally, however, the infection is restricted to the central nervous system.

LIFE CYCLE

N. fowleri has three stages in its life cycle. In the trophozoite stage the organism feeds and multiplies. This stage is found on mud and the surface of vegetation. The motile biflagellate stage is found in the surface layers of water. Finally, the organisms can also be found as cysts.

Both the trophozoite and biflagellate forms are potentially infectious for humans. Infection usually occurs during swimming. Infected water is inhaled into the nose and the pathogen then penetrates the nasal membranes and enters the cerebrospinal fluid by following the nasal nerves. The trophozoites then penetrate and feed on brain tissue.

CLINICAL FEATURES

N. fowleri causes primary amoebic meningoencephalitis (PAM). The incubation period is usually three to seven days. The initial symptoms are headache and a slight fever, which progressively gets worse over about three days. Vomiting, neck stiffness, increasing fever and severe headache lead to coma.

DIAGNOSIS

Diagnosis depends on examination of CSF. This is purulent, with no bacteria present. Motile trophozoites may be seen in a wet prep of the CSF, but care must be taken not to confuse them with motile white blood cells. Alternatively, a spun deposit of cells can be stained with acridine orange to show characteristic morphology.

TREATMENT

Treatment late in the course of an infection is probably futile. However, a few individuals have recovered when treatment was started early. Treatment included amphotericin, miconazole, or ketoconazole and rifampicin.

ENVIRONMENTAL DETECTION

Water samples for *Naegleria* are collected into jars after stirring up the water. Samples are cultured on a sterile agar plate which has been spread with a heat-killed *Escherichia coli* (HMSO 1989). The sample can be plated directly or first filtered through a membrane.

ECOLOGY

The natural habitat of *N. fowleri* is warm freshwater, and they have been isolated from lakes, rivers, swimming pools, sewage sludge, thermal effluents and drinking water (Fewtrell *et al.* 1994). For example, Wellings *et al.* (1977) found over 60% of Florida lakes to be positive. The optimum temperature for growth is 37–45 °C.

EPIDEMIOLOGY

Despite the finding that *N. fowleri* is common in many surface waters, human disease is, fortunately, rare. Visvesvara and Stehr-Green (1990) were able to find reports of only 144 cases of PAM in the world literature. Most cases were in the US (63), followed by Australia (19) and Czechoslovakia (18). The UK had three cases.

Up to 1970, 54 cases of PAM had been described worldwide. Of these 54 cases, 16 (30%) had occurred in the state of Virginia (Duma, Shumaker and Callicott 1971). All those affected had a history of swimming in one of three lakes located within a five-mile radius. The reason behind the link to these three lakes was unclear as there are many lakes in Virginia and *Naegleria* had been isolated from several of them.

Cain *et al.* (1981) reported the death from PAM of a young girl after swimming in a thermal spa-pool in Britain.

An outbreak of PAM affected five individuals, all of whom died, in Mexico during August and September 1990 (Lares-Villa *et al.* 1993). All five cases had been bathing or swimming in the same artificial canal in a warm, dessert valley. *Naegleria* was isolated from the canal water. All strains had identical isoenzyme patterns.

11   Cyanobacteria

Cyanobacteria, otherwise known as blue-green algae, are among the most ancient species known on this planet. Despite being implicated in both human and animal disease for over a century, it is only recently that interest in their potential to cause human disease has been rekindled. In the UK this renewed interest was a result of a highly publicized episode where a bloom led to the deaths of dogs and livestock.

MICROBIOLOGY

Despite being called algae by many workers, the cyanobacteria are true prokaryote bacteria. They belong to the class Photobacteria, photosynthetic bacteria that contain chlorophyll a but lack phycobilins. Rippka *et al.* (1979) classified the class into five subsections. Subsection I (order Chroococcales) contains unicellular genera that reproduce by binary fission or budding. Subsection II (order Pleurocapsales) also contains unicellular genera, but these genera can reproduce by multiple fission. Subsection III (order Oscillatoriales) grow in filaments with no cellular differentiation. Subsection IV (order Nostocales) grow as filaments, can produce heterocysts (specialized nitrogen fixing cells) and divide in only one plane. Subsection V (order Stigonematales) grow as filaments, can produce heterocysts and divide in more than one plane, so producing branching filaments.

A feature of cyanobacteria is that, because they are planktonic organisms and need to float, they possess gas vacuoles, which act as buoyancy aids.

PATHOGENESIS

Most illness related to cyanobacteria is thought to be mediated by toxins. Many species of cyanobacteria have been shown to produce one or more of a wide range of toxins (Figure 11.1). Cyanobacterial toxins include the hepatotoxins, the neurotoxins and lipopolysaccharide (LPS) endotoxins. One of the best reviews of cyanobacterial toxins is by Carmichael (1992).

Hepatotoxins are low molecular weight cyclic peptide toxins. The best known hepatotoxin is microcystin, which is a seven amino acid ring. Two of

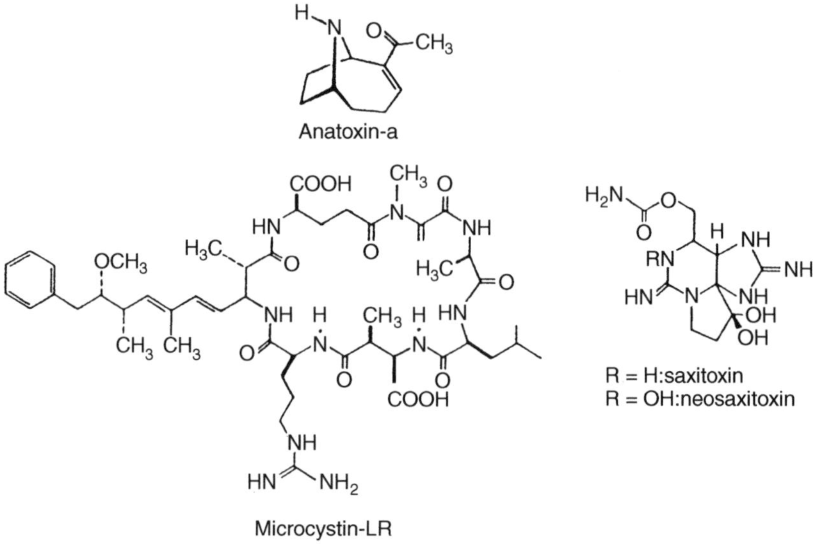

Figure 11.1 Examples of cyanobacterial toxins.

the amino acids are almost unique to microcystin. One is N-methyl-dehydro-alanine (Mdha) and the other 3-amino-9-methoxy-2,6,8-trimethyl-10-phenyl-deca-4,6-dienoic acid (ADDA). The many different varieties of microcystin differ in their L-amino acid components and the presence of certain methyl groups. Nodularin, a structurally distinct five amino acid ring hepatotoxin, is produced by cyanobacteria of the genus *Nodularia*.

Hepatotoxins are firstly absorbed through the ileum, before being transported to the liver. At the liver they are preferentially taken up by hepatocytes. Cyanobacterial hepatotoxins are extremely potent inhibitors of protein phosphatases types 1 and 2A (MacKintosh *et al.* 1995; Runnegar, Berndt and Kaplowitz 1995). Because of this effect on such important enzymes for cellular metabolism, it would not be surprising to discover that microcystins are carcinogens. Kirpenko, Sirenko and Kirpenko (1981) showed that sub-lethal doses of microcystin caused embryo-lethal, teratogenic and gonadotoxic effects in inbred laboratory rats. Effects were seen even after very low dosages, such as 0.0005 μg/kg/day. Higher doses, of 0.5 μg/kg/day, for six months in adults was associated with impaired sperm quality in males and oestrus disturbances in females. Chromosomal abnormalities in bone marrow cells were also increased. Falconer and Buckley (1989) showed that the consumption of small amounts of microcystin in drinking water enhanced the oncogenic effect of dimethylbenzanthracene on the development of skin cancers in mice. Using a rat liver model, Nishiwaki-Matsushima *et al.* (1992) reported that microcystin was the most potent liver carcinogen so far described.

The first cyanobacterial neurotoxin to be described was anatoxin-a (antx-a), isolated from *Anabaena* spp. It is a secondary amine, 2-acetyl-9-azabicyclo [4.2.1]non-2-ene, and a structural analogue of cocaine. It is an alkaloid neurotoxin and is reported to be the most potent nicotinic agonist so far described. Antx-a causes a depolarizing neuromuscular blockade.

Anatoxin-a(s) is a another neurotoxin associated initially with *Anabaena* spp. Antx-a(s) is an *N*-hydroxyguanidine methyl phosphate ester and acts as a potent cholinesterase inhibitor.

Saxitoxin and neosaxitoxin are also cyanobacterial neurotoxins. They are identical with the causal toxins of paralytic shellfish poisoning. These toxins have also been isolated from *Aphanizomenon flos-aquae*. They act by inhibiting nerve conduction by blocking sodium, but not potassium, transport across the axon membrane.

Cyanobacteria, like all Gram-negative bacteria, produce LPS as an important constituent of the cell wall. However, unlike LPS from other bacteria, cyanobacterial LPS lacks phosphate in the lipid A core. Compared to enterobacterial LPS, cyanobacterial LPS is about ten time less toxic in animal studies.

CLINICAL FEATURES

The clinical presentation of disease that implicates cyanobacteria is wide and varies from one report to another. The commonest clinical presentation is a self-limiting diarrhoea, which lasts for a few days. Erythematous skin rashes are also commonly described. Other clinical features are discussed during the discussion of epidemiology.

DIAGNOSIS

Diagnosis usually is one of exclusion. In other words, it rests on a history of contact with a cyanobacterial bloom with the absence of any diagnostic features or results of other disease. Rarely it may be possible to identify cyanobacterial cells in stomach contents or faeces. In people who develop allergic-type symptoms, a skin test may be helpful.

TREATMENT

No specific treatment is available. However, intense supportive therapy may be needed in some cases.

ENVIRONMENTAL DETECTION

Detection and identification of the cyanobacteria themselves is by the microscopic examination of water samples. The use of 0.5 ml counting chambers enables an easy semi-quantitative estimate of concentration.

Mostly methods for the detection of cyanobacterial toxins have been directed at microcystin. Methods for the detection of microcystin in water samples include a mouse bioassay. However, this is tending to give way to high-performance liquid chromatography (HPLC) as the preferred method (Codd *et al.* 1989). A rapid bioluminescence assay has also been developed (Lawton *et al.* 1990). Perhaps the most promising method for large-scale screening of water samples is that based on assaying water for anti-phosphatase activity (Edwards, Lawton and Codd 1994).

ECOLOGY

Cyanobacteria are widespread in aquatic environments. They are common in freshwater lakes and reservoirs and the intertidal zone of seashores, and can also be found on damp rocks, salt marshes, river beds and tree trunks. The definitive book on cyanobacterial ecology is that of Reynolds (1984), *The Ecology of Freshwater Phytoplankton.*

Cyanobacteria are most noticeable when they form scums on the water surface. However, this is not their preferred habitat. They normally live a planktonic existence and circulate at a depth that gives them their preferred level of light. Most toxic cyanobacteria grow best in warm, clear, eutrophic or hypertrophic waters that are not turbulent. Conditions limiting growth include low temperature (<10 °C), low phosphate concentration (<0.4 μg/l) and a high turbulence to light penetration ratio ($z_m/z_{eu} > 1.0$). The increasing number of blooms reported in temperate countries is thought to be related to increased phosphate load in many water bodies (Skulberg, Codd and Carmichael 1984; Codd, Bell and Brooks 1989). Blooms tend to form when bright, still weather follows overcast, stormy weather. During the stormy weather light levels are low and water turbulence high so that individual colonies have to increase their buoyancy to get the optimal amount of light for growth. When the turbulence ceases the colonies are now too buoyant and rise to the water surface.

EPIDEMIOLOGY

Recent reviews of human disease that have been associated with cyanobacteria include those of Carmichael *et al.* (1985) and Hunter (1991). Hunter classified reports of the epidemiology of human illness associated with cyanobacteria on the proposed route of intoxication: water contact, water consumption, fish consumption and airborne. In this book we are concerned with only the first two routes.

Drinking water associated outbreaks

Dean and Jones (1972) reported the epidemiological investigation of seasonal outbreaks of diarrhoea affecting US forces personnel on the Clark Air Base in the Philippines. These epidemics occurred during the hottest season of the year (March to July) and affected up to 6000 of the 36 000 Americans on the base. The epidemics stopped each year when the heavy rains came. All cases suffered from diarrhoea, and many had abdominal pain, nausea, weakness and fatigue. One-fifth of cases had illness lasting for more than two weeks, and in these, malabsorption occurred. Although the epidemiology was inconclusive, the authors suggested a temperature-dependent agent, possibly blue-green algae or bacteriophage, in the river water from which most of the drinking water was taken.

Patients attending a private dialysis clinic near Washington, DC, developed pyogenic reactions during a four-week period between July and August 1974 (Hindman *et al.* 1975). The authors documented 49 reactions in 23 patients characterized by chills, fever, myalgia, nausea and vomiting, and hypotension. High levels of endotoxin were detected in potable water supply to the clinic. On further investigation of the water supply, it was found that the epidemic coincided with a period of high blue-green algal bloom counts. When the algal counts declined, the outbreak stopped.

During 1975 an outbreak of gastroenteritis affected an estimated 5000 people supplied by a single reservoir in Sewickley, Pennsylvania, USA (Lippy and Erb 1976). Although clinically mild, this represented an attack rate of 62% in the population supplied from this reservoir. No microbial pathogen was implicated, but on examination of the reservoir, the remains of a bloom of *Schizothrix calicola* was obvious. Subsequent testing of this bloom in following years showed some mouse toxicity and endotoxin production (Carmichael *et al.* 1985).

Collins (1979) reported the results of an epidemiological investigation into a high birth defect rate that suggested a link to two drinking water reservoirs. Unfortunately, this study appears never to have been published in a peer-reviewed journal. Subsequent studies showed that the water was mutagenic in laboratory animals at the time of a cyanobacterial bloom (Collins *et al.* 1981).

In November 1979, an outbreak of disease affected 139 children and 10 adults of aboriginal descent in the Palm Island community, Queensland, Australia (Byth 1980). The illness began as an acute hepatitis with malaise, anorexia, vomiting and tender hepatomegaly. On presentation, 74% had glycosuria, 89% proteinuria, 20% haematuria and 53% ketonuria. During the next few days, 82% developed acidosis and hypokalaemia, often with severely abnormal serum electrolytes. Later, 39% developed diarrhoea, of whom 92%

passed frank blood. Recovery took between 4 and 26 days. There were no deaths. Laboratory investigations of cases found no pathogens or toxins. No illness was reported among people whose water supply was not connected to the general supply (Bourke *et al.* 1983). The Solomon Dam, which provided most of the water for the community, had developed a heavy cyanobacterial bloom the previous month, such that the local drinking water was discoloured and had a disagreeable odour and taste. The dam had been treated with copper sulphate five days before the start of the epidemic to kill the algae. Subsequent investigations of blooms on the Solomon Dam found that one of the main components of the bloom, *Cylindrospermopsis raciborskii*, causes major liver damage in mice, as well as affecting the kidneys, adrenals, intestines, and lungs (Hawkins *et al.* 1985). It should be noted that not everyone believes that the Palm Island Mystery Disease was algal. Prociv (1987) maintains that this outbreak was due to copper poisoning as a result of treatment of the bloom.

During a bloom of *Microcystis* on one reservoir in the city of Armidale, New South Wales, Falconer, Beresford and Runnegar (1983) conducted a retrospective study of liver enzyme results at the local hospital. Liver enzyme results from people living in the supply area of the Malpas Dam, the site of the bloom, were compared with those from people living in the surrounding countryside, who received their water from other sources. A biochemical marker of acute hepatitis, γ-glutamyl-transferase, was elevated in the population receiving their drinking water from the Malpas Dam at the time of the bloom compared to the control population and to times when no bloom was present. There was no difference in the prevalence of clinically obvious liver disease between the two populations.

El Saadi and Cameron (1993) identified 20 patients who had had 'oral intake' of Murray River water during a bloom of *Anabaena circinalis* in the summer of 1991–92. Symptoms included diarrhoea, vomiting, nausea, muscle weakness, sore throat, respiratory difficulty and headache. Of these 20 patients, 11 had contact within the house and 9 during water sport activity.

During 1988, an outbreak of gastroenteritis affected about 2000 people in the Paulo Afonso region of Brazil (Teixeira *et al.* 1993). The outbreak lasted for 42 days and was confined to Bahia State. There were 88 deaths. No *Salmonella*, *Shigella*, rotavirus or adenovirus was detected in the stools. Examinations of patients' blood for cholinesterase and heavy metals were also negative. Although no formal analytical epidemiological study was reported, most of the people involved drank piped water. The geographical distribution of cases corresponded to those communities that took their water from a new dam. The outbreak followed the flooding of the dam in early March. The only abnormal results were high levels of *Anabaena* and *Microcystis* in untreated dam water (1104–9755 standard cyanobacterial units per millilitre). The outbreak declined rapidly after copper sulphate treatment of the dam water to reduce cyanobacterial counts.

Outbreaks associated with water contact

Acute dermatitis has been described by several authors in individuals in contact with a variety of blue-green algae (Carmichael *et al.* 1985; Codd and Bell 1985). There have also been several case reports of individuals who repeatedly developed hay fever-like symptoms of rhinitis, conjunctivitis and asthma after swimming in waters with algal blooms (Billings 1981). In some of the reports these patients were subsequently shown to give positive skin tests against algal extracts. These case reports, therefore, suggest an allergic rather than a toxic effect, little different from illness associated with other environmental and plant allergens. It would appear that such illnesses are relatively common, though usually mild.

Billings (1981) reported two outbreaks of diarrhoea and vomiting in groups of children and adults 24–48 hours after bathing in two lakes in Pennsylvania, USA. In addition to gastroenteritis, patients also complained of fever, rash, sore throat, earache and conjunctivitis.

In 1989 two patients were admitted to hospital with fever, basal pneumonia, vomiting, sore throat and blistering around the mouth (Turner *et al.* 1990). These two patients were army recruits who had recently been on canoe exercises on Rudyard Reservoir, UK, while a bloom of *Microcystis aeruginosa* was present. Subsequently, eight other soldiers who had also been on the same canoe exercise were admitted to the medical centre at their barracks with similar symptoms.

In the UK, several sailboarders who had been on Rutland Water in Leicestershire during a bloom of *M. aeruginosa* in September 1989 complained of skin rashes, blistering inside the mouth and severe thirst (Codd and Beattie 1991).

Soong *et al.* (1992) described eight cases of skin, eye or respiratory symptoms developing in adults and children after contact with a bloom of *Nodularia* that occurred during 1991 on lakes near the Murray River, Australia. Four of these eight cases also suffered from respiratory symptoms, two with asthma, one with a sore throat and one with hay fever. Five had used affected water for showering, two for bathing and one for yabbying.

The following year El Saadi and Cameron (1993) also found similar symptoms in 18 individuals who had 'skin contact' with Murray River water during a bloom of *Anabaena circinalis*. Of these 18 people, 8 had participated in water sport activities and 11 had had domestic water contact.

Prospective epidemiological studies

Mortality due to primary liver cancer is particularly high (>30/100 000 person years) in the southeast coastal area of China. Several epidemiological studies have investigated the causes of this high prevalence in the most affected counties (Yeh 1989; Yu 1989; Zhu, Chen and Huang 1989). These studies have consistently shown that populations taking their water from ponds and ditches have a much higher incidence of primary liver cancer than those using river or well-water. No other risk factor could be identified for these differences between communities. Many of these ponds suffer from heavy cyanobacterial blooms (Carmichael et al. 1988). It must be noted, however, that the amount of contamination of the suspect water supplies is very great, so the implication for western water supplies is unclear.

Following reports of illness associated with blooms on or near the Murray River, El Saadi et al. (1995) conducted a more detailed prospective epidemiological study. In this study, 102 cases of gastroenteritis, 86 cases with dermatological symptoms and 132 controls were recruited from eight medical practices for a case-control epidemiological study. Patients with gastroenteritis, abdominal discomfort, vomiting or diarrhoea were more likely to drink chlorinated river water rather than rain or spring water, compared to controls (OR 1.96, CI 1.03–3.74). In the multiple logistic regression analysis this association was found to be even more significant (OR 2.37, CI 1.25–4.49). Cases of gastroenteritis were also more likely to use untreated river water for non-drinking domestic purposes (OR 6.67, CI 1.26–3.67). Furthermore, there was a correlation between the weekly mean log cyanobacterial cell counts in the river and the weekly proportions of patients presenting to medical practitioners with gastroenteritis ($r = 0.73$, $n = 10$, $p = 0.016$). Those patients presenting with dermatological symptoms, rash, itching or blistering of the mouth were more likely to have non-drinking domestic contact with untreated river water than with rain-water (OR 6.67, CI 1.15–46.61). Correlation between the weekly mean log cyanobacterial cell counts in the river and the weekly proportions of patients presenting to medical practitioners with dermatological symptoms did not achieve statistical significance ($r = 0.52$; $n = 10$, $p = 0.122$).

COMMENTS

When I reviewed the available literature on cyanobacterial disease in 1994, I stated that, although the cumulative evidence for human disease being linked to cyanobacteria in water was suggestive, the epidemiological studies taken by themselves were generally flawed (Hunter 1994). The study by El Saadi et al. (1995) is, however, much improved on previous studies. The evidence in favour of dermatological and gastrointestinal symptoms being related to cyanobacteria is now very strong.

The evidence for other symptom complexes, especially liver disease, remains to be proven. However, at the time of writing I am aware of news reports of multiple fatalities at a renal dialysis unit in South America which, allegedly, have been caused by liver failure associated with microcystin in the water supply.

12 Cholera and Other Vibrios

Cholera has the distinction of being the first disease to be shown to be water-borne by a proper epidemiological study. By his study of the epidemiology of cholera in east London, followed by his removing the handle from the Broad Street pump, John Snow became the founding father of modern epidemiology. He also did humanity one of the greatest of services in showing how one of the most feared of all diseases could be contained. Unfortunately, over a century later, cholera is still a major cause of death and disease worldwide, even if not in the western world. Perhaps the best review article on the clinical, epidemiological and ecological aspects of pathogenic vibrios in the past ten years is that by West (1989).

MICROBIOLOGY

Vibrio cholerae, the causative organism of cholera, is just one of at least 33 species in the genus *Vibrio*. Vibrios are short, Gram-negative, motile, comma-shaped bacilli. They are catalase-positive, ferment carbohydrates without producing gas and are usually oxidase positive.

V. cholerae can be classified on the basis of somatic O antigens. There are now known to be 139 O serotypes, of which just two have been responsible for epidemics of cholera, O1 and the recently described O139. *V. cholerae* O1 can be further divided serologically into three sub-types depending on the possession of three antigens, A, B and C: Ogawa (A,B), Inaba (A,C) and Hikojima (A,B,C). *V. cholerae* O1 can also be classified as one of two biotypes: classical and El Tor. The El Tor biotype is distinguished from the classical biotype in producing haemolysin, in haemagglutinating chicken or sheep red cells, and in its resistance to one of the cholera phages and to polymyxin B.

PATHOGENESIS

The infectious dose of cholera is high – 10^6–10^8 organisms. If gastric acidity is neutralized then the infectious dose falls to as low as 10^3 organisms.

The organism is not invasive but proliferates in the small intestine, where it penetrates the mucus barrier to attach to the mucosal surface. Once it starts to colonize the lining of the gut it secretes a potent enterotoxin. The enterotoxin is composed of five B subunits surrounding the A1 and A2 fragments. The B subunits of the toxin molecule bind to receptors on the cell surface, following which the A1 subunit penetrates the cell. A1 interferes with normal cellular metabolism by activating membrane bound adenylate cyclase, which causes an increase in the intracellular level of cyclic adenosine monophosphate (CAMP). This in turn affects ion transport in the villus and crypt cells so that there is increased secretion of chloride and inhibition of sodium uptake. This causes a massive loss of water and electrolytes into the gut, giving rise to the classic watery diarrhoea.

CLINICAL FEATURES

Clinical illness may only be present in about 20% of people infected with the El Tor biotype of *V. cholerae*. In those who become ill, the incubation period is normally between 1 and 3 days, though it can be up to 5 days. The main clinical feature is painless watery diarrhoea. In a mild case the patient may pass faeces 2–3 times per day for 5–7 days.

In the typical severe case onset is abrupt. Passage of copious water stool can be almost continuous. Within a matter of a few hours the stool becomes colourless, known as rice-water stool. The life-threatening effects of cholera are due to the rapid depletion of body fluids. Shock can develop within 4–12 hours, with death soon after. Complications include renal or cardiac failure due to the dehydration and metabolic acidosis due to the loss of bicarbonate in the stool.

DIAGNOSIS

In most cases the diagnosis can be made from the acute clinical presentation of watery diarrhoea and dehydration. Microscopic examination of fluid stool, using dark field or phase microscopy, may also be diagnostic. Vibrios may be seen in large numbers. They also have a characteristic darting motility, which is inhibited by specific sera.

Where possible, the diagnosis should be confirmed by culture of stool onto a selective medium such as thiosulphate citrate bile salt sucrose (TCBS) agar. *V. cholerae* produces yellow colonies. Isolation can be enhanced by pre-enriching the sample in alkaline peptone water. The diagnosis is confirmed by biochemical tests and slide agglutination to detect serotypes O1 and O139, the strains associated with cholera.

MANAGEMENT

Despite the sometimes grim prognosis of untreated cholera, the disease is remarkably easy to treat. Because all the main adverse effects of cholera follow from the fluid and electrolyte loss, treatment is aimed primarily at fluid and salt replacement. Most cases only require oral fluid replacement. The World Health Organization recommends a solution of glucose and salts made by the addition of 3.5 g NaCl, 2.5 g NaHCO$_3$, 1.5 g KCl and 20 g glucose to each litre of water. However, a simpler solution of one tablespoon sucrose and half a teaspoon of table salt per litre is also satisfactory in the short term and is easier to make. Intravenous fluid replacement therapy is only necessary in advanced dehydration or really severe diarrhoea.

Antimicrobials may shorten the duration of diarrhoea and so fluid loss, although their use is secondary to fluid replacement.

ENVIRONMENTAL DETECTION

The standard isolation from water samples is to add 100 ml to an equal volume of double-strength alkaline peptone water and incubate at 25 °C for 2 hours and then at 37 °C for 16–24 hours (Donovan and van Netten 1995). The enrichment culture is then subcultured on to TCBS agar for further incubation. Confirmation of the diagnosis is as described above for the detection of *V. cholerae* in faeces.

A monoclonal antibody-based method for the detection of cholera in water samples had been developed (al-Riyami, Haynes and Campbell 1991). This method is suitable for use in the field but only has a sensitivity of about 10^5 organisms per millilitre.

ECOLOGY

Man is the only known animal host of cholera. However, it has become increasingly clear in recent years that understanding *V. cholerae*'s survival in aquatic environments is central to understanding its epidemiology. In an excellent paper, West (1989) fully reviewed the distribution, survival and ecology of these organisms in the aquatic environment. This paper should be consulted for a fuller description of the ecology of *V. cholerae* and a list of many of the primary references up to 1989.

All pathogenic *Vibrio* spp. are halophilic and survive better in moderately saline waters. In solutions of differing salt concentrations, *V. cholerae* survived well at concentrations of between 0.25% and 3% (Miller, Drasar and Feachem 1982; Singleton *et al.* 1982). At salt concentrations between 0.01% and 0.1%

the organism declined rapidly. Thus, the natural distribution of *V. cholerae* in the environment tends to be limited to estuarine and inland coastal areas. Nevertheless, the organism can be isolated from freshwaters, where its survival may be linked to high organic loads. It has also been suggested that the survival of *V. cholerae* in freshwaters may be related to seasonal increases in salinity due to water stagnation and evaporation (Rhodes, Smith and Ogg 1986).

Temperatures of at least 10 °C for several consecutive weeks are also important for the survival of *V. cholerae* in the environment (Bockemuhl *et al.* 1986; Rhodes, Smith and Ogg 1986). Variation in temperature is probably responsible for seasonal variation in counts of *Vibrio* spp. in surface waters. During unfavourable periods *V. cholerae* will disappear from the water column. They can, however, still be isolated from sediments. Such benthic populations probably act as the seed to recolonize the water body during more favourable conditions (Williams and La Rock 1985).

More recent research has shown the importance of association with other aquatic organisms for survival of *V. cholerae*. For example, cyanobacterial blooms and freshwater amoebae may be important in supporting the maintenance of high levels of *V. cholerae* in waters (Thom, Warhurst and Drasar 1992; Epstein 1993; Islam, Drasar and Sack 1994).

EPIDEMIOLOGY

The epidemiology of cholera has been dominated by its tendency to spread throughout the world in waves or pandemics (Table 12.1 and Figure 12.1) (Crowcroft 1994). Each pandemic lasts for several years. The first six pandemics were due to the classical biotype of *V. cholerae* O1 and started in Bangladesh. The seventh, due to the El Tor biotype, started in 1961 in Indonesia. From there it spread to the Indian subcontinent, the USSR, Iran and Iraq during the early 1960s. During the 1970s it spread through Africa. In 1991 the pandemic reached South Africa. The eighth pandemic, the first due to a non-O1 strain, first appeared in 1991 in India and has spread more rapidly to Bangladesh, China, Thailand, Nepal and Malaysia.

The earlier pandemics spread slowly along main trade routes and were often associated with major migrations of whole populations. Global spread of the current pandemics reflects different social human ecology associated with international travel and trade (Levine and Levine 1994). For example, spread of *V. cholerae* to US coastal waters was probably related to water used for ballast in cargo ships (McCarthy and Khambaty 1994).

The main routes of cholera transmission are waterborne or foodborne. Several foodborne outbreaks have been described where the food was contaminated by infected food handlers or water or, in the case of seafood, was contaminated in its natural habitat (Roberts 1992). The relative

Table 12.1 The cholera pandemics. Adapted from Crowcroft (1994)

Pandemic	Organism	Origin	Duration	Affected regions
First	O1-Classical	Bangladesh	1817–1823	India, SE Asia, Middle East, East Africa
Second	O1-Classical	Bangladesh	1826–1851	India, SE Asia, Middle East, Africa, Europe, Americas
Third	O1-Classical	Bangladesh	1852–1859	India, SE Asia, Middle East, Africa, Europe, Americas
Fourth	O1-Classical	Bangladesh	1863–1879	India, SE Asia, Middle East, Africa, Europe, Americas
Fifth	O1-Classical	Bangladesh	1881–1896	India, SE Asia, Middle East, Africa, Europe, Americas
Sixth	O1-Classical	Bangladesh	1899–1923	India, SE Asia, Middle East, East Africa, Europe, Americas
Seventh	O1-El Tor	Indonesia	1961–	India, SE Asia, Middle East, Africa, Europe, Americas
Eighth	O139	India	1991–	India, SE Asia

importance of food and water in the transmission of disease can at times be difficult to determine. Direct person to person transmission of cholera is uncommon.

Water and the epidemiology of cholera

Unlike many of the other waterborne diseases described in this book, it is not so easy to separate prospective epidemiological studies from outbreak reports.

A study of the transmission of cholera in the Philippines showed that the relative importance of different modes of transmission can vary during the course of an outbreak (Philippines Cholera Committee 1970). Intensive epidemiological surveillance was combined with routine daily testing of water supplies. During the outbreak, 13 cases and 12 asymptomatic carriers, out of a population of 288, were identified over a six-week period in November and December 1967. Three cases and two carriers were identified before any water sample became positive. Person to person spread was the most likely route of transmission between these people. Most cases occurred during the week after one of the wells became positive. The drinking water from six of the houses was also found to be positive. In five of these houses cholera cases or carriers were identified, usually within a day or two of the first positive water sample.

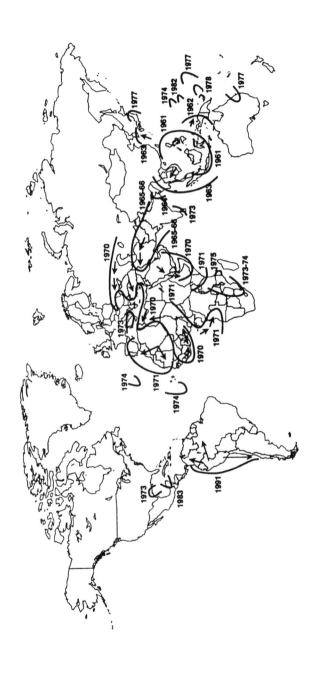

Figure 12.1 Global spread of the seventh cholera pandemic. Reproduced from Glass et al. (1991) Cholera in Africa: lessons on transmission. *Lancet* **338**: 791–795, by permission of The Lancet Ltd.

A study in an area of high incidence of cholera in Bangladesh looked at the protective effect of using sanitary pipe wells (Levine *et al.* 1976a). Paradoxically, the incidence of cholera was higher in families who used tube wells compared to those who did not, although this was not statistically significant. This lack of protective effect was probably because such families also tended to use unsafe water sources such as canals. Educated and wealthy families were found to have lower attack rates.

Investigations of differing incidences of cholera between different villages in Bangladesh over 11 years revealed a link with a cholera hospital (Levine *et al.* 1976b). The attack rate in an area close to the hospital was four or five times higher than in other areas. Before the hospital was built, no difference was noted. People living in the affected area used water that came from a canal into which effluent from the hospital was discharged. Within the affected area attack rates were higher in families that reported using the canal water ($p = 10^{-7}$).

From April to November 1974, a large outbreak of cholera affected several areas of Portugal (Blake *et al.* 1977a). There were 2467 bacteriologically confirmed cases who were hospitalized and 48 deaths. The most significant risk factor for the national outbreak was consumption of raw or semi-cooked shellfish. However, epidemiological investigations in the Lisbon district revealed that visitors to a local spa had a much higher attack rate (RR 10.3) (Blake *et al.* 1977b). *V. cholerae* was isolated from two springs that supplied water to the spa and a water bottling plant. A subsequent case-control study of culture-positive cases who did not attend the spa found an association with drinking non-carbonated bottled mineral water from the relevant plant (RR=12.0, $p = 0.003$). There was no link to carbonated water from the same source. The aquifer was limestone and the contamination could have come from sewage from local villages or ingress from a local river.

During September 1977 an explosive outbreak of cholera affected people living on the Gilbert Islands (Kuberski *et al.* 1979). From a population of only 8480, 420 were admitted to hospital. The attack rate was highest in families using the main water supply as opposed to private wells or rain-water. Although the outbreak was largely controlled by super-chlorination of the mains supply, cases continued to occur. Epidemiological investigations found an association with the consumption of seafood in these later cases.

All of the initial six cases of cholera during an epidemic in 1980 in South Africa drank water from an irrigation canal (Kustner *et al.* 1981). However, analytical epidemiology and microbiological investigations were negative. A subsequent outbreak affecting over 50 people the following year was investigated by a matched-pair case-control study (Sinclair *et al.* 1982). There was a significant ($p < 0.025$) association with drinking water from the Gumpies River and bought water ($p < 0.05$). Drinking treated water (chlorinated or boiled) was protective ($p < 0.05$). Indeed, no case drank treated water. Many people were forced to drink river water because draught had reduced stores of safe water.

Hughes *et al.* (1982) set out to investigate the reasons behind the failure, as described above, of tube wells to control cholera in Bangladesh. In neighbourhoods where cholera was present, 44% of surface waters were culture-positive for *V. cholerae* compared to only 2% of waters from control areas. Infection rates were higher in families using water from a source that yielded at least one culture-positive sample. Drinking and bathing in the same water as an index case of cholera were both independently associated with increased risk.

Starting in April 1982 for 16 weeks, 662 patients with cholera were admitted to hospital in Katsina, Nigeria (Umoh *et al.* 1983). The case fatality rate was 7.7%. Although *V. cholerae* was isolated from several wells, the strains were non-O1. It was noted that many pit latrines were situated very close to wells, with the probability of seepage of cholera from one to the other. The suggestion was made that water sellers probably facilitated the spread of this outbreak.

A prospective case-control study of cholera cases in Indonesia during July and August 1982 followed up 53 laboratory-confirmed cases of cholera (Glass *et al.* 1984). Ice was used more frequently by cases than by controls (RR=2.7, $p < 0.05$), with the use of chipped ice carrying the greatest risk (RR=3.8, $p < 0.02$). Chipped ice was sold by street vendors, who chipped the ice off a large block. Although not statistically significant, the use of river water also carried a large relative risk (5.0). *V. cholerae* O1 was isolated from nine Moore swabs from one river, but not from ice samples. However, *V. cholerae* non-O1 was isolated from 9 of 23 ice samples.

Chapman and Collocott (1985) reported their experience of screening children attending their paediatric outpatient clinic in 1983. Among 293 consecutive children they found 99 positive for *V. cholerae*. Information on water source was available on 112 patients, of whom 20 were cholera positive. Among cholera cases, 65% took their water from the river, compared to 52% of non-cholera cases. Only half of all cases, whether cholera positive or negative, treated their water in any way. Most that did not treat their water were not aware of the benefits of doing so. However, 12% of those who did not treat their water were aware of the benefits but could not afford to.

During an outbreak of cholera in Natal between November 1981 and January 1982, 154 patients from a single area were hospitalized (Sitas 1986). The author investigated the different attack rates among different settlement types. The incidence of cholera was higher in those that used unchlorinated water ($p < 0.0125$) and in the lower social class areas ($p < 0.0125$).

In Mali 1793 cases and 406 deaths due to cholera were reported during 1984 (Tauxe *et al.* 1988). Cholera cases in four villages were investigated in more detail. In two of these villages, a case-control study identified the route of transmission. In one village there was an association with drinking water from just one of 50 wells in the village (OR 6.0, $p = 0.03$). This well was in sandy soil and situated less than 10 m from three pit latrines. In another village, badly affected by a drought, cholera was associated with the consumption of leftover millet gruel (OR 13, $p = 0.02$).

Two separate episodes of cholera occurred in Kelantan, Malaysia during 1990 (Isa, Othman and Ishak 1990). Although no analytical epidemiology was done, waterborne spread was suggested by the observation that the incidence was higher in the riverine villages. Foodborne spread was also suggested by the finding of cholera in food vendors and the subsequent identification of two clusters of cases related to these food handlers.

Between March and May 1988, 951 cases of cholera were identified in a refugee camp in Malawi (Moren et al. 1991). The case fatality rate was 3.3%. A matched case-control study was done on the first 51 cases. Cases were more likely to drink water from shallow wells rather than from boreholes (OR 4.5, CI 1.0–20.8). Cases were also more likely to have contact with the market where the outbreak first developed (OR 3.5, CI 0.7–16.8).

The seventh pandemic of cholera eventually arrived in South America in January 1991. In little over a year, more than 533 000 cases and 4700 deaths had been reported from 19 countries on that continent. One of the first studies of the epidemiology of cholera to be reported from South America was done in the city of Trujillo, Peru (Swerdlow et al. 1992a). By the end of March 1991, 16 400 cases of suspected cholera and 71 deaths had been reported in the province of Trujillo. A matched case-control study was done of 46 cases and 65 symptom-free controls. Cases were more likely to have drunk unboiled water within the 3 days before the onset of illness (OR 3.1, CI 1.3–3.7), drunk from a container into which the hand had been dipped (OR 42, CI 1.2–14.9) and attended a fiesta (OR 3.6, CI 1.1–11.1). During the study several water samples were taken. Total and faecal coliforms were very low in well-water, generally high in house tap-water and very high in samples from water containers.

Piura, another city in Peru, also experienced the full brunt of the pandemic (Ries et al. 1992). By the end of March 1991, 7922 cases and 17 deaths had occurred. In a similar study of 50 cases and 100 matched controls, risk factors were identified as: drinking unboiled water (OR 3.9, CI 1.7–8.9), drinking beverages from street vendors (OR 14.6, CI 4.2–51.2), eating food from street vendors (OR 24.0, CI 3.0–19.1), eating rice more than 3 hours old without reheating (OR 3.1, CI 1.2–8.4) and putting hands in a drinking vessel (OR 2.6, 1.2–5.9). In a multiple linear logistic regression analysis, drinking unboiled water, drinking a beverage from a street vendor and putting hands into a water storage vessel remained as significant independent factors. To test the beverage from street vendors hypothesis further, those cases who had drunk from a street vendor were matched with controls who had also drunk such beverages. Although cases and controls consumed similar amount of street beverage, cases were more likely to have had ice with their drinks (OR 4.0, CI 1.1–18.3). Testing of the water supply revealed inadequate or non-existent chlorination. Faecal coliforms were isolated from several water samples and *V. cholerae* isolated from two. Inspection of the ice factories revealed poor conditions, allowed because the ice was not intended for human consumption.

About 30 000 cholera cases and 500 deaths were reported in Columbia between 5 March 1991 and 1 September 1992 (Cardenas *et al.* 1993). The city of Riohacha reported 548 cases out of a population of 68 000. A cross-sectional survey found significant associations between consumption of municipal water drinking water and cholera (OR 5.7, CI 1.2–41.1) and diarrhoea (OR 3.3, CI 1.1–11.2). Drinking bottled water was found to be protective. A case-control study also found an association of cholera with drinking municipal water (OR 3.6, CI 1.3–10.1) and with a shortage of water in the home (OR 3.6, CI 0.8–16.4). The water supply to the city was from both surface water and wells. Sewage contamination of the supply was known to occur as a result of cracked pipes and low pressure in the distribution system combined with too close a proximity to sewage systems.

A further case-controlled study of cholera in a Peru city in 1991 interviewed 50 cases and 100 controls (Mujica *et al.* 1994). In Iquitos, a city in the Amazonian region, 2767 cases and 33 deaths, out of a population of 280 000, had occurred by 1 June. Risk factors were: drinking unboiled water (OR 2.9, CI 1.3–6.4), eating unreheated cooked rice (OR 2.1, CI 1.0-4.5) and eating unwashed fruits or vegetables (OR 8.0, CI 2.2–28.9). Consumption of toronja drink (prepared from the juice of a citrus fruit like a grapefruit with added water and sugar) was found to be protective (OR 0.4, CI 0.2–0.7). This negative association was present even though untreated water was used in making the toronja drink. The protective effect of this drink was undoubtedly due to its low pH of 4.0, which is sufficiently low to be vibriocidal. Recommending toronja drink would be a cheap, readily available way to prevent cholera.

In Ecuador during 1991, 46 320 cases of cholera and 697 deaths were reported. A study undertaken in Guayaquil, Ecuador, in July 1991 interviewed 63 cases and 126 controls (Weber *et al.* 1994). This found that drinking unboiled water (OR 4.0, CI 1.8–7.5), drinking a beverage from a street vendor (OR 2.8, CI 1.3-5.9), eating raw seafood (OR 3.4, CI 1.4–11.5) and eating cooked crab (OR 5.1, CI 1.4–19.2) were associated with illness. Always boiling drinking water at home (OR 0.5, CI 0.2–0.9) and having soap in the kitchen (OR 0.3, CI 0.2–0.8) or bathroom (OR 0.4, CI 0.2–0.9) were found to be protective. This same study found that 15 of 33 isolates studied were multiply resistant to antibiotics including chloramphenicol, doxycycline, kanamycin, streptomycin, sulfisoxazole, tetracycline, and trimethoprim/sulfamethoxazole. It was noted that the proportion of multi-drug resistant strains had increased since the start of the pandemic in South America.

An outbreak of cholera affected a large number of Mozambican refugees in southern Malawi from June to September 1988 (Hatch *et al.* 1994). At its peak, 10–15 cases of suspect cholera were admitted to hospital each day.

During the first two weeks of the outbreak, 51 cases were interviewed as part of a case-control study. Multivariate analysis found the following independent risk factors: having two (OR 9.7, CI 2.1–44.9) or more than two (OR 38.2, CI 7.2–202.0) children under 5 years old in the home and being resident in the transit centre (OR 17.6, CI 3.6–85.9). Owning water containers (OR 0.02, CI 0.003–0.12) and cooking pots (OR 0.3, CI 0.12–0.7) were both protective. Indeed, there was an inverse relationship between the risk of cholera and the number of cooking pots or water containers. It was suggested that the relationship with water containers was because people with few water containers did not have ready access to clean drinking water.

Another South American study later that same year, this time in rural El Salvador, was undertaken following a nationwide door to door education campaign (Quick et al. 1995). The education programme had been designed to encourage the population to wash their hands with soap, boil or chlorinate drinking water, keep drinking water containers covered, wash produce, and eat cooked food and all seafood hot. The case-controlled study found that eating cold cooked or raw seafood at home (OR 7.0, CI 1.4–35.0), and drinking water outside of the home (OR 8.8, CI 1.7–44.6) were associated with disease. Knowledge of how to prevent cholera (OR 0.2, CI 0.1–0.8), eating rice (OR 0.2, CI 0.1–0.8), and using soap always or almost always to wash hands (OR 0.3, CI 0.1–1.0) were protective.

A study of 103 confirmed cholera cases admitted to the Delhi Infectious Diseases Hospital found that most cases were in children under ten years or housewives (Singh et al. 1995a). All cases were either illiterate or only educated up to primary school level. About 96% of cases stored drinking water in wide-mouthed containers such as buckets and more than 90% were in the habit of drawing water by dipping cups into these containers. None of the cases washed their hands with soap and water before preparing or eating food, though 40% claimed to wash with soap and water after defecation. The authors noted that the results of routine water testing for the year of the study showed that only 54% of stored water was fit for human consumption compared to 94% of piped water and only 18% of water from shallow tube wells.

Coppo et al. (1995) reported the results of a cholera surveillance scheme in Somalia, Horn of Africa, from 1983 to 1990. Stains of V. cholerae O1 were only isolated during a cholera epidemic in 1985 and 1986. The attack rate during this epidemic was 3–3.5/1000 population and the case fatality rate was 13%. The epidemic had its main early focus in a refugee camp near the Ethiopian border. In the first seven days there were at least 2600 cases in the camp and 700 deaths. As the epidemic spread to nearby towns two case-control studies were done to elucidate its epidemiology. One study found that 13 of 18 cases and only 4 of 32 matched controls in Hawlwadaag drank unboiled water from a certain unprotected well (OR 12.0, CI 3.57–40.37). In another larger study of two villages it was not possible to demonstrate an association between cholera and drinking river water. Although the original strain was not resistant to antibiotics, it soon gave rise to two antibiotic-resistant derivatives. The predominant derivative was resistant to ampicillin, kanamycin, streptomycin, sulphonamide and tetracycline. Later in the epidemic the resistant strains were themselves replaced by sensitive strains.

COMMENTS

Cholera was the earliest infectious diseases to be linked to a water source. It was also one of the earliest to have the microbe identified. Yet it remains one of the few diseases that has the potential to cause rapid large-scale fatalities among populations where public health systems fail.

Despite the many years of effort in studying *V. cholerae*, there remain significant uncertainties; for example, the role of viable but non-culturable organisms in the epidemiology of the disease and the finding that the infectious dose as demonstrated by experiment is much higher than that normally found in implicated waters.

Nevertheless, the outlook is not all gloomy. The study by Quick *et al.* (1995) shows that health education and simple personal hygiene such as washing with soap can be significantly protective.

VIBRIO VULNIFICUS

V. vulnificus is an aquatic vibrio that has caused considerable interest in recent years. There are two main presentations of the disease. The first is that of a rapidly progressive septicaemia with a high fatality associated with the consumption of contaminated shellfish. The other is wound infection following contamination of a wound sustained in the water or before. These wound infections can also progress to a spreading necrotic cellulitis, which may be rapidly fatal. The virulence of the organism is thought to rest in its capsule, which impairs normal host defences. The organism also produces various proteolytic and cytolytic toxins responsible for tissue destruction.

A nested PCR method for detection in water samples has been described (Arias, Garay and Aznar 1995). This was able to detect as few as 12 cells in artificially inoculated samples.

V. vulnificus has been identified in estuarine waters throughout the world (Kaysner *et al.* 1987; Myatt and Davis 1989; Amaro *et al.* 1992; O'Neill, Jones and Grimes 1992; Veenstra *et al.* 1994). The organism prefers water and does not survive well below 8.5 °C or at salinities above 30 ppt (Kaspar and Tamplin 1993). Like other vibrios, *V. vulnificus* can exist as a viable but non-culturable form (Oliver 1995). This may be how the organism survives the winter.

Armstrong, Lake and Miller (1983) reviewed hospital records in Virginia and identified 18 patients with extraintestinal infections caused by halophilic vibrios. Primary septicaemia due to *V. vulnificus* was the cause in three, while 15 had soft tissue infection. Most of the soft tissue infections followed injuries that had become contaminated by seawater.

Not all cases of infection due to *V. vulnificus* are associated with seawater. Tacket *et al.* (1984) described two cases of soft tissue infection that followed contact with brackish inland waters.

Klontz *et al.* (1988) reported on infection in 62 patients in Florida between 1981 and 1987. Primary septicaemia was seen in 38 patients, of whom 55% died; wound infection in 17, of whom 24% died; and gastroenteritis in 7 patients.

A case-control study was done on 19 patients with infection and three times as many matched controls (Johnston, Becker and McFarland 1985). Patients with a wound infection were more likely to have had a puncture wound when handling fresh seafood or been exposed to salt water. Risk factors for septicaemia were: having eaten raw oysters, having underlying liver disease, haematopoietic disorders, chronic renal insufficiency, using immunosuppressive drugs and having a history of heavy alcohol consumption.

From May 1985 to July 1990, 27 patients were identified as suffering from a *V. vulnificus* infection in Taiwan (Chuang *et al.* 1992). One patient had two episodes of infection. Fifteen presented with a wound infection, of whom seven also had septicaemia. Four of these seven died, while only one of the eight presenting with wound infection alone died. Four cases were linked to injuries in a saltwater fish pond, one to exposure of abraded skin to saltwater, two to injuries from crabs and three to injuries from seafood; one patient was a fisherman.

In 1989 four US gulf states conducted a coordinated surveillance scheme for vibrio disease (Levine, Griffin and the Gulf Coast *Vibrio* Working Group 1993). They identified 18 infections due to *V. vulnificus*, of which 7 were primary septicaemia, 3 gastroenteritis and 8 wound infections. Four patients died. All patients with septicaemia had a known underlying illness.

Penman *et al.* (1995) described six wound infections associated with Mississippi gulf coastal waters during the three months from June to August 1993. Five cases were admitted to hospital and two underwent surgery. Two died from septicaemia.

13 Typhoid and Paratyphoid Fevers and Other Salmonella Infections

Typhoid is a disease of great historical interest to the water industry because, in the early part of the twentieth century, it was the commonest known cause of waterborne outbreaks in both the UK and the USA. Much water legislation and practice dating back to the early and mid-20th century was aimed at preventing this disease. Although now uncommon in the western world, it is still a major problem in many less wealthy countries. When outbreaks occur they can still cause many deaths in affected individuals.

MICROBIOLOGY

Salmonella spp. are members of the family Enterobacteriaceae. They are Gram-negative, non-spore forming, facultative anaerobic bacilli. Most produce acid and gas from the fermentation of sugars; some produce only acid. Most are motile. There is currently only one species recognized, *S. cholerae-suis*, although this is divided into seven sub-types (Table 13.1). *S. cholerae-suis* subspecies *cholerae-suis* contains the vast majority of serotypes responsible for human disease. Kaufmann and White further subdivided salmonellae based on their somatic 'O' and flagella 'H' antigens. Serogroups are based on the O antigens, while serotypes are based on the combination of O and H antigens. Most of those serotypes of human significance are given a serotype name. Thus, *S. enteritidis* is in fact *S. cholerae-suis* subspecies *cholerae-suis* serogroup 9 (previously known as serogroup D), serotype *enteritidis*. Important serotypes can now be further subdivided based on phage typing schemes. Genetic fingerprinting methods are also being used more frequently.

Typhoid fever is caused by infection due to *S. typhi*, a serogroup 9 (or D) organism. *S. typhi* does not produce gas from sugars. Paratyphoid is due to A similar infection with *S. paratyphi* serogroups 2, 4 or 7 (A, B or C).

PATHOGENICITY

For those salmonellae that give rise to diarrhoeal illness, disease is caused by invasion of the superficial layers of the lower part of the small intestine. This

Table 13.1 Subspecies of *Salmonella cholerae-suis*

Subgroup number	Subgroup name
I	*cholerae-suis*
II	*salamae*
IIIa	*arizonae*
IIIb	*diarizonae*
IV	*houtenae*
V	*bongori*
VI	*indica*

invasion then stimulates an inflammatory response, which gives rise to fluid loss by release of prostaglandins, which activate cyclic adenosine mono-phosphate (cAMP). Sometimes even in species that normally only cause diarrhoea, infection is not restricted to the superficial layers of the gut, and deeper invasion occurs. This penetration can lead to systemic spread with septicaemia, meningitis, and abscess formation at distant sites. Based on volunteer experiments, it was thought that the infectious dose for non-typhoidal salmonellosis was of the order of 10^9 organisms. However, evidence from many recent outbreaks suggests that the infectious dose is certainly below 1000 and possibly below 10 organisms.

The pathogenesis for typhoid and the other enteric fevers is rather different. After passing through the stomach, the organism penetrates the lining of the small bowel. The organisms then pass to the mesenteric lymph nodes, where they multiply. As the bacterial load grows, the organisms are released into the bloodstream to infect any organ. In particular, the gall bladder is infected from the liver or bloodstream. From the gall bladder the intestine is infected a second time, but in greater numbers. This second infection can be so severe that perforation of the intestine occurs. This also causes an increase in the excretion of the infective agent in the stool, so propagating the infection. As few as 10^3 organisms can cause a typhoid infection. An important virulence factor is the capsular Vi antigen, which protects the organism from phagocytes.

CLINICAL FEATURES

The incubation period for salmonella gastroenteritis is usually 12–49 hours although it can be shorter or extend up to seven days. The predominant feature is diarrhoea, which is usually watery but contains blood in up to 30% of cases. Colicky abdominal pain and fever are also common. Nausea and mild vomiting may also be present. Usually the disease is self-limiting, with recovery within a couple of days, although it can persist for up to a couple of weeks or more. In a small proportion of immunocompetent cases (<5%), features of invasion can be seen with positive blood cultures and/or secondary complications such as meningitis, osteomyelitis or endocarditis. Occasionally fluid loss can be so severe that acute renal failure develops. After recovery faecal carriage may persist for up to 12 weeks. Less than 10% of patients are reported to be carriers for longer than that.

The incubation period for typhoid is usually 10–14 days (range 5–23 days), although it can vary widely from outbreak to outbreak. Disease onset is insidious, with fever, malaise, aches and pains, and flu-like symptoms. Over the first week or so, fever increases in a step-wise fashion. Abdominal pain is seen in 20–40% of cases. Patients may have diarrhoea or constipation. As the illness progresses patients may develop delirium. Rose spots, delicate rose-pink macular or papular spots, develop in up to 50% of white adults. Untreated fatality rates can be as high as 15%, but are about 1% after antibiotic therapy. In those who survive, weakness, debilitation and weight loss may persist for months. Death is usually due to one of the various complications associated with typhoid fever. These include: massive intestinal haemorrhage and perforation of the gut; pericarditis, orchitis, and splenic or liver abscesses. Between 1 and 3% of patients become chronic carriers.

DIAGNOSIS

Diagnosis of both gastrointestinal and typhoidal disease rests on the culture of the responsible pathogen from faeces or blood culture. Culture from faeces has to be in a selective medium such as deoxycholate citrate agar directly and after enrichment in selenite broth. Confirmation of identity is based on biochemical and serological agglutination reactions.

For typhoid, the Widal test has been used for many years. This is based on the demonstration of the ability of the patient's serum to agglutinate killed stains of salmonellae carrying the appropriate O and H antigens. The test is rarely used these days because it is relatively non-specific to *S. typhi*, and becomes positive after vaccination. *S. typhi* lipopolysaccharide antigen may also be detected in the serum and urine of patients using enzyme-linked immunosorbent assay (ELISA) or counterimmuno-electrophoresis.

TREATMENT

Treatment of salmonella gastroenteritis is usually supportive. Antibiotics are rarely necessary. However, in severe or prolonged disease, one of the newer quinolones such as ciprofloxacin may be valuable. Ciprofloxacin may also have a role in clearing long-term carriage in the few circumstances where this is necessary.

The antibiotic drugs of choice for typhoid are now ciprofloxacin and chloramphenicol. Co-trimoxazole or amoxycillin are potential alternatives. There are several vaccines available with effectiveness against typhoid.

ENVIRONMENTAL DETECTION

The isolation of salmonellae, including *S. typhi*, from water involves concentration by filtration followed by enrichment in buffered peptone water (BPW) to enhance resuscitation of stressed organisms (HMSO 1994). The BPW is then subcultured into selenite broth for *S. typhi* or Rappaport Vassiliadis broth for other salmonellae. Finally, the broths are subcultured onto selective agar such as xylose lysine desoxycholate agar, brilliant green agar or bismuth sulphite agar. Colonies with the appropriate appearance are then identified using standard biochemical and serological methods. Morinigo *et al.* (1993) have reported the results of a comparative study of enrichment broths for detecting salmonellae in water.

Recent alternative methods for the detection of *Salmonella* spp. including *S. typhi* in water samples include the use of polymerase chain reaction (Way *et al.* 1993) and fluorescent-antibody methods (Desmonts *et al.* 1990). These methods are effective at detecting the viable but non-culturable forms.

ECOLOGY

Salmonellae are primary pathogens of the intestinal tracts of animals. Therefore, their distribution in the environment mirrors the distribution of animal faecal contamination. Indeed, few surface waters appear free from contamination (Hooper 1970; Claudon *et al.* 1971; Garcia-Villanova, Cueto and Bolanos 1987; Kueh and Grohmann 1989; Fewtrell *et al.* 1994; Khalil *et al.* 1994). *S. typhi* and *S. paratyphi* only colonize humans. Their ecology is, therefore, intimately linked to the distribution of human sewage. *S. typhi* has also been isolated from water and sewage when cases of enteric fever were being reported from nearby populations. However, in none of the outbreaks described below was *S. typhi* isolated from the drinking water. This is perhaps not surprising given the long incubation period of the disease.

EPIDEMIOLOGY

Although common during the first half of the twentieth century, typhoid and paratyphoid are now uncommon in the western world. Nevertheless the disease is still very common elsewhere, affecting an estimated 12.5 million people each year. Indeed, most cases presenting in the UK and USA are now imported.

The preference of *S. typhi* and *S. paratyphi* for humans means that the organisms are only spread faecal-orally, usually via contaminated food or water. Direct person to person spread is uncommon. Foodborne typhoid has had a somewhat notorious history. The most infamous case was a cook called Mary Mallon (Typhoid Mary). She was a typhoid carrier who disobeyed medical instructions to cease her work. She directly infected 53 people, of whom 5 died, and was probably responsible for an outbreak that ultimately affected over 1000 people. She spent the last 15 years of her life in quarantine.

Waterborne outbreaks of non-typhoidal salmonellosis

Despite their widespread distribution in the water environment, non-typhoidal salmonellae rarely cause waterborne outbreaks. A very large waterborne outbreak affecting 16 000 people was reported from California in 1966 (Greenberg and Ongerth 1966). Since then I can find evidence of only one waterborne outbreak. This outbreak affected a church group who attended a rural camp on Trinidad in 1976 (Koplan *et al.* 1978). Of 73 children and 15 adults attending a camp in northern Trinidad, 48 were admitted to hospital on a single day with diarrhoea, fever and vomiting. Further investigations revealed that 63 (76%) people out of 83 who replied had suffered a similar illness. *S. arechevalata* was cultured from the stools of 45 cases and 11 symptomless contacts. Food preference questionnaires showed no significant association. Two food items were positive for the epidemic stain, as was the kitchen tap on two occasions. Both food items had been mixed with tap-water. The water supply to the kitchen came from water collected on building roofs. Examination of the roofs showed then to be heavily contaminated with dried and fresh bird droppings. It was suggested that recent rainfall had washed salmonellae off the roof and into the drinking water supply.

Waterborne outbreaks of typhoid

After a four-week voyage from Southampton, a British liner sailed into Vancouver on the morning of 14 January 1970 (Davies *et al.* 1972). On board were 17 crewmen and 3 passengers who were ill suffering from typhoid. During this outbreak 83 passengers and crew were admitted to hospital with typhoid or suspect typhoid. One individual died. Of 1565 passengers and 607 crew, 11 (0.7%) passengers and 42 (7.0%) crew were diagnosed as having typhoid. The attack rate in the European crew (8.5%) was more than twice that in the Goan crew (4.1%), probably reflecting increased immunity in the non-Europeans. Among the passengers, the attack rate was much lower in first class (0.1%) than in tourist class (1.3%). In a case-control study there was a significant relationship between the average number of glasses of water consumed each day and an increased risk of disease. The attack rate was 0% in those not drinking unboiled water and 69.2% in those drinking five or more glasses per day. Interestingly, drinking beer was found to be protective. Faecal coliforms were isolated from the some of the ship's drinking water. Inspection of the ship found several unhygienic practices in the kitchens. It was suggested that the source of infection was probably one or more typhoid carriers and that faecal contamination of the affected tanks occurred during maintenance work in dock.

An outbreak of chloramphenicol-resistant typhoid in Mexico in 1972 affected 83 and killed 6 (Gonzalez-Cortes *et al.* 1973). It was discovered that, shortly before the outbreak started, the mains water supply failed because of a defective pump. Although trucks delivered water to the village, many people took their drinking water from a canal. The attack rate was much higher in those taking their water from the canal (26.1% versus 7%) ($p = 0.007$). Inspection of the canal found heavy faecal soiling on the banks upstream of the village and pipes discharging raw sewage into the canal in the village.

During February and March 1973, 225 cases of typhoid occurred among 1795 residents of a labour camp for migrant workers in Dade County, Florida (Feldman *et al.* 1974). The index case was a young girl who developed typhoid fever two weeks before the main outbreak. A simple cohort study showed that the risk of hospitalization increased with increasing daily water consumption ($p = 8 \times 10^{-5}$). The water supply came from two wells and was then chlorinated by a single chlorinator. Routine testing of the water before the outbreak had found coliforms, after which the local public health department had demanded the replacement of the chlorinator. Studies using fluorescein dye found that surface water could gain access to either well. Although fluorescein dye did not appear in well-water after flushing down toilets, faults in the sewage system were identified, as were naturally made channels in the subsurface limestone. Faecal material was found in the camp's water storage tank. The hatch on the tank lid had been unlocked.

Perhaps the world's largest waterborne outbreak of typhoid fever occurred in Sangli Town, Maharashtra State, India, between December 1975 and February 1976 (Sathe *et al.* 1983). Out of a population of some 135 000 an estimated 9000 people were affected. The water supply was from two wells on the banks of a nearby river. The water was treated by rapid sand filtration and chlorination by chlorine gas. However, the water treatment works had no reserve gas cylinder so during times when this was away being refilled bleaching powder was used. An underground sewerage system was not then in operation and most sewage drained by surface gutters into a stream that entered the main river near one of the wells. To prevent direct contamination of the well area the stream carrying the sewage was dammed. The accumulated sewage was then fed down a ditch to enter the main river further downstream. Some of this faecally contaminated water was also pumped onto rice fields after the monsoon rains. Because of a prolonged monsoon, sewage was not pumped onto the fields and so overflowed onto the well area. Such an overflow choked the filter beds in the treatment works, leading to raw water entering the supply.

An outbreak of typhoid followed a waterborne outbreak of dysentery in northern Israel in 1985 (Egoz et al. 1988). The outbreak affected 77 people, of whom 75 were hospitalized. The affected communities were supplied with unchlorinated well-water. One of the wells was subsequently found to be heavily contaminated with faecal coliforms. This well was sunk in relatively porous ground and was only 7 m from a fractured main sewage pipe.

During July and August 1983, 52 patients were admitted to hospital suffering from typhoid in the Chu-Tung township, Taiwan (King et al. 1989). A subsequent community survey suggested an overall attack rate of confirmed and presumptive typhoid of 9.4 per 1000. Thus, over 500 people were probably affected. A case-control study of early cases found that the most significant risk factor was drinking tap-water (OR 5.36, $p = 0.02$). Drinking from the river or from wells (OR 0.09, $p = 0.02$) and poor kitchen hygiene (OR 0.12, $p = 0.002$) appeared protective. In a similar study of late cases the association with tap-water was no longer present. Risk factors for later cases were crowded living conditions (OR 3.81, $p = 0.008$), poor garbage handling (OR 2.56, $p = 0.01$) and poor kitchen hygiene (OR 3.18, $p = 0.05$). This difference in epidemiology illustrates an important point. An outbreak that starts as a waterborne one may then spread from person to person. If epidemiological analysis does not distinguish early from late cases, the importance of the waterborne route may be missed. The risk factors associated with the late cases were those that indicated poverty and poor personal hygiene. Faecal coliforms were isolated from about one-quarter of drinking water samples. S. typhi was not isolated from any water sample. How the water supply came to be contaminated was not clear.

Early in April 1988, an outbreak of multi-drug resistant typhoid fever affected a town in the Kashmir valley (Kamili et al. 1993); 230 cases were identified. It was discovered that in the area where cases were occurring, the water filtration plant was not working and consequently the water supply was intermittent. Intermittent supply was allowing faecal contamination as pressure drop in the pipes created a partial vacuum and sucked contaminated material through cracks in the pipes.

During May 1992, 81 cases of bacteriologically confirmed typhoid fever occurred in Tabuk City, northwestern Saudi Arabia (Al-Qarawi et al. 1995). In a case-control study purchasing water by the gallon from a private reverse osmosis desalination station was associated with increased risk of disease (OR 2.58, CI 1.25–5.39). Furthermore, this increased risk was associated with just one well (OR 7.05, CI 2.51–20.71). Drinking municipal water was protective (OR 0.42, CI 0.17–0.90). It was noted that the private company providing the implicated water had not changed its filter for two years and did not chlorinate the water. Furthermore, the aquifer from which the affected water was extracted lay beneath a depression in the ground in which the city sewage collected. It was suggested that the sewage was taken into the aquifer because of over-extraction.

Epidemiological studies of sporadic disease

Bahl (1976) reported a study of the incidence of typhoid in Lusaka, Zambia before and after the provision of pipe water was extended to urban and peri-urban self-help settlements (squatter camps). During 1973, as a result of fund raising campaigns by the local residents, pipe water was supplied for the first time. There was a dramatic reduction in the incidence of typhoid from a peak of 13 per 100 000 in 1971, to 6 in 1972, 3 in 1973, 0.9 in 1974 and 0.8 in 1975. Although there was also a decline in the incidence of diarrhoeal disease from 338 per 1000 population in 1972 to 212 per 1000 in 1975, this was less dramatic.

Stroffolini et al. (1992) reported a case-control study on endemic typhoid fever in the Neapolitan area of Italy, done during the first six months of 1990. Raw shellfish was eaten by 76.5% of cases (OR 13.3, CI 5.5–32.8). Although cases were more likely to have drunk non-potable water, this did not achieve statistical significance (OR 2.7, CI 0.7–11.1).

14 Shigellosis (Bacillary Dysentery)

Dysentery is a term that was first use by Hippocrates to refer to the frequent passage of stools containing blood and mucus. It was not until this century that bacillary dysentery caused predominantly by *Shigella* spp. and amoebic dysentery were first distinguished from each other. Worldwide, shigella infections probably infect over 2 000 000 people and cause the death of approximately 650 000 each year (Lindberg and Pal 1993).

MICROBIOLOGY

Shigella spp. are Gram-negative non-motile bacilli that are members of the Enterobacteriaceae. Shigella are distinguished from other enterobacteria and from each other on the basis of biochemical and serological characteristics. There are four subgroups, A to D. Group A are all *Sh. dysenteriae*, of which there are 10 serotypes, 1–10. Usually only types 1 and 2 cause disease. *Sh. dysenteriae* serotype 1 was previously known as *Sh. shigae*. Group B organisms, known as *Sh. flexneri*, differ from group A in that they ferment mannitol. There are 13 serotypes and sub-types. Group C organisms, of which there are 15 serotypes, are biochemically similar to Group B strains in that they ferment mannitol but are antigenically distinct. They are named *Sh. boydii*. There is only one serotype of Group D, *Sh. sonnei*. This also ferments mannitol but, unlike other groups, is also a late lactose fermenter.

PATHOGENICITY

Shigella spp. are restricted to causing disease in humans and primates, although there have been occasional reports of the disease in dogs. They are among the most infectious intestinal pathogens known and can cause disease in healthy adults with the administration of fewer than 200 viable organisms (DuPont *et al.* 1989).

Virulent *Shigella* spp. produce disease by invasion and subsequent destruction of the superficial intestinal mucosa. Invasiveness seems to be related to the presence of a 140-MDa plasmid (Hale, Oaks and Formal 1985). *Sh.*

dysenteriae serotype 1 (*Sh. shigae*) differs from other strains in that it produces a heat-labile neurotoxin that causes paralysis and death in mice and rabbits. This serotype, along with some strains of *Sh. flexneri* and *Sh. sonnei*, also produce a heat-labile enterotoxin which causes a bloody fluid secretion in the rabbit ileal loop. The mechanism for this secretion is not the same as that of cholera toxin.

In the early stages of infection there are large numbers of the organism in the faeces (up to 10^9 viable organisms per gram). Shigellosis is, therefore, highly infectious by the faecal–oral route.

CLINICAL FEATURES

In most cases the incubation period of shigellosis is about 2–3 days, with an upper limit of about 7 days. The nature and severity of the clinical disease varies depending on the infecting strain.

The illness due to *Sh. sonnei* is usually relatively mild and self-limiting. Many cases of infection have no symptoms. Those with diarrhoea usually settle within a couple of days. Occasionally, diarrhoea is more severe and accompanied by vomiting, which can lead to dehydration. Systemic features of fever, meningism and abdominal pain may then occur. In rare cases the clinical presentation can be even more severe, with sudden onset of severe diarrhoea, vomiting, fever and headache, leading to marked dehydration and prostration.

Illness due to the other groups of *Shigella* spp. is usually more severe than that caused by *Sh. sonnei* and the diarrhoea can persist for up to a week, the stool eventually being mostly mucus with varying amounts of blood. Tenesmus, a painful straining to empty the bowels, is often a feature. Systemic symptoms of malaise, fever, headache, generalized pains and rigors may be present.

More severe, fulminating disease is usually associated with *Sh. dysenteriae* type 1. Patients can either present with an acute cholera-type illness, with the passage of profuse watery diarrhoea, or with a gangrenous form. This latter form is associated with severe abdominal pain and the passage of stools containing altered blood and necrotic mucosa (lining of the bowel wall). In both forms of this fulminating disease there is rapid collapse. Death is the usual outcome.

Haemorrhoids as a result of straining are common and rectal prolapse can also occur following shigella infections. Post-infection joint disease can include Reiter's syndrome and a symmetrical arthritis usually affecting the knees or ankles. Reiter's syndrome presents with as polyarthritis affecting the smaller joints, with conjunctivitis, skin rash, urethritis and mucocutaneous lesions predominantly affecting the mouth and genitals. Haemolytic–uraemic syndrome occurs in about 10% of infections with *Sh. dysenteriae* type 1.

DIAGNOSIS

Diagnosis is usually made by culture of a stool sample onto a selective medium such as deoxycholate citrate agar.

TREATMENT

Most mild cases of shigella infection are self-limiting and require no therapy other than oral fluids. Those more severely ill will require intravenous fluid replacement. Specific antimicrobial therapy has been used, with variable and probably only minimal effect in most cases. Antimicrobial therapy is complicated by the rapid development of resistance to any antimicrobial regularly used. Antibiotics should be reserved for only the most seriously ill and if possible after antibiotics sensitivity testing has been done.

ENVIRONMENTAL DETECTION

The fist step in the isolation of *Shigella* spp. from water is concentration, usually by filtration (HMSO 1994). The filters are then incubated in enrichment broth (usually modified Hajna GN Enrichment Broth), following which the broth is then subcultured on to both modified deoxycholate citrate agar and Hektoen agar. Polymerase chain reaction methods with gene probes and fluorescent antibody methods have been shown to identify viable but non-culturable *Shigella* spp. (Bej *et al.* 1991; Josephson, Gerba and Pepper, 1993; Islam *et al.* 1993).

ECOLOGY

As man is the only known host, the distribution of *Shigella* spp. in the environment reflects human faecal contamination. *Shigella* spp. have been isolated from some water supply systems in tropical countries. Using standard culture methodology, a study in Lahore, Pakistan, found positive isolations in 5% of water sampled from an upper middle class area, 3% of samples from rivers and canals and 10% of samples from a hospital water system (Khalil *et al.* 1994). Water sampled from a village, a peri-urban slum and a market were negative.

Studies on the survival of *Shigella* spp. have given differing results. Mitscherlich and Marth (1984) reported that *Sh. sonnei* could survive more than 100 days in freshwater, and Popovitch and Bondarenko (1982) reported survival of *Sh. sonnei* and *Sh. flexneri* of up to about 50 days at 25 °C. By contrast, El-Sharkawi *et al.* (1989) found survival of *Sh. flexneri* for only 4–7 days at 25–35 °C. Even when no longer culturable, *Sh. dysenteriae* type 1, and probably other *Shigella* spp., can remain alive and potentially infectious in a viable but non-culturable state (Islam *et al.* 1993).

EPIDEMIOLOGY

Shigella infections occur worldwide. In the industrialized countries such as the USA and the UK, *Sh. sonnei* predominates. In these countries the infection is usually a disease of childhood and is transmitted almost entirely by person to person spread. The incidence of the disease declines markedly in the five and over age groups as personal hygiene improves. Outbreaks often occur in schools, where they can be extremely difficult to control. Shigella infections can also be venereally transmitted by oral–anal contact in male homosexuals.

In tropical countries the various serotypes of *Sh. flexneri* and *Sh. dysenteriae* predominate, although *Sh. boydii* and *Sh. sonnei* are also found. As in the developed world, direct person to person spread of bacillary dysentery is probably the predominant mode of transmission, although foodborne and waterborne spread are also common. Flies are thought to be important for transmission of the disease in those countries where human excrement is left in the open (Khalil *et al.* 1994).

Drinking water outbreaks

An outbreak of *Sh. flexneri* 6 on a Caribbean cruise liner affected 90% of 650 passengers and 35% of 299 crew in June 1973 (Merson *et al.* 1975). Epidemiological analysis linked the outbreak to drinking water and ice. There was a significant association between attack rate and the customary daily consumption of water and iced beverages. The ship's water had elevated faecal coliform counts. It was not discovered how the drinking water had come to be contaminated.

In November 1972, 194 pupils at a public school developed *Sh. sonnei* infection resistant to multiple antibiotics (Baine *et al.* 1975). The organism was isolated from the water supply.

There were 434 cases and 28 deaths among a population of 1318 on a coral island in the Bay of Bengal due to *Sh. dysenteriae* type 1 over a three-month period (Rahaman *et al.* 1975). The outbreak abated once the water supply was chlorinated.

In Florida, between January and March 1974, an outbreak of shigellosis affected 1200 people in a community of 6500 (Weissman *et al.* 1976). An epidemiological study showed consumption of tap-water to be a risk factor.

One of the wells was continuously contaminated by faecal material from a nearby septic tank. There had also been a failure of chlorination for 48 hours in January.

During October 1974, 62 out of a crew of 91 on a work train developed shigellosis (White and Pedersen 1976). Epidemiology implicated unchlorinated lake water, which was stored in tanks, as the source.

In May 1980 a private school in Rio de Janeiro experienced an outbreak of diarrhoea (Sutmoller *et al.* 1982). During the outbreak period 812 (70.6%) students had a period of absence. A questionnaire survey was returned from 487, of whom 386 (79.3%) reported having gastroenteritis. Approximately 55% of cases occurred within just two days. Stool examination revealed both *Sh. sonnei* and rotavirus infections. Investigations showed that the school was accidentally pumping water from a shallow well that was poorly protected and known to contain high coliform counts. This supply was only chlorinated by hand.

Multi-drug resistant *Sh. dysenteriae* type 1 was responsible for an explosive outbreak in a southern Indian village during October and November 1972 (Mathan *et al.* 1984). There were 546 cases (overall attack rate 26.6/100), of whom 6 died. Paradoxically, the poorest parts of the village were relatively spared from disease, reflecting the fact that they did not have access to the common piped water supply but relied on shallow wells near their homes. Despite the fact that the village well was hyperchlorinated the day before the outbreak team arrived, evidence of faecal pollution, including *Salmonella* spp. but not *Shigella* spp., was identified in stored water.

One unusual waterborne outbreak affected UK travellers returning from holiday in Soviet Central Asia (McEvoy *et al.* 1984). After reports of illness in people returning to several UK airports after visits to Tashkent, Bukhara and Samarkand, 71 individuals were identified, of whom 65 completed a postal questionnaire. Of these 46 (70%) were ill with features of gastroenteritis. Four separate pathogens were identified from faecal culture: *Sh. flexneri*, *Sh. sonnei*, *Salmonella lexington* and *Campylobacter* sp. The most significant association with clinical illness was with the consumption of bottled mineral water in Samarkand ($p = 1.5 \times 10^{-5}$).

During the summer of 1979 diarrhoeal illness affected an estimated 1850 people who had camped at a private campsite in Arizona (Starko *et al.* 1986). Illness was significantly associated with staying at this site rather than any of the neighbouring sites ($p < 0.0001$), with drinking water at the campsite ($p < 0.0001$) and with drinking larger quantities of this water ($p < 0.001$). The investigators found that the water supply to the campsite had been developed over several years and that no records existed of its design and maintenance requirements. Treated sewage was used for irrigation purposes on the site. The same type and colour pipe was used for both the potable water supply and the irrigation system. Addition of fluorescein dye to the sewage treatment plant led to intense staining of the potable water. Subsequent excavation

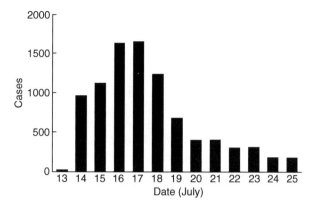

Figure 14.1 Epidemic curve of an outbreak of waterborne *Shigella sonnei* infection during July 1985 showing the number of visits to clinics due to acute gastroenteritis each day. Adapted from Egoz *et al.* 1991. A waterborne *Shigella sonnei* outbreak. *J. Infection* **22**: 89 with kind permission.

showed a direct cross connection between the sewage system and the drinking water system.

An outbreak of *Sh. sonnei* affected 146 resident of one village on Crete over a one-month period from 11 December 1990 (Samonis *et al.* 1994). All strains had a similar antibiotic susceptibility pattern and those strains that were examined had the same plasmid profile. The outbreak affected 30% of children under 12 and 4% of adults. The peak of the outbreak was prolonged over a five-day period, 11 days after the index case. None of the three fountains supplying water to the village was found to contain *Sh. sonnei* though one had 20 faecal coliforms per 100 millilitres. This fountain was sited lower down a valley than a sewage outflow. Although the authors postulated waterborne spread, the evidence for this is rather uncertain. Indeed, the authors reported that the children under 12 years old were more likely to be primary cases (the first case in a family) than secondary cases. By contrast, adults were equally likely to be primary or secondary cases.

More than 8000 cases of gastroenteritis affected four communities in northern Israel with a combined population of 101 000 in 1985 (Egoz *et al.* 1991). By the end of the second day, almost 1000 cases had occurred (Table 14.1). One 5-year-old boy died and 90 other patients were admitted to hospital. *Sh. sonnei* was isolated from 49% of stool samples tested, suggesting that other pathogens may have also been present. Such a large-scale, abrupt-onset outbreak could only be waterborne. All four communities were supplied with water from the same numerous wells with many interconnections in the distribution system. This water was not routinely chlorinated. One of the wells was subsequently found to be heavily contaminated with faecal coliforms. This well was sunk in relatively porous ground and was only 7 m from a main sewage pipe serving a town of 17 000 inhabitants. This pipe was fractured in several places, probably as a result of roadworks. A waterborne outbreak of typhoid in these same communities occurred later the same month.

In 1991 an outbreak of multi-resistant *Sh. flexneri* 2a occurred in northern Thailand (Swaddiwudhipong, Karintraratana and Kavinum 1995). Alerted by an increase in hospital admissions, the authors undertook an active case-finding exercise, which included a review of hospital admissions and visits to nearby villages. Altogether, 242 cases of diarrhoeal illness were identified, 65% of which were clustered between 6 and 10 August. A case-control study revealed drinking unboiled pipe water as a significant risk factor (OR 3.7). Two water distribution systems supplied the area. The attack rate affecting people drinking from system A was found to be 7% compared to only 0.1% for people drinking from system B. The water source for system A was raw river water, from which faecal coliforms were cultured. The tap-water in system A had no residual chlorine and faecal coliforms were present, compared to system B, which had chlorine and no faecal coliforms. Apparently system A was not being chlorinated because of a shortage of chemicals. People living near the water intake for system A admitted dumping faecal waste into the river. Interestingly, attack rates diminished with increasing distance from the water intake.

Two factors are responsible for all drinking water outbreaks of shigellosis. The first is human faecal contamination and the second is inadequate chlorination.

Recreational water outbreaks

An outbreak of shigellosis associated with recreational water contact occurred in 1974 among people who had been swimming in an 8-km stretch of the Mississippi River (Rosenberg *et al.* 1976). A neighbourhood case-control study among residents of Dubuque, Iowa, found a significant association with swimming ($p < 0.0001$). A survey was also undertaken among 60 families who had stayed in a camping park. This also found a significant association with swimming ($p < 0.0001$). Among swimmers, getting water in the mouth and being under 20 years old were both associated with illness. The affected stretch was below a sewage works. Bacteriological analysis showed faecal coliform counts of up to 5 000 000 per 100 ml just below the sewage works and 400 000 per 100 ml at the camping park's swimming area. *Sh. sonnei* was isolated from the river water.

An outbreak of gastroenteritis due to *Sh. sonnei* in Oklahoma during June 1982 was traced to a single lake (Makintubee, Mallonee and Istre 1987). In a case-control study, 14 of 17 cases had visited the lake compared to only 3 of 17 controls. In a cohort study of 85 people who had visited the lake the risk of disease increased with exposure to lake water. None of 9 people who did not swim was ill, compared to 17% of those who waded, 20% who had their head under water but no water in their mouths and 62% who had water in their mouths ($p = 1.6 \times 10^{-5}$). It was discovered that three boys had been swimming in the lake while still suffering from diarrhoea.

Within one week of attending a man-made lake in Los Angeles county over the Labour Day weekend in 1985, 68 persons reported diarrhoeal illness (Sorvillo *et al.* 1988). *Sh. sonnei* was isolated from 29 cases and *Sh. boydii* from 4. Swallowing water, but not immersion in water without swallowing, and age under 15 years were both found to be significantly associated with disease. The authors suggested that the increased usage of the lake over the holiday period was responsible for the contamination.

A case-control study of 65 cases of shigellosis after attending a lake in Michigan during July 1989 found significant associations with swimming in the lake (OR 11.43, CI 2.62–57.17), having the head under water (OR 12.43, CI 3.73–43.48) and being in the water for more than one hour (OR 4.97, CI 1.69–14.89) (Blostein 1991). During the summer of 1991, simultaneous outbreaks of *E. coli* O157:H7 and *Sh. sonnei* were traced to a lakeside park in Oregon (Keene *et al.* 1994). A total of 38 cases of shigellosis were identified, all involving people who swam in the lake ($p < 0.001$). No external sources of faecal pollution were identified and the source of infection was assumed to be other bathers.

All five recreational waterborne outbreaks were associated with swimming in unchlorinated surface waters.

Epidemiological studies of endemic disease

Rajasekaran, Dutt and Pisharoti (1977) reported a prospective study of 1091 children under 5 years old living within one of five Indian villages. The children were visited twice a week for a year and any diarrhoeal stool examined for *Shigella* spp. The incidence of laboratory-confirmed shigellosis was highest in villages where water was taken from a street tap (12.52/100 population), next highest in those taking their water from a well (8.76/100) and lowest in those taking their water from a tap within the house (4.72/100) ($p = 0.001$).

A prospective study was done to assess the factors leading to secondary cases in 47 families in which one case of *Sh. dysenteriae* type 1 had occurred (Khan, Curlin and Huq 1979). The overall infection rate in family contacts was 20.4%. Infection rates were higher in males (25.5%) than in females (16.7%) and in children under 9 years (29.4%) compared to those older (13.0%). The most significant factor affecting subsequent infection was the source of water, those only using water with a closed source having lower attack rates than those using water from a variety of non-closed sources. The next most important factor was whether the family had access to a sanitary or open latrine. Also, poverty was found to be important.

Khan and Shahidullah (1980) compared the epidemiology of *Sh. dysenteriae* and *Sh. flexneri* in Dacca. For both pathogens the infection rate was higher in families taking water from a mixture of open and closed sources, including ponds, rather than from a single closed source such as a tap or tube well. However, another study, also in Bangladesh (Boyce *et al.* 1982), found that drinking surface water was not a risk factor for shigella infection.

Reporting their experience of monitoring shigellosis in Dacca for 14 years from 1969 to 1982, Khan *et al.* (1985) noted that those areas of Dacca with good water supplies had fewer admissions to hospital due to shigellosis despite the fact that these districts were much closer to the hospital.

A case-control study of the epidemiology of antimicrobial-resistant epidemic *Sh. dysenteriae* type 1 in Zambia identified 42 cases and 84 controls (Tuttle *et al.* 1995). Identified independent risk factors included a family member with dysentery (OR 3.6, CI 1.4–9.5) and drinking water by dipping the hand into the water jug (OR 2.8, CI 1.1–6.8). It was suggested that this habit of dipping the hand into the water was responsible for contaminating the water. An effective control measure was to make water vessels with small necks.

15 Campylobacteriosis

Although known as a veterinary pathogen for many years, the importance of campylobacter as a cause of human disease was not recognized until the late 1970s (Skirrow 1977). Since then it has become recognized as the most common bacterial cause of gastroenteritis in the western world.

MICROBIOLOGY

Campylobacters are slender, spirally curved, motile, Gram-negative bacilli. They are strictly microaerophilic, non-saccharolytic and oxidase positive. They do not produce acid from carbohydrates. There are two main subgroups of campylobacter. Subgroup 1 consists of *C. coli*, *C. jejuni*, *C. laridis* and *C. upsaliensis*. Subgroup 2 consists of *C. fetus*, *C. hyointestinalis*, *C. concisus*, *C. mucosalis* and *C. sputorum*. Subgroup 1 are also called thermophilic campylobacters in that they are able to grow at 43 °C. Of the subgroup 1 species, *C. jejuni* has two subspecies, *C. jejuni* subsp. *jejuni* and *C. jejuni* subsp. *doylei*. Table 15.1 shows the distinguishing characteristics of the subgroup 1 species and subspecies. A simple biotyping scheme exists for *C. jejuni*, *C. coli* and *C. laridis* based on DNAase production and a rapid H_2S test.

PATHOGENICITY

Although species from both subgroups can cause human disease, subgroup 1 species are by far the more important as a cause of gastroenteritis in humans. Of the subgroup 1 species, *C. jejuni* is the commonest cause of gastroenteritis, but *C. coli* is also important. Subgroup 2 species are primarily pathogens of animals, although occasional human infections have been reported.

Human volunteer experiments have shown that the infective dose of campylobacter is as low as 500 organisms, although most natural infections probably require at least 10^4 organisms. *Campylobacter* spp. are sensitive to stomach acid and so infection will be enhanced by the buffering effect of foods.

C. jejuni grows well in human bile so the site of initial colonization is the upper small intestine. However, non-specific tissue damage can be seen

Table 15.1 Distinguishing features of subgroup one *Campylobacter* spp.

Species	Growth at 43 °C	Hippurate hydrolysis	Nitrate reductase	Growth in 1.5% NaCl	Growth on 0.04% TTC agar	H$_2$S production in TSI medium
C. jejuni subsp. jejuni	+	+	+	–	+	+/–
C. jejuni subsp. doylei	–	+	–	–	–	–
C. coli	+	–	+	–	+	+
C. laridis	+	–	+	+	+/–	+
C. upsaliensis	+	–	+	–	–	–

throughout the small and large intestines. The exact mechanism for this tissue damage is unclear, although demonstration of bacteraemia in some cases suggests invasion as one mechanism. Some enterotoxins have also been demonstrated but their presence does not seem to correlate with virulence.

CLINICAL FEATURES

Campylobacter infection due to *C. jejuni* has an incubation period of 2–4 days with a range of 1–7 days. Diarrhoea is the most frequent symptom. The diarrhoea is usually watery, occasionally bloody and can be quite severe. There may also be pus in the faeces. Cramping abdominal pain is also a major feature. Indeed, this pain may be the most prominent, or even the only, feature, and has been so severe as to suggest an intra-abdominal emergency. Camplylobacteriosis can mimic appendicitis, acute Crohn's disease and ulcerative colitis. Fever and malaise are also features. The illness usually lasts for about 2–3 days, although in up to 20% of cases it will last for over a week. In another 10% there is relapse. There have also been some reports of the disease lasting for many months or years.

Complications of campylobacter enteritis include septicaemia, septic abortion, acute cholecystitis, pancreatitis and cystitis. Reactive arthritis can occur up to several weeks after the initial infection. Finally, up to 40% of cases of Guillain–Barré syndrome follow a campylobacter infection.

Infections due to *C. fetus* subsp. *fetus* are much less common. Diarrhoea is less of a feature, while systemic illness, such as septicaemia, meningitis, phlebitis and abscess formation, is more common. Septic arthritis, peritonitis, salpingitis, lung abscess, empyema, cellulitis, osteomyelitis, cholecystitis and cystitis have all been described. The remaining campylobacters are more similar to *C. jejuni* in their clinical presentation.

DIAGNOSIS

Diagnosis is made by culture of faeces on a selective agar, usually commercial campylobacter medium containing special supplements. Incubation has to be carried out in a microaerophilic atmosphere. Diagnosis is based on the demonstration of a characteristic colonial morphology, oxidase positivity and microscopic appearance.

TREATMENT

As with all diarrhoeal illness, fluid and electrolyte replacement is essential. Both erythromycin and ciprofloxacin have been shown to have useful clinical effects. However, most cases recover spontaneously without specific anti-microbial therapy. Indeed, many will be well on the way to recovery by the time the diagnosis has been made. Antibiotics should be reserved for those who are showing no signs of improvement when the laboratory result is available or after one week.

ENVIRONMENTAL DETECTION

The isolation of thermophilic campylobacters from water supplies depends on filtration of the sample through a 0.2 μm pore size filter, which is then incubated in Preston enrichment broth (PEB) with only a very small air space for 48 hours at 42 °C (HMSO 1994). The broth is subcultured to Preston selective agar or its blood-free modification. Colonies are identified as already discussed.

As would be expected for a recently described pathogen, there are a number of papers describing and comparing alternate methods for the isolation of campylobacter from water samples (Blaser and Cody 1986; Humphrey 1986; Agulla *et al.* 1987; Bolton *et al.* 1987; Humphrey 1989; Jacob and Stelzer 1992; Korhonen and Martikainen 1990). Filtration appears to be about twice as effective at detecting campylobacter in river water than a multiple tube method (Bolton *et al.* 1987).

PCR methods for the detection of both *C. jejuni* and *C. coli* in water samples have been developed (Kirk and Rowe 1994). Kirk and Rowe (1994) estimated that if 100 ml volumes were used the sensitivity of the method would be approximately two campylobacter cells per litre.

ECOLOGY

Campylobacter spp. are very common organisms, being found in many environments and in the gastrointestinal tracts of a wide range of birds and animals. They have frequently been isolated from surface water and occasionally from drinking water.

Bolton *et al.* (1987) studied the distribution of thermophilic campylobacters in a single river system over a 12-month period. They found that 43% of samples were positive, but counts and isolation rates were lower in rural areas and in fast-flowing stretches. Counts were highest below a sewage works. The peak incidence was obtained in late autumn, possibly because of increased rainfall washing faecal material off fields and into the river. This seasonal variation has also been noted by other authors (Carter *et al.* 1987; Brennhovd, Kapperud and Langeland 1992).

Stelzer *et al.* (1989) found campylobacter, usually at low count, in 82.1% of moderately polluted river water. However, counts were generally low. In line with the known association between poultry and campylobacter, counts were higher in the river near a poultry farm and where waterfowl were present. There was a significant correlation between campylobacter counts and total coliform counts.

In Norway campylobacter was isolated from 43.8% of surface water samples (Brennhovd, Kapperud and Langeland 1992). In a survey of canals in Bangkok, Dhamabutra, Kamol-Rathanakul and Pienthaweechai (1992) isolated campylobacters from 116 of 156 water samples, although all strains were either *C. cryaerophila* or *C. cryaerophila*-like organisms of uncertain human significance. Pollution rates were higher in those waters with the greatest microbiological evidence of faecal pollution. *C. jejuni* was detected in 6.3% of river water samples and from no seawater samples in the Pesaro-Urbino area of Italy over the years 1985–1992 (Baffone *et al.* 1995). In this same study *C. coli* was isolated from 25% of river water samples and from no seawater samples.

Skjerve and Brennhovd (1992) used a multiple logistic regression model to show that the probability of detecting *Campylobacter* spp. in surface water samples was independently related to the faecal coliform counts and water temperature.

Jones, Betaieb and Telford (1990) estimated the concentration of campylobacters in fresh sewage sludge to be 200–5000 per 100 ml, with a peak in May and June to mirror the incidence in the community. Baffone *et al.* (1995) reported isolating *C. jejuni* from 0.5% of domestic sewage samples; *C. coli* was isolated from 2.6% of domestic sewage samples.

During a year-long study of campylobacters in a large public water supply, 14 strains were isolated from 891 samples (Megraud and Serceau 1990). All but one were isolated from untreated water and of these 13, 11 were associated with faecal indicator bacteria. None was thermophilic and therefore of public health significance. Brennhovd, Kapperud and Langeland (1992) did not detect any campylobacters in samples from 100 different drinking water wells in Norway.

Campylobacters can exist in a viable but non-culturable state from which they can still cause illness in suckling mice (Rollins and Colwell 1986; Jones, Sutcliffe and Curry 1991).

Campylobacters can be cultured from water for up to four weeks at 4 °C but only for four days at 25 °C (Fewtrell *et al.* 1994). Survival is best in drinking water and declines in river water and sewage. Decline in numbers is also more rapid in the light.

EPIDEMIOLOGY

In the UK campylobacters are the most frequently reported cause of gastroenteritis. Campylobacteriosis is a zoonosis, and humans may become infected by a direct or indirect contact with animals (Skirrow 1991). Person to person transmission is relatively uncommon. People who work with animals, such as farmers, veterinarians, slaughterhouse workers, poultry processors and butchers, rapidly become immune as a result of repeated infection. People can become infected from their pets. Indirect transmission is reported to occur through milk, water and food.

Waterborne outbreaks

The first waterborne outbreak of campylobacter to be identified occurred the year after Skirrow reported his method of selectively culturing the organism. Approximately 3000 cases of diarrhoea in Bennington, Vermont, were reported in June 1978 (Vogt et al. 1982a). This represented 19% of the population. In a cohort survey, there was a strong statistical association with drinking unboiled mains water in four of five areas surveyed. The water was chlorinated but unfiltered surface water. An environmental survey of the water distribution system showed several possible causes. The most likely was the finding of deficient sewerage systems located near the main water intake point. There were also large quantities of animal waste around the brook from which the water was extracted. In the period before the outbreak there had been especially heavy rains.

The second recorded outbreak was in Sweden in October 1980 (Mentzing 1981). Over 380 people consulted their family doctors because of diarrhoea. Most cases occurred over just three days. *C. jejuni* was isolated from 221 of 263 faecal samples. Attack rates did not differ markedly between the different age and sex groups. The epidemic area corresponded with a water supply zone, and several out-of-district cases had drunk unboiled tap-water. The water supply was from two deep wells; the water was sand filtered but not chlorinated. In the week before the outbreak there had been complaints of low water pressure in the mains. The author suggested that back siphoning, either from a factory, from garden hoses or from toilets that were flushed with river water to reduce water charges, could explain the contamination.

A more prolonged outbreak of waterborne campylobacter was described in a British boarding school over a period of eight weeks (Palmer et al. 1983). During May and June 1983, 234 pupils and 23 staff developed abdominal pain and/or diarrhoea. A survey of staff members showed a strong association with drinking water from School House. However, there was no significant association of illness and drinking water among pupils, although illness was lowest in those pupils who lived in houses not supplied with water from School House. Campylobacter of the same serotype was isolated from two samples of the water storage tank for School House. The water supply was from a private borehole and was stored in an open-top tank. It was not chlorinated. The open-top tank was in a tower with roosting birds, which could easily defecate into the tank.

During July 1982, 150 of 512 inhabitants of a kibbutz near Jerusalem developed diarrhoea, and *C. jejuni* was isolated from 10 of 42 stool samples examined (Rogol *et al.* 1983). The outbreak started the day after the main reservoir to the kibbutz was taken out of service. The temporary reservoir was small, stagnant, open to animals and unchlorinated. Infants in the kibbutz nursery, which had a filtered water supply, were not affected.

An outbreak during May 1983 in Greenville, Florida, affected an estimated 865 people (Sacks *et al.* 1986). Within the affected area there was an 879% increase in sales of antidiarrhoeal medicines compared to May 1982. The attack rate within the city limits was 56% compared to 9% outside. An epidemiological survey showed a relative risk of 12.39 (CI 6.80–22.59) in those who drank Greenville water. Furthermore, there was a highly significant ($p < 0.0001$) linear trend in the association between illness and the amount of water drunk per day, rising from 7.7% in people drinking one glass per day to 76.5% in those drinking three or more. The water supply was from a well which was pre-chlorinated, aerated over an open-top settling tank, passed through two sand filters, chlorinated a second time and then passed to an underground cistern before distribution. The pre-chlorinator had failed in mid-April, allowing an algal scum to develop on the settling tank. Three days before the start of the outbreak the post-chlorination injector also failed. The investigators cultured cloacal swabs taken from birds captured around the treatment plant. Although *Campylobacter* spp. were isolated from the birds, these were of different types to the outbreak strain.

A waterborne outbreak due to *C. laridis* affected 162 cases at a power station in Canada in March 1985 (Broczyk *et al.* 1987). The mains water had been accidentally contaminated with water from Lake Ontario due to a faulty plumbing connection.

Nineteen cases occurred over two weeks in a small town in a cattle and sheep farming area of New Zealand in March 1986 (Brieseman 1987). The normal rate of notification had been about one per month. The outbreak had followed some heavy rains, after which the potable water supply had become discoloured. The water supply was abstracted from the nearby river. It was the policy only to chlorinate the supply when river flow rates were high. On this occasion there had been a few hours' delay in starting the chlorination.

In Finland, 75 of 88 conscript soldiers developed diarrhoea, abdominal pain, malaise and fever during July and August 1987 (Aho *et al.* 1989). Campylobacter was isolated from 37 out of 63 men investigated. Two days before the outbreak the men were on manoeuvres in hot weather. Each man consumed up to 4 litres of water from a stream before dinner. *C. jejuni* of the same serotype as the human strain was isolated from the stream.

During November and December 1986, 32 patients and 62 staff members developed gastroenteritis at a hospital for rheumatic disease in Finland (Rautelin *et al.* 1990). Campylobacter of the same strain was isolated from the water distribution system. Water was extracted from a private borehole, filtered and chlorinated. Earlier work on the distribution system or remaining leaks in the pipe from the borehole may have allowed the contamination.

In an outbreak in northern Norway, 59% of the affected population developed gastroenteritis (Melby *et al.* 1990). A questionnaire revealed that all those with gastroenteritis drank untreated water from an unfenced reservoir shortly after flooding due to heavy spring rainfall. None of the responders who denied drinking this water was ill. Although *C. jejuni* was isolated from water samples, it was of a different serotype to the human strains.

June 1987 saw an outbreak of gastroenteritis affect a small rural community in Canada (Alary and Nadeau 1990). Approximately 50 cases were identified. There was a significant association with drinking 10 or more glasses of water per day. The water supply was from collected surface water that was not subsequently treated. The sites where the water was collected were found to be poorly designed and badly protected.

Yet another rural community served by an unchlorinated water supply suffered an outbreak of campylobacter (Millson *et al.* 1991) in which 241 cases were documented, although there were suggestions that many more were affected. A case-control study showed a significant association with the amount of untreated water drunk each day. An especially heavy snowfall during the previous winter had led to a heavy spring runoff just before the start of the outbreak.

Approximately 680 out of a population of 1000 developed gastroenteritis in a Norwegian community during one month, although the majority of cases occurred over ten days (Melby *et al.* 1991). Campylobacter was isolated from patients and tap-water. The water supply was from three upland lakes. It was untreated. A sheep path ran along one of the lakes. During the spring melt, flooding was able to wash faeces from the path into the reservoir.

An outbreak of campylobacter enteritis affected 44 staff and campers at a camp and convention centre near Christchurch, New Zealand, in August 1989 (Stehr-Green *et al.* 1991). In a cohort study cases were more likely to have drunk two or more cups of unboiled water per day than unaffected individuals (100% versus 58%, $p < 0.01$). The water supply was taken from four wells and was neither filtered nor chlorinated. Presumptive and faecal coliforms, up to 92/100 ml, were present in all water samples examined. The outbreak occurred a few days after heavy rains, and it was suggested that the rains had washed excreta into the wells from farm animals grazing in the surrounding fields. The outbreak was terminated by the introduction of a water treatment system.

All 14 of these outbreaks were associated with the consumption of untreated or inadequately treated water. At least 11 were associated with non-chlorinated water or chlorination failures. Most were also associated with water in rural areas, supporting the suggestion that the disease is primarily a zoonosis and waterborne outbreaks follow animal faecal contamination of unchlorinated supplies.

Prospective studies of endemic disease

A prospective study of cases of gastroenteritis was undertaken during the summer months among persons in the Grand Teton National Park area of Wyoming (Taylor *et al.* 1983). Campylobacter was isolated from 21 cases between June and August 1980 and from 41 cases during the same period in the following year. There were a wide variety of serotypes. The only risk factor compared to matched controls was drinking untreated surface water in the month before illness (RR 5.0, $p = 0.018$ for 1980; RR 4.8, $p < 0.005$ for 1981). The authors also reported a variety of different serotypes of campylobacter from water and animal specimens.

A prospective study of laboratory-confirmed campylobacteriosis in Colorado in the summer of 1981 analysed 40 sporadic case with 71 matched neighbourhood controls. (Hopkins, Olmsted and Istre 1984). Cases were more likely than controls to have drunk untreated surface water (OR 10.74, CI 1.93–59.84), to have drunk raw milk (OR 6.93, CI 1.03–46.8) or to have cats in the house (OR 3.21, CI 1.25–8.28). Cases were less likely to have eaten chicken, but more likely to have eaten undercooked chicken (OR 6.27, CI 0.90–43.84).

In rural Lesotho, southern Africa, a study of diarrhoeal morbidity found no association in the incidence of campylobacter between children in families who exclusively used an improved water supply or supplemented it with the traditional contaminated water source (Esrey *et al.* 1988). There were, however, fewer cases of giardiasis in those families exclusively using the improved supply.

Two Liberian communities were compared in a study of faecal colonization of children aged between 6 and 59 months (Molbak, Hojlyng and Gaarslev 1988). One community was an urban slum and the other was rural. It was found that 44.9% of children from the slum were excreting campylobacter compared to 28.4% from the rural area. Colonization was much lower in children who were still breast-feeding. Among children in the rural area, the carriage rate was highest in those drinking stagnant water (35%) compared to 32% in those drinking from a shallow well, 21% in those drinking from an improved well and 19% in those drinking from a hand pump. In the urban slum carriage rate was 45.8% in those using public standpipes, compared to 38.2% among those with a private household tap.

A cohort of 111 children in the Central African Republic was followed from birth until two years old (Georges-Courbot *et al.* 1990); 1.6 diarrhoeal episodes were recorded per child per year. Campylobacter was isolated from 11.7% of diarrhoeal episodes. The isolation of campylobacter was associated with the absence of a piped water supply (OR 13.41, CI 1.65–51.2) and keeping poultry in the home (OR 2.5, CI 1.08–5.54) but not with keeping dogs or goats.

In an Egyptian study of campylobacter in young children, the authors found that 16.8% of 880 children presenting with diarrhoea were stool positive

(Pazzaglia *et al.* 1993). These children were recruited for the study from admissions to two hospitals. The prevalence of *Campylobacter* spp. in a control group of 1079 healthy children was 6.4%. Campylobacter infections were more prevalent during the rainy season ($p = 0.001$). Keeping fowl, such as chickens, pigeons or ducks, in the home was associated with campylobacter diarrhoea ($p = 0.003$). Having an outside source of drinking water was also associated with an increased risk of campylobacter disease for admissions to one hospital ($p = 0.029$) but not the other.

A case-control study of 100 sporadic cases of campylobacter infection in the Christchurch area of New Zealand took place during the summer of 1992–93 (Ikram *et al.* 1994). Eating poultry at a friend's house (OR 3.18, CI 1.0–10.73, $p = 0.03$) or at a barbecue (OR 3.00, CI 0.99–9.34, $p = 0.03$) or eating undercooked chicken (OR 4.94, CI 1.03-23.62, $p = 0.05$) were all associated with increased risk of infection. Drinking water was also associated with an increased risk, although this did not achieve statistical significance (OR 2.7, CI 0.89–8.33, $p = 0.09$).

In a large case-control survey of 598 sporadic cases of campylobacter in England and Wales, drinking untreated surface water (OR 4.16, CI 1.45–11.9), occupational exposure to raw meat (OR 9.37, CI 2.03–43.3) and having a family pet with diarrhoea (OR 2.39, CI 1.09–5.25) were all independent risk factors (Adak *et al.* 1995). Handling or eating any whole chicken with giblets in the domestic kitchen and occupational contact with livestock were found to be associated with a decreased risk. This latter finding may be related to pre-existing immunity.

Despite the observation that all reported waterborne outbreaks of campylobacter infection have come from wealthy Western nations, the evidence from several of the prospective studies has shown that the disease is far more common in tropical countries. The absence of reported outbreaks in such countries could be explained by the lack of diagnostic facilities for this fastidious organism or because endemic disease is so common that identifying outbreaks is difficult.

16 Escherichia coli

Escherichia coli is well known to water microbiologists as a marker for faecal pollution. Although it has been known for many years that some strains of *E. coli* can cause disease in humans, it has only been in recent years that the importance of this organism as a cause of waterborne outbreaks in its own right has increased. Most important in this regard is the recent appearance of waterborne outbreaks of haemorrhagic colitis due to *E. coli* O157:H7.

MICROBIOLOGY

E. coli are motile, Gram-negative, non-spore-forming bacilli that produce acid and gas from lactose at 37 and 44 °C. They are widely distributed in the guts of animals. Strains can be serotyped based on the presence of different O antigens.

PATHOGENICITY

E. coli are capable of causing many diseases, including urinary tract infections, meningitis and septicaemia. However, in the context of waterborne disease we are essentially interested only in the associations of the organism with gastroenteritis. The mechanism by which *E. coli* causes diarrhoea varies between strains, and strains can be grouped depending on which mechanism is used by a particular strain.

Enterotoxigenic *E. coli* (ETEC) adhere to the gut wall by colonization factors. They produce two enterotoxins, a heat-stable toxin (ST) and a heat-labile (LT) oligopeptide toxin. ST is almost identical to cholera toxin. Both toxins are cell-associated and so can only act on short distances from the parent organism. Both also work in a similar way. The toxins enter the cell and affect its metabolism by increasing the concentrations of cyclic guanine monophosphate (cGMP) in the case of ST or cyclic adenine monophosphate (cAMP) for LT. This affects electrolyte transport, with excessive loss of fluid by the cell. The pathogenesis of the other modes of action are less well understood.

Enteropathogenic *E. coli* (EPEC) has a pathogenesis that is still not fully understood. What is known is that the organism possesses a plasmid encoded adherence factor that enables it to bind to the enterocytes by means of a special pilus. EPEC produce a characteristic lesion with microcolonies surrounded by an area of damaged microvilli.

Enteroinvasive *E. coli* (EIEC) resemble *Shigella* spp. in that they bind specifically to enterocytes of the large intestine before being taken into the cells. Once inside the enteroctye they multiply before destroying the cell and spreading to neighbouring cells, thereby causing extensive tissue damage and inflammation.

Enterohaemorrhagic *E. coli* (EHEC) were previously called verocytotoxic *E. coli*. EHEC posses a fimbrial-mediated adherence factor, as in EPEC, which assists in binding to cell walls. EHEC also produce a shiga-like toxin that is cytotoxic for Vero cells. This toxin is thought to be the mechanism for the pathogenesis of haemolytic uraemic syndrome. It is known that the kidney possesses receptors for this toxin. The commonest EHEC is O157.

Enteroaggregative *E. coli* (EAggEC) show a characteristic aggregative pattern of adherence to Hep-2 cells in tissue culture. A plasmid encoded heat-stable enterotoxin and fimbriae are the responsible virulence factors.

Diffuse adherence *E. coli* (DAEC) also adhere to Hep-2 cells but in a more diffuse pattern than is seen in EaggEC. This adherence is also due to fimbriae.

CLINICAL FEATURES

The clinical features and epidemiology of intestinal disease due the various groups of *E. coli* differ with the differing pathogenic mechanisms. The incubation period is usually one or two days, although it can be up to five days.

ETEC cause a dehydrating diarrhoea in children, which can be difficult to distinguish from mild cholera. It is also a common cause of traveller's diarrhoea. EIEC produces a disease similar to shigella dysentery. In infants EPEC can cause fever and watery mucoid diarrhoea. EaggEC can cause persistent diarrhoea, lasting for up to 14 days or longer in developing countries. No volunteer studies have demonstrated illness with DEAC. However, one field study suggested an association with prolonged diarrhoea.

EHEC is associated with haemorrhagic colitis. Diarrhoea quickly becomes bloody and abdominal pain develops. Recovery is usually within 7–10 days. A proportion of cases progress to haemolytic uraemic syndrome, particularly in children. Features include rising serum urea and creatinine, anaemia and thrombocytopenia.

DIAGNOSIS

Most cases of *E. coli* diarrhoea are relatively non-specific and few laboratories would routinely investigate diarrhoeal faeces for their presence. The exception is EHEC. Diagnosis is based on clinical presentation and culture of faeces using a modified sorbitol MacConkey agar. A positive isolation is confirmed by biochemical tests and agglutination by specific O157 antiserum. A serological test has been developed.

TREATMENT

Very few cases of E. coli diarrhoea would require anything other than symptomatic or supportive treatment. Quinolones such as ciprofloxacin may be of benefit in severe or prolonged illness. There is uncertainty as to whether the use of quinolones in EHEC will prevent the development of haemolytic uraemic syndrome.

Up to half of patients with haemolytic uraemic syndrome will require renal dialysis.

ENVIRONMENTAL DETECTION

E. coli is the indicator organism of faecal contamination used in water bacteriology. To a water bacteriologist E. coli is a member of the Enterobacteriaceae which ferments lactose or mannitol at 44 °C with the production of acid and usually gas within 24 hours, and which produces indole from tryptophan (HMSO 1994). This definition must not be taken as an accurate measure of the taxonomic species. Counts of E. coli in water are made by filtering 100 ml and then incubating the filter on membrane laryl sulphate broth. Alternatively, counts can be estimated from the multiple tube method using minerals-modified glutamate medium. Given the importance of the organism to water quality monitoring, it is not surprising that the literature has many papers comparing different media formulations and methods for isolation of E. coli in water. An identification method for E. coli that is gaining ground is the demonstration of β-glucuronidase activity using the flurogenic substrate 4-methylumbelliferyl beta-D-glucuronide (MUG) (Shadix and Rice 1991).

The colilert system is also becoming a frequent alternative to the standard methods in several countries. This method is based on culture in a defined substrate, which develops a yellow colour if coliforms are present and fluorescence if E. coli is present. It gives very good correlation with multiple tube methods and membrane filtration methods in both raw and treated waters (Edberg, Allen and Smith 1988, 1989; Lewis and Mak 1989; Edberg et al. 1990; Olson et al. 1991). A modification of the method has been shown to be effective on marine waters (Palmer et al. 1993a). The method has also been automated (Lewis and Mak 1989).

Other methods include one based on direct impedance technology (Colquhoun, Tims and Fricker, 1995). Polymerase chain reaction methods have been developed and used by several authors (Bej, McCarty and Atlas 1991; Bej *et al.* 1991; Tsai, Palmer and Sangermano 1993; Fricker and Fricker 1994; Tamanai-Shacoori *et al.* 1994). Gale and Broberg (1994) described a commercial gene probe assay kit for confirming positive tubes in the multiple tube method.

For the detection of *E. coli* O157, the filter is incubated in modified buffered peptone water followed by subculture to modified sorbitol MacConkey agar (HMSO 1994). Pyle, Broadaway and McFeters (1995) have described a rapid method based on incubation with cyanoditolyl tetrazolium chloride to detect respiratory activity with a modified fluorescent antibody.

ECOLOGY

E. coli is a widely distributed organism in the guts of most mammalian species. Its isolation in environmental samples usually indicates faecal contamination. It can be isolated, therefore, from virtually all surface waters, both inland and coastal.

There is some suggestion that *E. coli* can survive and grow in pristine waters in the tropics without any faecal contamination (Rivera, Hazen and Toranzos 1988). If this is the case, it calls into doubt the value of relying on *E. coli* as a marker of faecal pollution in tropical countries.

E. coli can survive in sterile river water for at least 260 days with little change in viability (Flint 1987). However, survival is reduced in the presence of other bacteria and in sunlight (Kapuscinski and Mitchell 1981; Barcina *et al.* 1989).

EPIDEMIOLOGY

Like many other enteropathogens, *E. coli* can be spread directly from one person (or animal) to another or indirectly via contamination of food, water or the environment.

Waterborne outbreaks of enterotoxigenic *E. coli*

During June and July 1975 an outbreak of gastroenteritis affected more than 2000 staff and visitors to an American National Park in Oregon (Rosenberg *et al.* 1977). Enterotoxigenic *E. coli* were isolated from 20 (16.7%) of 120 rectal swabs examined. No other bacterial pathogen was isolated. Positive results were obtained from 17 of 40 people who had diarrhoea at the time of sampling but from only 3 of 80 people who had already recovered. In an epidemiological survey there was a strong correlation between illness and drinking park water in park staff and visitors ($p < 10^{-5}$). The only group in whom there was no association with drinking water was visitors on 7–9 July when chlorination of the water supply was being more closely monitored. Water came from a shallow spring and was chlorinated, but there was no systematic monitoring of chlorine levels throughout the distribution system. In May three of four routine samples were deemed to be unsatisfactory because of coliforms. A sewage overflow was discovered some 2000 feet uphill from the spring and fluorescein tests showed contamination of the park water supply from this source.

An outbreak of gastroenteritis affected 251 passengers and 51 crew on a Mediterranean cruise (O'Mahony *et al.* 1986). Enterotoxigenic *E. coli* was isolated from 13 of 22 passengers and 6 of 13 crew sampled. In a case-control study, consumption of tap-water was the only risk factor associated with increased risk ($p = 0.01$). Faecal coliforms were isolated from tap-water. Inspection by a water engineer found defects that could explain contamination, including possible faulty chlorination and faulty covers, possibly allowing bilge water into the water tanks.

Drinking water associated outbreaks of *E. coli* O157

Neill, Agosti and Rosen (1985) reported two cases of haemolytic uraemic syndrome in adults following infection with *E. coli* O157:H7. Although the source was not definitively identified, both had drunk untreated water, the first after an accidental fall into a lake and the second from a stream that served her log cabin.

The first outbreak of infection due to *E. coli* O157:H7 strongly linked to the consumption of drinking water occurred in Burdine Township, Missouri between 15 December 1989 and 20 January 1990 (Swerdlow *et al.* 1992b). The population of the township was 3126, of whom 243 developed the illness. Of these 243 cases, 86 developed bloody diarrhoea, 36 were hospitalized and 4 died. In a case-control study based on 53 cases, the only significant factor was that cases drank more cups of municipal water per day (7.9) than did controls (6.1) ($p = 0.04$). In a household survey, 99% of homes in the city boundary used municipal water compared to none of those outside the city boundary. During the peak of the outbreak residents within the city boundary were much likelier to have diarrhoea (7.7% versus 2.8%, $p = 0.01$). If the analysis was restricted to those with bloody diarrhoea the association with residence within the city boundary was increased (3.6% versus 0.2%, $p = 0.001$). Among those who lived outside the city, cases drank more cups of municipal water per day than those who were well (1.4 versus 0.4, $p = 0.08$). The water supply to the city came from two deep groundwater sources. It was noted that two mains water breaks had occurred on the 23 and 26 December, after the start of the outbreak but before its main peak. The sewage system was inadequate and sewage overflow often resulted. Sewage overflows could cross drinking water mains. The outbreak was also of interest because a computer model was used to show that potentially contaminated water from either mains break would reach 85% of the cases of bloody diarrhoea. *E. coli* O157:H7 was not isolated from water.

An outbreak of *E. coli* O157:H7 in Grampian, Scotland, affected four people during the hot summer of 1990 (Dev, Main and Gould 1991). All four (three boys aged 4, 8 and 9 and one women aged 20) developed haemorrhagic colitis. Faecal coliforms, but not *E. coli* O157, were present in large numbers in the drinking water supplied to the cases' homes. The village normally took its water from a reservoir situated on a hillock in the village. However, because of the hot weather this supply was low, so water from two subsidiary reservoirs was being used. One of these was found to be fed from a source that resembled a field-drain system, which may have been contaminated by cattle slurry.

During October 1992 a large outbreak of bloody diarrhoea affected thousands of individuals in South Africa and Swaziland (Isaacson *et al.* 1993). There were fatalities and cases of renal failure. *E. coli* O157 was isolated from 22.5% of 89 stool samples. The authors stated that epidemiological investigations implicated waterborne spread. In some areas cases were mainly men who drank surface water in the fields, while women and children who drank borehole water were spared. *E. coli* O157 was isolated from 14.3% of 42 samples of cattle dung and 18.4% of 76 randomly collected water samples. The underlying problem seems to have been cattle carcasses and dung washed into rivers and dams by heavy rains after a period of drought.

Recreational water associated outbreaks

In the summer of 1991 an outbreak of bloody diarrhoea affected people who had swum in a lake in Oregon (Keene *et al.* 1994). Two different pathogens were identified. *Shigella sonnei* was identified as the cause in 38 cases and *E. coli* O157:H7 in 21. Seven of the *E. coli* infected individuals were admitted to hospital, of whom three developed haemolytic uraemic syndrome. In a case-control study the most significant factor was swimming in the lake ($p <$ 0.001). Among swimmers, illness was associated with swallowing lake water ($p <$ 0.002). No specific source of pollution was identified and the authors assumed that the source was other bathers.

In the summer of 1993, *E. coli* O157 infected six children in an area of southwest London (Hildebrand *et al.* 1996). Three children developed haemolytic uraemic syndrome, of whom one died. Four of the six cases had visited outdoor paddling pools within 10 days of becoming ill. Three had visited the same pool, probably on the same day. Inspection of the pools found that, although written guidelines were available, these were not being followed by many of the park keepers. Half of waters sampled had no detectable chlorine levels and *E. coli* (not O157) was isolated from 40%.

Epidemiological studies of sporadic disease

Echeverria *et al.* (1984) used highly sensitive DNA hybridization techniques to detect ETEC in children and their homes in Thailand. From February to July 1982, 221 children with diarrhoea attending a children's hospital in Bangkok were recruited into the study. ETEC were identified in 30 (14%) of these children. ETEC were found significantly more often in environmental samples (water, food and mothers' hands) from the homes of cases and neighbours of cases than in homes not associated with ETEC infection (8/369 versus 3/2290; *p* < 0.001).

EPEC were isolated from 67 (18%) of 406 children admitted to hospital with diarrhoea in Rio de Janeiro in 1987–88 (Regua *et al.* 1990). Strains from a variety of different serogroups were isolated, the commonest being O111 (33%). Fifteen (22.4%) children with EPEC had no mains water supply, compared to 42 (13.5%) of EPEC-negative children (*p* = 0.089). Twenty-five (37.3%) EPEC-positive children lived in homes without a drainage system compared to 93 (30.0%) EPEC-negative children (*p* = 0.248).

In a cross-sectional survey of Ecuadorian children aged 7–10 months, Brussow, Rahim and Freire (1992) correlated the presence of antibodies against ETEC with demographic and hygienic factors. Out of 74 children, 37 (50%) were antibody-positive, indicating current or past infection. Significant association was found with low quality drinking water (70% versus 41%, *p* = 0.043). There was no association with the state of the sanitation system.

A case-control study of cases of diarrhoea in Sao Paulo, Brazil, was conducted during 1986 (Blake *et al.* 1993). Cases were children less than 12 months old with diarrhoea who had been taken to the emergency room of a municipal hospital. Controls were children taken to the emergency room who did not have diarrhoea. From 500 case-control pairs, 97 were excluded because of the isolation of more than one pathogen from the case or the isolation of a pathogen from the control, leaving 403 pairs for analysis. Adherence factor positive (EAF+) EPEC were isolated from 89 (22.1%) case infants, rotavirus from 46 (11.4%), ETEC from 18 (4.5%), *Shigella* sp. from 16 (4.0%), *Salmonella* sp. from 14 (3.5%), EAF− EPEC from 10 (2.5%), *Campylobacter* sp. from 7 (1.7%) and EIEC from 5 (1.2%). No pathogen was isolated from the remaining 49.1%. In a multivariate logistic regression analysis, it was found that boiling household drinking water (OR 0.4, *p* < 0.0001) was protective. Prior hospitalization (OR 3.4, *p* < 0.001), prior diarrhoea in another household member (OR 4.4, *p* < 0.01), day care (OR 2.0, *p* < 0.05) and low income (OR 1.8, *p* < 0.02) were associated with increased risk. When the analyses were restricted to individual pathogens statistical significance could not be achieved because of small numbers, although boiling drinking water seemed to be protective for all pathogens.

The incidence of diarrhoeal disease due to *E. coli* was studied in children in poor communities in Santiago, Chile (Levine *et al.* 1993). Two cohorts of children were studied. The first cohort was a group of mixed ages up to 47 months old. These children were followed until they were 60 months old. The second cohort was of newborns, who were studied until they were 24 months old. The home of each child was visited twice a week to enquire about any diarrhoeal illness. When an episode of diarrhoea was detected, a stool specimen or rectal swab was taken for culture. A stool culture was also taken from a matched asymptomatic member of the cohort as a control. After initial culture of stool samples on MacConkey agar the different, individual colonies of *E. coli* were identified using DNA probes. Unlike in previous studies, the authors looked for all six categories of *E. coli*. In the mixed-age cohort, 1178 episodes of diarrhoea were detected in the 340 children over 30 months (1.39 episodes/children.years). In this cohort ETEC was much more likely to be isolated from cases than from controls (12.3% versus 7.0%, $p = 3.9 \times 10^{-6}$) as was DAEC (16.6% versus 11.9%, $p = 0.0024$). EPEC was isolated from 4.3%, EIEC from 2.8%, EHEC from 1.5% and EAggEC from 16.2% although these were not significantly different to controls. The incidence rate in the newborn cohort was higher (2.76 episodes/children.years). In the newborn cohort only ETEC were significantly more associated with diarrhoea ($p = 0.003$), although there was a significant association of EPEC with diarrhoea in children under 11 months ($p = 0.02$). Although this study was not specifically concerned with elucidating the link between *E. coli* diarrhoea and waterborne disease, I have discussed it in some detail because of its indication of the importance of these pathogens in poorer communities in tropical countries. Nevertheless, the authors noted that despite the provision of bacteriologically safe water to this community, transmission of *E. coli* pathogens was still continuing, although at lower levels than in communities without such a supply.

17   Yersinia Infections

The genus *Yersinia* is better known for the species *Y. pestis*, the causative agent of plague, known in medieval times as the black death. Plague is still a threat in many parts of the world but fortunately does not appear to spread by a waterborne route. Other *Yersinia* spp. have been implicated in waterborne spread and outbreaks.

MICROBIOLOGY

Yersinia spp. are members of the Enterobacteriaceae and, as such, are Gram-negative, facultatively anaerobic, non-spore-forming bacilli. They are non-motile at 37 °C but some species are motile at 22 °C. They ferment carbohydrates with the production of acid but rarely gas.

There are currently four *Yersinia* spp. accepted within the genus: *Y. pestis*, *Y. pseudotuberculosis*, *Y. enterocolitica* and *Y. ruckeri*. However, *Y. enterocolitica* is very biochemically and serologically heterogeneous and there is currently some debate over whether this is a single species. It is probably best practice to refer to the *Y. enterocolitica* group. Within this group there exist five biogroups of *Y. enterocolitica sensu stricto*: *Y. aldovae*, *Y. frederiksenii*, *Y. intermedia*, *Y. kristensenii* and *Y. enterocolitica*-like (XI). The differing species are distinguished from each other on the basis of various biochemical reactions.

Six serotypes and four sub-types of *Y. pseudotuberculosis* and more than 50 serotypes of *Y. enterocolitica* have been described.

Both *Y. pseudotuberculosis* and *Y. enterocolitica* group organisms have been associated with waterborne outbreaks, and the rest of this chapter is restricted to a discussion of these organisms.

PATHOGENESIS

The infective dose is probably high, up to 10^9 organisms. The exact pathogenic mechanisms are not fully understood. Infection of the terminal ileum leads to ulceration and inflammation of the mesenteric lymph nodes. Pathogenic strains are resistant to serum complement, can penetrate human epithelial cells and are cytotoxic.

CLINICAL FEATURES

The incubation period for both species is between 3 and 7 days.

Y. enterocolitica mainly affects children under five years old. In this age group it causes fever, diarrhoea and abdominal pain, which lasts for about one to three weeks. In some cases rectal bleeding and perforation of the small bowel may occur. In patients over five years old the clinical picture may be indistinguishable from that caused by *Y. pseudotuberculosis*, as described below. Erythema nodosum is seen in up to 30% of cases. In adults, reactive polyarthritis may occur in 10–30% of individuals, especially in those patients who are HLA-B27 antigen positive. Septicaemia is uncommon and when it occurs is usually seen in the elderly or in individuals with pre-existing disease. Patients with septicaemia may develop abscesses in the liver or spleen and may develop osteomyelitis.

Y. pseudotuberculosis most commonly causes a mesenteric adenitis, which can be indistinguishable from acute appendicitis. If the patient is operated on, the appendix appears normal, but mesenteric lymph nodes are enlarged and the terminal ileum may appear inflamed. Septicaemia is rare.

DIAGNOSIS

The diagnosis may be made by culture of the relevant pathogen from faeces, mesenteric lymph nodes, pharyngeal exudate, peritoneal fluid or blood culture. Culture for these organisms from faeces is not routinely carried out in most laboratories. A yersinia selective agar is available for culture of *Y. enterocolitica* from faeces. Positive cultures are confirmed by biochemical and serological investigations.

Serological tests are available for diagnosis, although they only become positive after two to three weeks.

TREATMENT

The role of specific antibiotic therapy for any infection other than septicaemia is unclear. Even with antibiotic therapy the mortality with septicaemia is up to 75%. By the time the diagnosis is considered most patients are well on the way to recovery. Tetracyclines have been recommended as the preferred antibiotic, and good responses have been seen with ciprofloxacin.

ENVIRONMENTAL DETECTION

The currently recommended method for the isolation of *Yersinia* spp. is based on filtration followed by incubation of the filter in Tris-buffered peptone at

9 °C for two weeks (HMSO 1994). Prior to culture on cefsulodin irgasan novobiocin agar, the enrichment broth is mixed with a solution of potassium hydroxide in saline. Confirmation of typical colonies is by the demonstration of motility and biochemical reactions. Escudero *et al.* (1994) compared five different enrichment media and five plating media for the detection of *Yersinia* spp. from river and lake water. They found that yeast extract-Bengal rose-broth with bile-oxalate-sorbose broth was the best enrichment medium and MacConkey agar the best plating media.

Some authors have described a selective isolation method using HeLa cell lines (Fukushima, Hoshina and Gomyoda, 1994).

A PCR method for the detection of pathogenic *Y. enterocolitica* in water samples has been described (Kapperud *et al.* 1993). The authors also described a concentration step based on immunomagnetic separation using magnetic particles covered with antibodies to *Y. enterocolitica* serogroup O:3. The PCR was able to detect all pathogenic serogroups (O:3, O:5,27, O:8, O:9, O:13 and O:21). If the sample was pre-enriched overnight in a non-selective medium, the detection limit was 2 colony forming units (CFU) per gram.

ECOLOGY

Yersinia spp. have been isolated from a wide range of animal and environmental samples, although many of these environmental strains are of uncertain significance. Strains have been isolated from water supplies during the investigation of outbreaks.

Aleksic and Bockemuhl (1988) reported on 416 strains of *Yersinia* spp. that had been isolated from well-water and drinking water plants in the Federal Republic of Germany over the years 1982–1987. Of these 82% were *Y. enterocolitica*, 11% were *Y. intermedia*, 5.8% were *Y. frederiksenii* and 1.2% were *Y. kristensenii*. None of the strains isolated was of serogroups commonly associated with human disease and none was positive in virulence tests.

Various authors have described the isolation of *Yersinia* spp. from surface water samples. Isolation rates are usually less than 10% with the exception of Japanese studies. There does not appear to be any relationship with markers of faecal pollution. In an Italian study, 26 strains were isolated from 120 samples of river water (Massa *et al.* 1988). Of these, 12 were identified as *Y. enterocolitica*, two as *Y. frederiksenii* and one each as *Y. kristensenii* and *Y. aldovae*. There were also five atypical strains. Regular samples of surface water sources in Norway over a 14-month period found just four (4.2%) *Yersinia* spp. isolates, all four being non-pathogenic (Brennhovd, Kapperud and Langeland 1992). In a one-year study of three rivers and two lakes in Argentina, *Yersinia* spp. were isolated from 7.14% of samples but none demonstrated virulence (Escudero *et al.* 1994). Using their isolation method based on HeLa cell cultures, Fukushima *et al.* (1995)

reported isolating *Y. pseudotuberculosis* from 25.7% of river samples in Japan but from no similar sample from Germany. On the other hand, Lombin *et al.* (1986) were unable to demonstrate the isolation of *Y. enterocolitica* from any sample from 250 wells, 118 ponds and 34 streams around Zaria in northern Nigeria.

EPIDEMIOLOGY

Yersiniosis has a worldwide distribution. Outbreaks and sporadic cases have been linked to contact with wild and domestic animals, food and milk, and person to person spread.

Outbreaks associated with drinking water

Perhaps the first alleged waterborne outbreak of yersiniosis to be described was at a ski lodge in Montana in 1974 (Eden *et al.* 1977). The outbreak first came to light when about 30 of a party of 50 individuals who had just returned from a skiing trip experienced gastroenteritis. In the initial investigations, the authors surveyed 86 employees, of whom 65 (76%) had a similar illness. They also conducted a telephone survey of approximately 10% of guests who had at the stayed at the resort during December 1974 and early January 1975. Of 317 guests on whom information was obtained, 129 (41%) had been ill. The median interval between arrival at the resort and the onset of symptoms was 57 hours and the duration of symptoms was 18 hours. No pathogen was cultured from any acute faecal specimen. There was a significant association between drinking water and illness ($p = 0.0001$). The risk increased with increasing daily consumption. The water supply came from wells and was neither disinfected nor filtered before the outbreak. Culture of the water revealed low levels of coliform contamination and *Y. enterocolitica* (Highsmith *et al.* 1977). *Y. enterocolitica* was not isolated from any specimen, although stool samples were only examined for this pathogen several weeks after the outbreak. Serum samples from employees did not show any activity against yersinia antigens.

Thompson and Gravel (1986) described two cases of gastroenteritis in a family. *Y. enterocolitica* serogroup O:3 was isolated from both patients and from the well from which the family took its drinking water.

Inoue *et al.* (1988) described three outbreaks of *Y. pseudotuberculosis* that occurred in Japan between 1982 and 1984. One of the outbreaks was foodborne. The other two occurred in remote mountain areas. In one outbreak 260 (18.5%) people out of 1402 were affected. The attack rate was low in adults (7.5%) and high in all children's age groups (70.6%). In the other outbreak, 11 (64.7%) out of 17 children in a village were affected.

Y. pseudotuberculosis was isolated from 35 (13%) of 267 stool samples in the first outbreak and one of four in the second. Stains identical to those isolated from clinical samples were isolated from 5.9% of mountain stream water samples in the area of the first outbreak and from two (16.7%) samples of well-water from the second.

A 24-year-old resident hospital doctor presented with a ten-week history of loose, frequent bowel motions, malaise and weight loss (Cafferkey *et al.* 1993). The only potential pathogen isolated was *Y. frederiksenii*, which was detected on three separate occasions. Faecal samples were obtained from 9 other medical residents, 25 student nurses and 25 inpatients. Three of the nine medical residents were also positive for *Y. frederiksenii*, but no nurse or inpatient was positive. At the time of the initial investigation the authors suspected unpasteurized milk as the cause. However, two months later they investigated the storage water roof tanks following an unrelated complaint over water quality. It was discovered that the water tank supplying the medical residences was uncovered and that much debris had collected in the tank. A pure growth of *Y. enterocolitica* was isolated from the water.

Prospective epidemiological studies

Ostroff *et al.* (1994) conducted a prospective case-control study of patients from whom *Y. enterocolitica* had been isolated from faeces. The study was done in and around Oslo, Norway. Two age-, sex- and geographically-matched controls were identified for each case. Sixty-seven patients were enrolled in the study, all of whom had an enteric infection. In the univariate analysis, cases were more likely to prefer meat raw or rare (OR 3.58, CI 1.52–8.44), to have eaten raw minced meat (OR 7.59, CI 1.44–55.95) and to have drunk untreated water (OR 2.76, CI 1.19–6.43). Cases were less likely to clean their kitchen work surfaces with soap and water (OR 0.41, CI 0.18–0.90). In addition, various meats were associated with infection. In the multivariate analysis the variables that remained independently significant were consumption of pork ($p = 0.02$), consumption of sausage ($p = 0.03$), drinking untreated water ($p = 0.02$) and a preference for eating undercooked meats ($p = 0.01$).

In another Norwegian study, Saebø *et al.* (1994) examined sera from 755 Norwegian military recruits. They found that 56 (7.4%) had IgG antibodies against *Y. enterocolitica* serogroup O:3. Demographic data was obtained from all recruits, and drinking water from a private well (OR 3.40, CI 1.49–7.73), being a resident of Oslo City (OR 2.99, CI 1.37–6.56) and living in Eastern Norway (OR 2.25, CI 1.17–4.30) were all found to be independently associated with having a positive serological result. The only medical condition that was associated with positivity was a history of having had a previous abdominal operation.

COMMENTS

The evidence from the outbreaks supporting a waterborne route of spread for *Yersinia* spp. is at best circumstantial. The large outbreak in Montana in 1974 (Eden *et al.* 1977) occurred before many of the more common waterborne pathogens such as cryptosporidium or Norwalk virus were recognized as potential waterborne agents. Therefore, in the absence of isolation from stool or demonstration of a rise in antibody levels, the cause of this outbreak must remain uncertain. Insufficient analytical epidemiology was presented in the reports of the other proposed waterborne outbreaks to enable adequate assessment of the role of drinking water. Nevertheless, the two prospective studies from Norway (Ostroff *et al.* 1994; Saebø *et al.* 1994) do provide fairly convincing evidence that *Y. enterocolitica*, at least in Norway, is a waterborne pathogen.

18 Plesiomonas Infections

Plesiomonas shigelloides was first described in 1947, though since then it has been placed into several genera, including *Pseudomonas, Aeromonas* and *Vibrio*. It was not until 1962 that the genus was named; even now its taxonomy is uncertain and future reassignments can not be ruled out. To match its uncertain taxonomy, its potential to cause disease in humans is still debated.

MICROBIOLOGY

Plesiomonads are members of the family Vibrionaceae. They are motile, Gram-negative, facultatively anaerobic and non-spore-forming bacilli, which are oxidase and catalase positive. *P. shigelloides* is the only species in the genus. They grow on deoxycholate and MacConkey agars but not on TCBS. Some 50 somatic 'O' antigens and 17 flagella 'H' antigens have been described. Several of the O antigens cross-react with O antigens of different *Shigella* spp.

PATHOGENESIS

No pathogenic mechanism for causing human diarrhoea is known. Volunteer and animal studies have been unable to reproduce disease.

CLINICAL FEATURES

The clinical presentation of gastroenteritis associated with *P. shigelloides* varies from mild to severe mucoid and bloody diarrhoea. In some reports the diarrhoea is predominantly secretory, while in others it appears invasive.

There are also a few reports of extra-intestinal disease, including bacteraemia, osteomyelitis, septic arthritis and meningitis.

DIAGNOSIS

Diagnosis is from culture of faeces or other clinical material. The organism grows well on MacConkey or deoxycholate citrate agar, where it can be mistaken for a *Shigella* sp. Confirmation is by biochemical reactions.

TREATMENT

Specific antibacterial therapy may be indicated in severe or extra-intestinal disease, but must be guided by the results of antimicrobial sensitivity tests.

ENVIRONMENTAL DETECTION

No recommended method for the isolation of *P. shigelloides* from waters is given in the UK water microbiology methods book (HMSO 1994). Medema and Schets (1993) compared inositol brilliant green agar with *Plesiomonas* agar and found that although both agars gave a similar percentage of positive results, only 30% of samples positive on at least one agar were positive on both. They concluded that the two media were complementary. In a recent study of the environmental distribution of *P. shigelloides*, de Mondino, Nunes and Ricciardi (1995) used culture on inositol brilliant green bile salt agar, directly and after enrichment in alkaline peptone water.

ECOLOGY

P. shigelloides appears to be common in many freshwater environments. During their investigation of two possible waterborne outbreaks in Japan, Tsukamoto *et al.* (1978) examined 342 samples of water and mud from ponds, rivers and shallow streams. They isolated *P. shigelloides* from 38.6% of these samples. Kwaga *et al.* (1988) reported isolating *P. shigelloides* from 7.4% of pond water samples and 0.6% of well-water samples in Zaria, Nigeria. A survey of the ecosystems in five ponds in Dacca, Bangladesh, over one year found *P. shigelloides* in 20.8% of hydrophyte, 13.3% of water, 18.3% of phytoplankton and 29.2% of sediment samples (Islam, Alam and Khan 1991).

De Mondino, Nunes and Ricciardi (1995) sampled four saltwater and two freshwater sites in and around Rio de Janeiro City. They sampled each site on four occasions over six months. Of the 24 samples collected, 4 were positive for *P. shigelloides*, 2 of 16 saltwaters and 2 of 8 freshwaters. Ten strains were isolated from saltwater, and then only after enrichment, while 36 strains were isolated from freshwater, two of which came up without enrichment.

Following an outbreak of illness associated with *P. shigelloides*, in the Netherlands, Medema and Schets (1993) studied the distribution of the organism in Dutch recreational waters. *P. shigelloides* was present in 30 of 42 freshwater samples but in no seawater sample. All samples were taken during July and August. Log counts of *P. shigelloides* were most highly correlated with log counts of *E. coli* ($r = 0.59$, $p < 0.001$) and with chlorophyll a concentrations ($r = 0.55$, $p < 0.001$). The latter is a surrogate marker of trophic state. Whether the association with these other markers reflects increased growth because of increased nutrient availability or increased seeding in pollutants is unclear.

EPIDEMIOLOGY

The only published outbreaks of waterborne disease linked to *P. shigelloides* both occurred in Osaka, Japan (Tsukamoto *et al*. 1978). The first outbreak affected 978 of 2141 people who had stayed at a youth centre between 5 and 10 August 1973. *P. shigelloides* was isolated from 21 acute diarrhoeal samples and from 1 of 8 tap-water samples. Three serovars (O17:H2 17 strains, O22:H3 4 strains and O8:H5 1 strain) were isolated from human samples. The tap-water sample yielded O17:H2. *P. shigelloides* was also isolated from water samples taken from the water treatment plant. The second outbreak affected 24 of 35 individuals on a sightseeing tour between 18 and 20 October 1974. Three of eight faecal samples were positive for *P. shigelloides* serovar O24:H5. It is not clear why the authors decided this second outbreak was waterborne.

A survey of *P. shigelloides* positive stool samples in Vancouver between August 1986 and December 1987 identified 30 patients (Kain and Kelly 1989). The authors interviewed all patients or their physicians and control patients without a positive stool. Cases were more likely to have abdominal pain ($p = 0.02$) and a prolonged illness lasting for more than two weeks ($p < 0.02$). Cases were more likely to have travelled abroad than controls (71% versus 10%, $p < 0.001$). Information on the consumption of seafood or untreated water was only available for 21 cases and none of the controls. Overall, 95% of cases reported consumption of untreated water and 95% reported consumption of seafood.

The evidence linking Plesiomonas to waterborne outbreaks of disease is still circumstantial. No analytical epidemiological evidence in favour of a waterborne source has been presented to date.

19 Aeromonas Infections

Although *Aeromonas* spp. have been known for some time their role as a primary cause of gastroenteritis has only attracted renewed interest in recent years. Nevertheless, uncertainty still remains over the pathogenicity, ecology and epidemiology of *Aeromonas* spp. Much of this confusion may be because of remaining difficulties in the taxonomy of the genus.

MICROBIOLOGY

Aeromonas spp. are members of the family Vibrionaceae. They are Gram-negative, non-spore-forming, facultatively anaerobic bacilli. The taxonomy of this genus is still a subject of debate. There is one non-motile species, *A. salmonicida*, which is usually unable to grow at temperatures above 30 °C. It is an important fish pathogen but has not been isolated from human clinical specimens. There are currently thought to be three species of motile aeromonads, *A. hydrophila*, *A. caviae* and *A. sobria*. They are distinguished from each other on the basis of biochemical reactions. All of the motile aeromonads grow well at 30 °C and most at 37 °C. This chapter is restricted to discussing the motile *Aeromonas* spp.

PATHOGENESIS

The pathogenesis of Aeromonas-associated diarrhoea is unclear. A variety of potential toxins have been described, including: a cytotoxic β-haemolysin, which causes fluid accumulation in suckling mice, an extracellular cytotonic entero-toxin, which causes fluid accumulation in rabbits and rats but not in suckling mice, a cytotonic enterotoxin, which cross-reacts with cholera toxin and causes fluid accumulation in suckling mice, an enteroinvasive factor demonstrable in Hep-2 cells, and a variety of haemagglutinins, proteases and elastases.

CLINICAL FEATURES

The motile *Aeromonas* spp. occasionally cause soft tissue infections. *A. hydrophila* is the most likely to do so. Often a history of trauma followed by exposure to contaminated water is obtained. Interestingly, *A. hydrophila* is a symbiotic commensal of the leech, providing enzymes to assist the leach digest its blood meal. Infection develops in up to 20% of patients who have been treated by leeches. Bacteraemia is rare and is usually seen only in patients with pre-existing immunosuppressive disease. Most cases of bacteraemia are due to *A. sobria*.

The clinical features of Aeromonas diarrhoea are varied. Patients usually present with mild, self-limiting diarrhoea. However, a proportion go on to develop fever, abdominal pain and bloody diarrhoea. Diarrhoea can occasionally be protracted, and a small proportion of adults go on to develop a chronic colitis. Most cases of diarrhoea are associated with *A. caviae*.

DIAGNOSIS

Aeromonas can be isolated by culture of faeces on ampicillin containing blood agar. Confirmation is by biochemical tests.

TREATMENT

Clinical improvement has been reported when antibiotics to which the organism is sensitive have been given. Correct choice of antibiotic depends on the results of sensitivity tests.

ENVIRONMENTAL DETECTION

The tentative method for the isolation of *Aeromonas* spp. from water is to filter the sample and then culture the filter on ampicillin–dextrin agar (ADA) (HMSO 1994). All oxidase positive, yellow colonies are presumptive *Aeromonas* spp. Further confirmation is by biochemical analysis. Work is still being reported on suggestions for new isolation media and on the comparison of selective isolation media and culture conditions (Havelaar, During and Versteegh 1987; Arcos *et al.* 1988; Cunliffe and Adcock 1989; Ribas *et al.* 1991; Bernagozzi *et al.* 1994; Papapetropoulou, Rodopoulou and Giannoulaki 1995).

ECOLOGY

Aeromonas spp. are ubiquitous in the aquatic environment, being present rather more commonly than faecal coliforms (Fewtrell *et al.* 1994). Nakano *et al.* (1990) studied the distribution of *Aeromonas* spp. in aquatic environments over one year. They identified 2444 isolates. *A. hydrophila* was the predominant species in clean riverine samples, while *A. sobria* was predominantly isolated from stagnant waters. *A. caviae* was more commonly isolated from marine waters. Several workers have studied the relationship between counts of *Aeromonas* spp. and markers of pollution. In one such study, estuarine water counts of *A. hydrophila* were correlated with total viable counts and counts of coliforms and faecal coliforms, and negatively correlated with salinity and dissolved oxygen (Kaper *et al.* 1981). In freshwaters the association between faecal coliforms and *Aeromonas* spp. appears only with microbiological evidence of high levels of faecal pollution (Araujo *et al.* 1989).

Parveen, Islam and Huq (1995) reported a study of the environmental distribution of *Aeromonas* spp. in Bangladesh. *Aeromonas* spp. were isolated from all samples throughout the year. The peak counts in surface water were in the warmer months (April and May), while peak counts were seen in sediment in March and August. *Aeromonas* spp. were isolated from aquatic plants, the highest counts being seen in the winter months.

As will be seen in the section on epidemiology, *Aeromonas* spp. have also been isolated from chlorinated waters samples that comply with existing standards. Burke *et al.* (1984) intensively monitored the Perth, Australia, water distribution system each week for a year starting in November 1981. This was a chlorinated supply that met current microbiological standards. In total, 3224 samples were examined during the study. *Aeromonas* spp. were isolated from almost all raw water samples from surface sources, but only rarely from raw groundwater. Counts in raw surface water showed a marked seasonal variation, with the highest counts being seen in summer months. Immediately after chlorination *Aeromonas* spp. were detected on just 36 occasions and counts were lower than those in raw surface water. Samples from the service reservoirs showed counts similar to those found in raw surface water. Before leaving the service reservoirs, water was once again chlorinated and a decline in counts of *Aeromonas* spp. was noted. However, counts from various sites in the distribution network after the service reservoirs showed counts similar to those in raw surface water. Clearly chlorination has only a temporary effect on counts of *Aeromonas* spp. and there is regrowth in the distribution system.

Aeromonas spp. have also been isolated from some brands of bottled mineral waters (Hunter 1993). These have been waters with relatively high bioavailable carbon.

EPIDEMIOLOGY

I am unaware of any outbreaks of Aeromonas-associated disease linked to either drinking water or recreational water contact. As the epidemiology of gastrointestinal infections and extra-intestinal infections varies I will discuss these separately.

Gastrointestinal infections

In the study by Burke *et al.* (1984) discussed above, the authors noted a seasonal variation in counts of *Aeromonas* spp. from raw surface water and from various points in the distribution system. They were able to demonstrate a very close correlation between mean temperature of water samples, counts of aeromonads and the isolation of *Aeromonas* spp. from diarrhoeal stools. On a smaller scale Picard and Goullet (1987) also found a seasonal correlation between counts of Aeromonas in a hospital water supply in France and isolations from the hospital's patients.

Holmberg *et al.* (1986) reported a case-control study of 34 patients from whom *A. hydrophila* had been isolated. The patients came from across the US. Two controls were identified from the same areas as the patients. Of the 34 patients, six had other gastrointestinal pathologies as well. Of the remaining 28, 20 had diarrhoea, 17 had abdominal cramps, 10 had vomiting, 5 had dehydration and 5 had fever. Blood was seen in the stool of only two. Disease was more prolonged in adults (median duration 42 days) than in children (18 days). There was a strong association with drinking untreated water (OR 20.91, CI 3.17–887.9). Although not statistically significant, more patients than controls had been swimming in freshwater ponds or streams (11.8% versus 2.9%).

A study in the Netherlands investigated 137 patients, from whom *Aeromonas* spp. had been isolated from faeces (Kuijper *et al.* 1989). The authors tested strains for cytotoxigenic potential. They then compared patients' clinical details and risk factors in patients from whom a cytotoxigenic strain had been isolated with those whose strain had been non-cytotoxigenic. Patients whose strain was cytotoxigenic were more likely to have gastro-enteritis of acute onset and with vomiting. Diarrhoea was more likely to be prolonged. The occurrence of cytotoxigenic strains was also strongly associated with surface water contact such as swimming, surfing or fishing during the week prior to the onset of illness (OR 7.54, $p < 0.005$) and with foreign travel (OR 4.89, $p < 0.05$).

Also in the Netherlands, Havelaar *et al.* (1992) typed 187 strains of *Aeromonas* spp. from human diarrhoeal stools and 263 strains from drinking water. They used three different typing methods: biotyping using several biochemical tests, serotyping, and the analysis of cell wall fatty acid methyl esters by gas-liquid chromatography. Using cluster analysis and principal component analysis they were able to demonstrate that strains from human infections were, generally, very similar to strains from drinking water, thereby supporting a drinking water hypothesis.

Hänninen and Siitonen (1995) also compared the typing results of strains isolated from human infections and strains isolated from drinking water. This time the authors used chromosomal DNA ribotyping. In contrast to the findings in the previous study, the authors found little similarity between human and drinking water isolates.

Extra-intestinal infections

Voss, Rhodes and Johnson (1992) reported on a series of 28 patients in New Zealand from whom *Aeromonas* spp. were isolated from a wound or soft tissue infection between November 1985 and November 1989. Of these 28 patients, 23 (82%) gave a history of an acute open or penetrating injury. In 13 cases the original injury had occurred in lake or river water. Of ten patients with a pure infection, seven had a water-related injury.

In another series of patients with extra-intestinal infection, this time in tropical Queensland, Australia, 52 cases were identified during 1991 (Kelly, Koehler and Ashdown 1993). Of these infections, 6 were acquired in hospital and the remaining 46 were community-acquired. *A. hydrophila* was the commonest species isolated (71%) and *A. sobria* the second most common (25%). The disease was disproportionately common in aborigines. In 27 of the community-acquired infections, there was a history of trauma and in 17 (63%) of these the patient had been in contact with fresh water at the time of injury.

COMMENTS

As far as I can find, there have been no outbreaks of Aeromonas infection linked to water. Nevertheless, the case-control study by Holmberg *et al.* (1986) and the study by Kuijper *et al.* (1989) both provide convincing evidence in favour of a waterborne route for gastroenteritis. These studies are supported by the observation of temporal correlations between counts in drinking water and the incidence of human disease. The similarity of phenotypes between isolates from human infection and drinking water demonstrated by Havelaar *et al.* (1992) also provides good circumstantial evidence. That Hänninen and Siitonen (1995) were unable to demonstrate a similar association in Finland may suggest that some water supplies are colonized with strains pathogenic to humans while others are not. If this is the case then a potent area for future research would be to determine what factors in a water supply influence the strain types likely to colonize it.

20 Pseudomonas Infections

The genus *Pseudomonas* is extremely large with several potential pathogenic species. One species, *P. aeruginosa*, has the distinction of being one of the few bacteria specifically mentioned in water quality legislation.

MICROBIOLOGY

Pseudomonads are strictly aerobic, non-spore-forming, Gram-negative bacilli. They derive energy from carbohydrates by oxidation and not fermentation. They are oxidase and catalase positive. Most are motile with the aid of one or more polar flagella. Growth will occur in many different media. There are over 100 species of *Pseudomonas* currently recognized.

Many species are saprophytic, being present in soils and aquatic environments. Others are pathogenic only for plants. Yet others are conditionally pathogenic.

The most significant human pathogen is *P. aeruginosa*, which is able to grow at 41 °C and produces a blue-green pigment called pyocyanin. *P. aeruginosa* possesses O and H antigens, which form the basis of serogrouping and serotyping schemes. In the UK, serogroups O6 and O11 predominate in clinical specimens.

PATHOGENESIS

The pathogenesis of the various clinical syndromes associated with *P. aeruginosa* differs with the syndrome and source of infection. The organism rarely causes disease in an otherwise healthy individual unless some insult to the host has predisposed him or her to infection. For example, pseudomonal folliculitis tends to occur only in waterlogged skin after immersion in water. Pseudomonal otitis will only affect people who have some pre-existing ear problem or after repeated immersion in water to remove the protective wax coating of the external ear canal.

P. aeruginosa can also produce a variety of toxins, such as extracellular proteolytic enzymes and haemolysins, which are important in the formation of local lesions, exotoxins A and S, which can inhibit cellular protein production, and endotoxins. While the resistance of *P. aeruginosa* to many antibiotic agents is not a virulence factor *per se*, it certainly makes treatment of many infections difficult.

CLINICAL FEATURES

P. aeruginosa can affect many different body systems and cause a variety of clinical syndromes. For example the organism has been the cause of endocarditis, respiratory infection (particularly in children with cystic fibrosis), bacteraemia, meningitis and brain abscess, and ear, eye, bone and joint, urinary tract, gastrointestinal, and skin and soft tissue infections. Of these the most significant to the water epidemiologist are skin and ear infections. The most characteristic water-related skin rash is folliculitis.

Pseudomonal folliculitis presents as a rash, which starts as erythematous or urticarial about 18–24 hours after contact with water. This can then develop into a folliculitis. Fever and itching are uncommon. The infection is usually self-limiting. Pseudomonal otitis externa presents as a purulent discharge from the ear. The ear may also be itchy or painful. Inspection of the ear canal shows it to be inflamed and full of debris. Occasionally, the infection becomes invasive, and unless promptly treated it can cause local destruction of the ear canal and may be fatal. This condition, known as malignant otitis externa, is more common in elderly diabetics and the immunosuppressed.

DIAGNOSIS

Laboratory diagnosis of *P. aeruginosa* is by culture of swabs of or material from affected lesions. Most *Pseudomonas* spp. grow well on many laboratory media, including MacConkey agar.

TREATMENT

P. aeruginosa is resistant to many antimicrobial agents, and specific therapy should, wherever possible, be based on laboratory sensitivity data. Antimicrobials such as ciprofloxacin have been a significant advance in providing an oral antibiotic effective against *P. aeruginosa*.

ENVIRONMENTAL DETECTION

Routine isolation of *P. aeruginosa* from water is either by multiple tube methods, using asparagine broth and ethanol, or by membrane filtration using modified King's A broth (HMSO 1994). Provision positive isolates are confirmed by culture on milk agar with cetrimide. *P. aeruginosa* causes clearing in the medium. Pigment will also be produced.

De Vicente *et al.* (1986) reported a study comparing various media for isolation of *P. aeruginosa* from water. They concluded that mPA-D was preferable for river water and mPA-E for seawater.

Polymerase chain reactions methods have also been reported for the detection of *P. aeruginosa* in water. A PCR test reported by Khan and Cerniglia (1994) was able to detect as few as five cells in 10 ml of water.

ECOLOGY

P. aeruginosa is distributed widely in the natural and man-made aquatic environment. It has been isolated frequently from both fresh and seawaters (Fewtrell *et al.* 1994). For example, in Israel, the organism was found in 44.8% of 652 seawater samples from 34 beaches (Yoshpe-Purer and Golderman 1987). Mates (1992) found the organism in 14% of water samples from Mediterranean beaches. In 31% of those samples positive for pseudomonads, faecal coliforms were found only in low numbers (<10/100 ml).

A survey of drinking water samples in Greece found *P. aeruginosa* in eight (9%) of 88 tap-water samples and 20 (18.8%) of 106 bottled waters (Papapetropoulou *et al.* 1994). Grundmann *et al.* (1993) isolated *P. aeruginosa* from tap-water in a special-care baby unit, one area where the organism could potentially cause serious disease.

Grobe, Wingender and Truper (1995) reported that 10 of 81 strains of *P. aeruginosa* isolated from water or surfaces in contact with water were mucoid. They suggested that the production of excess slime material was important in the attachment to surfaces in aquatic environments.

P. aeruginosa has been isolated from innumerable spa-pools (see below). An early study found *P. aeruginosa* in 62.5% of samples from 24 different spa-pools (Kush and Hoadley 1980). Price and Ahearn (1988) reported its isolation from seven commercial and two residential spas. None of the commercial spas had been consistently maintained at appropriate disinfection levels. More recently, Hollyoak, Boyd and Freeman (1995) reported that *P. aeruginosa* was isolated from all 16 whirlpool baths in a survey of nursing homes. Cleaning and maintenance practices were variable.

Most spa-pools use either chlorine- or bromine-based disinfectants. Klenner and Webber (1979) showed that chlorine was a better disinfectant in spa-pools than chlorine-bromine-hydantoin. Shaw (1984) also showed that chlorination was superior to bromine in controlling *P. aeruginosa* in spa-pools. He reported that during the investigation of one outbreak, *P. aeruginosa* could be isolated from the water despite it having a total residual bromine level of 5 mg/l and a pH of 7.5. Shaw then conducted a retrospective comparison of the results of routine microbiological analyses of spas in Alberta. In adequately maintained spa-pools, as measured by a plate count of <1 CFU/ml, *P. aeruginosa* was isolated from 5% of bromine-disinfected pools and 0.8% of chlorine-disinfected pools. In those pools where the plate count was in the range 1– 200 CFU/ml the counts were 16% and 6%, and for plate counts >200 CFU/ml 38% and 17%, respectively. As a result of this work Alberta removed approval of bromine-based disinfectants for use in spa-pools, and the prevalence of spa-pool associated skin disease fell (Shaw 1987).

EPIDEMIOLOGY

Outbreaks of pseudomonal skin infections

Before progressing, I need to clarify terminology, as some confusion exists. In this chapter I use the term **spa-pool** to indicate any pool that remains filled and has some mechanism to generate turbulence in the water. Spa-pools are typically able to hold several individuals. I use the term **whirlpool** to indicate a bath fitted with hydrojet circulation and/or air induction bubble systems. Whirlpool baths typically hold only one individual and are emptied between uses.

Reported outbreaks of pseudomonal dermatitis or folliculitis associated with the use of spa-pools or swimming pools are numerous. Between 1985 and 1994 there were 48 outbreaks of skin disease, due to or compatible with *P. aeruginosa*, reported to the American CDC as being associated with spa-pools or hot tubs (St Louis 1988; Levine, Stephenson and Craun 1990; Herwaldt *et al.* 1991; Moore *et al.* 1993; Kramer *et al.* 1996). During the same time there were four outbreaks linked to swimming pools. These outbreaks affected 1078 individuals. Outbreaks of pseudomonal skin disease associated with spa-pool baths or hot tubs are apparently common. Indeed, there is a considerable number of outbreak reports in the literature. Discussing each report would add very little value for the reader. Consequently, I discuss only a very few of these papers.

Ratnam *et al.* (1986) reported an outbreak of folliculitis affecting guests at a hotel in St John's, Newfoundland, Canada, in 1984. Of 36 people who had used the hotel's spa-pool, 26 (72%) developed pseudomonal folliculitis. *P. aeruginosa* was isolated from the spa-pool at counts of up to 340 000 colonies/ 100 ml. The disinfectant in use for the spa-pool was bromine. As well as reporting on their outbreak, the authors undertook a very thorough review of the world literature up to that time. They were able to find 36 reports of pseudomonal folliculitis, affecting over 1000 people, associated with swimming pools, spa-pools or hot tubs. These outbreaks were due to several different serotypes. In these 36 reports spa-pools were implicated on 23 occasions, swimming pools on 7 occasions and hot tubs on 7. On three of these occasions both a spa-pool and a swimming pool were implicated in the same outbreak. Also implicated were a physiotherapy pool and a water slide. The earliest report was in 1972, probably reflecting the recent fashion for spa-pools. The interested reader should refer to this paper for publication details of the reports reviewed.

Although reported rather less commonly, other more severe illnesses are associated with outbreaks of follicular dermatitis. For example, Kosatsky and Kleeman (1985) reported an outbreak of folliculitis in 10 of 14 participants in a hot-tub party. The risk of illness depended on the duration of use of the hot tub; the median duration of affected individuals was 120 minutes while that of non-affected people was 25 minutes ($p = 0.023$). The index case presented with indurated subcutaneous swellings on the plantar surfaces of her feet. She also had indurated and tender Montgomery's follicles in the areolae of both breasts. Five other individuals also suffered from indurated Montgomery's follicles, three of whom also had axillary lymphadenopathy. Almost half of the cases reported fever and chills.

Insler and Gore (1986) described an outbreak of folliculitis that affected 12 of 17 healthy people who had used a particular hot tub. In one case, a woman who normally used extended-wear soft contact lenses, the patient also suffered from pseudomonal keratitis.

Penn and Kain (1990) reported an outbreak of pseudomonal folliculitis affecting six (75%) of eight people who had used a new spa-pool in British Columbia. The disinfectant was bromine and although bromine levels were not routinely measured, the manufacturer's disinfection protocol was strictly followed. Based on a combination of their experience and a review of the literature, the authors suggested that while outbreaks of pseudomonal disease were unlikely to occur in an adequately maintained chlorinated spa-pool, outbreaks still occurred in well-maintained bromine-disinfected spa-pools.

One relatively recent development, at least in the UK, has been the increased use of whirlpool baths. These are like ordinary baths except that they are fitted with hydrojet circulation and/or air induction bubble systems. They have become quite popular in nursing homes. Hollyoak, Allison and Summers (1995) described an outbreak of *P. aeruginosa* wound infection associated with such a bath in a nursing home. During one week pseudomonal wound infection was diagnosed in 4 of 24 residents of the home who had used the bath. No wound infections were identified in 7 residents who had not used the bath. Samples of water that had been agitated in the bath for ten minutes grew *P. aeruginosa* at a count of greater than 180 colonies/100 ml. The staff of the nursing home had no cleaning or disinfection instructions for the bath. Furthermore, the bath had not been serviced regularly.

Outbreaks of folliculitis and other disease linked to spa-pools are likely to be under-reported because the infection in many people is mild and self-limiting or the association with water contact not suspected. Even if outbreaks are identified, few countries other than the USA have surveillance systems in place that monitor this disease. The main outstanding issue is the continued use of bromine as a disinfectant by many spa-pool owners. I have already referred to the comments of Penn and Kain (1990) and work by Shaw (1984) about the potential for disease in bromine-disinfected spa-pools. I would agree with these authors and others (Penny 1991) that, for a variety of reasons, chlorine remains the best disinfectant for spa-pools and swimming pools.

Otitis externa

A telephone survey of residents near a lake in Georgia was conducted during 1972 (Hoadley and Knight 1975). Of 82 swimmers, 6 (7.3%) reported a chronic ear problem compared to 5 (3.1%) of 162 non-swimmers ($p = 0.189$). From 1970 to 1974 the authors also reported on the results of laboratory examination of ear swabs from patients with otitis externa. *P. aeruginosa* was isolated from the ears of 77.6% of 89 swimmers and 33.3% of 21 non-swimmers with otitis ($p = 0.0002$). In controls without otitis *P. aeruginosa* was isolated from 10.5% of 38 swimmers and 14.3% of 21 non-swimmers.

Reid and Porter (1981) described an outbreak of otitis externa in two squads of competitive swimmers. The 25 members of squad A trained twice a day. *P. aeruginosa* was isolated from one or both ears of 18 members of squad A. All but two of these people complained of ear discomfort. Even among the seven members from whom *P. aeruginosa* was not isolated, three complained of recent ear problems. Only one of 54 members of squad B yielded a positive culture. He also complained of a painful, discharging ear. Squad B only used the pool once a day. More than one serotype was isolated from the swimmers. It was noted that chlorine levels were at their lowest in the morning, when squad A trained.

Over a one-year period, 1980–1981, over 300 visitors to a Dutch recreational park developed otitis externa (Havelaar, Bosman and Borst 1983). *P. aeruginosa* was isolated from 23 of 28 ear swabs, 7 of 20 spa water samples and from several other environmental samples. The highest counts of environmental isolates were from the spas. *P. aeruginosa* was not isolated from any water sample with a free chlorine sample above 0.5 mg/l. The outbreak was controlled by installing better chlorination equipment.

Seyfried and Cook (1984) reported on studies undertaken from 1974 to 1977 at five Ontario lakes. They reported that infection rates were highest in those individuals who swam in the lakes with the highest counts of *P. aeruginosa* and in those who reported swimming at least five time a week.

Two case-control studies have also looked at the risk of swimming in freshwater for otitis externa. In the US, Springer and Shapiro (1985) identified 105 cases, who presented to their local emergency department with otitis externa. Of these cases 76.2% had been swimming during the previous week compared to only 53.1% of 239 controls (OR 2.82, CI 1.64–4.94). Swimming in freshwater compared to treated water was also found to be a risk factor (OR 1.93, CI 1.08–3.45). There was also a significant trend for the prevalence of otitis with an increasing number of recent freshwater swims ($p < 0.001$).

Van Asperen *et al.* (1995) reported a similar study of 164 cases and 216 controls in the Netherlands. This time cases were identified by local general practitioners. Swimming in the previous two weeks was strongly associated with disease (OR 4.9, CI 2.3–10.6), as was a history of recurrent ear disease (OR 16.4, CI 5.0–53.6). When swimming was categorized as to the type of water, swimming in a freshwater lake was a risk factor (OR 15.5, CI 4.9–49.2, adjusted for recurrent disease) but swimming in a swimming pool, a river or the sea was not (OR 2.2, CI 0.7–6.7). *P. aeruginosa* was isolated from 83% of ear swabs from cases and 4% of ear swabs from controls.

Other water-related infections with *P. aeruginosa*

Salmen *et al.* (1983) described three cases of urinary tract infection due to *P. aeruginosa* with onset within 48 hours of use of a spa-pool. Two cases were in teenage girls and the other in an adult male. The two teenagers had used a private spa-pool. The adult male had had an erection and had ejaculated while in a hotel spa-pool. *P. aeruginosa* was isolated from both spas. Rose *et al.* (1983) described a pseudomonal pneumonia in an adult male who had used a private spa-pool the evening before onset of symptoms. The man was a heavy smoker. *P. aeruginosa* was isolated from the pool.

21 Melioidosis

Melioidosis is a tropical disease caused by the organism *Burkholderia pseudomallei*. This species was until recently classified as belonging to the genus *Pseudomonas*. The disease is distributed through the tropics and has spread into southern Europe. The areas of highest incidence are southeast Asia, especially Thailand, and parts of northern Australia.

MICROBIOLOGY

Like the closely-related genus *Pseudomonas*, *Burkholderia* are strictly aerobic, non-spore-forming, oxidase and catalase positive, Gram-negative bacilli. *B. mallei* is an obligate animal parasite, but the other species in the genus are environmental organisms. *Burkholderia* spp. are distinguished from *Pseudomonas* spp. by accumulating poly-β-hydroxybutyrate and lacking pigment. *B. pseudomallei* and the closely related *B. mallei* produce ammonia from arginine and amylase, unlike other members of the genus. *B. mallei* is the only species not possessing flagella.

PATHOGENESIS

Melioidosis, due to infection by *B. pseudomallei*, causes purulent abscesses, which can affect several body systems. These abscesses can become very large, and neighbouring abscesses can merge. Septicemic invasion may also occur.

CLINICAL FEATURES

The clinical presentation of melioidosis is varied (Kanai and Dejsirilert 1988; Leelarasamee and Bovornkitti 1989; Dance 1991). Serological surveys in certain parts of Thailand suggest that asymptomatic infections may be common. Latency may also occur so that the incubation period may be as short as two days or as long as 26 years. Clinically melioidosis may present as an acute localized suppurative lesion, an acute pulmonary or septicaemic illness or as a chronic suppurative infection.

DIAGNOSIS

Laboratory diagnosis of *B. pseudomallei* is by culture of swabs of or material from affected lesions. Both species grow well on many laboratory media, including MacConkey agar. Various serological tests, such as agglutination and complement fixation tests, are available. Demonstration of a rising titre is probably diagnostic. However, the results of single sera are difficult to interpret.

TREATMENT

B. pseudomallei is resistant to many antimicrobial agents, and specific therapy should wherever possible be based on laboratory sensitivity data.

ENVIRONMENTAL DETECTION

B. pseudomallei may be isolated from environmental samples using the media described by Ashdown (1979).

ECOLOGY

B. pseudomallei is an environmental organism that is distributed widely in soil and water of certain regions (Leelarasamee and Bovornkitti 1989; Dance 1991). It is particularly common in the northeast of Thailand, where it is associated with rice paddy fields. Isolation rates are higher during the rainy season and in still rather than running water. The organism can survive for many months in moist and shaded areas.

EPIDEMIOLOGY

Melioidosis is usually acquired by contamination of a skin abrasion or ulcer by water or soil. Useful review of the epidemiology and clinical features of melioidosis have been published by Kanai and Dejsirilert (1988), Leelarasamee and Bovornkitti (1989) and Dance (1991). I will restrict my discussion to those papers that have been published since these reviews.

From November 1990 to June 1991 there was a significant increase in the diagnosis of acute melioidosis in the Northern Territory, Australia (1993). Of 33 cases diagnosed during that time 25 were from Darwin, the capital city. The crude attack rate was 52/100 000 residents. Alcoholic (RR 6.7, CI 2.9–15.2) and diabetic (RR 12.9, CI 5.1–32.7) patients were at increased risk. A case-control study was unable to identify an environmental source for the outbreak. However, an environmental survey identified *B. pseudomallei* in 4% of soil samples and 9% of surface water samples.

Suputtamongkol *et al.* (1994) reported a study of the epidemiology of melioidosis in northeast Thailand over the years 1987–1991. They calculated rates based on diagnosed culture-positive cases and population data from recent censuses. The average incidence rates was 4.4/100 000, with the highest rate being 6.1. The disease was more common in males and in the 40–60 year age groups. The majority of patients had a pre-existing disease, of which diabetes was the commonest. There was a strong seasonal correlation with rainfall ($r = 0.7$, CI 0.5–0.9) and individuals who were occupationally exposed to soil and water (mainly rice farmers) were also at greater risk. This was most notable in the 40–59 year age group (RR 4.1, CI 2.4–6.9).

22 Legionnaires' Disease

The world first became aware of Legionnaires' disease after the 58th annual convention of the American Legion held in Philadelphia during July 1976 (Fraser *et al.* 1977). There were 182 cases of pneumonia, of which 29 were fatal. At the time of the outbreak there was almost a state of hysteria in the local press, with suggestions of foul play and foreign agents. Although it was soon shown to be due to a novel and entirely natural pathogen, the disease still exerts a major effect on the public's psyche when outbreaks occur.

MICROBIOLOGY

Legionella spp. are short, but occasionally filamentous, Gram-negative aerobic bacilli. Most species are motile. The bacteria require cysteine and iron for primary growth. The optimum temperature for growth is 35 °C (range 20–40 °C). About 40 species have now been described, but only 12 have been associated with disease in humans (Table 22.1). Several species have distinct lipopolysaccharide-based serogroups, *L. pneumophila* having 14.

PATHOGENESIS

Legionella spp. are thought to enter the lung by direct inhalation of aerosols. The infective dose is unknown, although air sampling during one outbreak suggested that a dose as low as one colony forming unit per 50 litres of air could still cause disease (Breiman *et al.* 1990). Aspiration down to the alveoli is presumably more likely in those individuals whose respiratory tract is damaged by pre-existing disease or smoking. Legionella are known to replicate within alveolar macrophages. Once pneumonia develops, the main form of defence is cellular immunity. For example, interferon-γ activated monocytes decrease the growth rate of intracellular organisms and natural killer cells will kill infected mononuclear cells.

Table 22.1 Species of legionella associated with disease in humans

Species	Number of serogroups	Illness
L. pneumophila	14	Pneumonia, Pontiac fever
L. anisa	1	Pneumonia
L. bozemanii	2	Pneumonia
L. cincinnatiensis	1	Pneumonia
L. dumoffii	1	Pneumonia
L. feeleii	2	Pneumonia, Pontiac fever
L. gormanii	1	Pneumonia
L. hackeliae	2	Pneumonia
L. longbeachae	2	Pneumonia
L. macaechernii	1	Pneumonia
L. micdadei	1	Pneumonia, Pontiac fever
L. wadsworthii	1	Pneumonia

CLINICAL FEATURES

The range of illness caused by legionellae is broad, the two typical disease syndromes being Legionnaires' disease and Pontiac fever.

Legionnaires' disease usually affects individuals with a pre-existing illness, such as diabetes, chronic lung or cardiac disease, smokers or the elderly. It has an incubation period of 2–10 days, after which there is fever, cough and prostration. Sputum may become blood streaked and there may be pleuritic pain. The pneumonia is not characteristic on chest X-ray. The severity of the illness typically reaches a peak after about 5 days, with high fever, severe prostration and mental confusion. Diarrhoea may be seen in up to half of cases. If the patient survives, recovery is slow. Complications include respiratory and renal failure.

Pontiac fever is a self-limiting influenza-like illness characterized by malaise, myalgia, fever, chills and headache. The incubation period is only one to two days. Attack rates are typically high and otherwise healthy individuals are affected. Pneumonia is absent.

DIAGNOSIS

Laboratory diagnosis in the acute stage of the disease rests on culture of the organism from sputum, bronchial secretions or lung biopsy. Culture should be on blood agar or a commercial legionella medium. However, culture is slow and only 80–90% sensitive. Other tests for diagnosis include the serological demonstration of seroconversion or high convalescent titres to specific *Legionella* spp. or serogroups, direct fluorescent antibody, urinary antigen or the use of DNA probes.

TREATMENT

Because of the difficulties in obtaining an early laboratory diagnosis, treatment should be started on the basis of clinical suspicion. The antimicrobial therapy of choice should be erythromycin in higher doses than usually given. Ciprofloxacin or rifampicin may added to the erythromycin to speed recovery. Pontiac fever patients recover without specific therapy.

ENVIRONMENTAL DETECTION

The most usual method for detection of *Legionella* spp. in water is by filtration, after which the filters are cut up and vortexed in 10 ml peptone saline diluent to resuspend the bacteria. This diluent is then centrifuged and 100 μl amounts of the deposit inoculated onto a legionella-selective agar (Collins, Lyne and Grange 1995). Highly contaminated samples can be treated by heating the deposit at 50 °C for 30 minutes or suspension in acid buffer.

Kusnetsov *et al.* (1994) reported a study of the comparison of various culture methods for the detection of *Legionella* spp. in water samples. They found that no one method was best in all situations, but depended on the type of water being analysed. Reinthaler *et al.* (1993) also found little difference between culture media.

If samples negative for *Legionella* spp. but positive for amoebae are incubated at 35 °C and recultured the detection rate can increase substantially (Sanden *et al.* 1992).

Alary and Joly (1992) compared direct immunofluorescence with culture for the detection of *Legionella* spp. in domestic homes. Compared to culture, immunofluorescence had a sensitivity of only 16.7–21.1% and specificity of 76.7–88.3%. They concluded that the latter technique was not adequate for detection of *Legionella* spp. in water. By contrast, a study of cooling tower waters found direct counting of bacteria by immunofluorescence to be more sensitive than culture (Yamamoto, Hashimoto and Ezaki 1993).

A polymerase chain reaction method for the detection of *Legionella* spp. in water samples has been described which has a greater than 50% sensitivity increase over culture and is considerably quicker (Catalan *et al.* 1994). In another study using PCR and culture methods to detect *Legionella* spp. in hospital waters, neither was found to be more sensitive (Maiwald *et al.* 1994). Of 78 samples tested, 57 (73%) were positive by both methods, 9 (11.5%) were positive by culture and negative by PCR and 9 (11.5%) were positive by PCR and negative by culture, all but 2 being positive by one method or the other. PCR also appears to be a reliable method for cooling tower waters (Koide *et al.* 1993; Yamamoto, Hashimoto and Ezaki 1993; Chang *et al.* 1995).

ECOLOGY

Legionella spp. are naturally aquatic organisms. They have been isolated from natural freshwaters, including rivers, streams, lakes, puddles and mud. They have also been isolated from waters in human environments and aquatic environments polluted by man such as thermal effluents, cooling tower waters, pluming systems and sewage-contaminated coastal waters (Fewtrell *et al.* 1994).

A study found *Legionella* spp. in raw and treated sewage and in ocean receiving waters five miles offshore, but not in seawater closer to the shore (Palmer *et al.* 1993b). Counts of legionella did not change during sewage treatment.

Alary and Joly (1991) took hot water samples from various points in private homes including showerheads, taps and water heaters. They found that 30% of homes had culture-positive *Legionella* spp. in at least one sample. *Legionella* spp. were not isolated from any of 33 oil or gas water heaters, but positive cultures were obtained from 39% of electric water heaters ($p <$ 0.0001). Logistic regression of risk factors for colonization of electric water heaters were: location of the home in an older part of the city ($p <$ 0.0001), owning an old water heater ($p = 0.003$) and having a low water temperature ($p = 0.05$). Contamination of peripheral outlets such as taps and showerheads was only associated with water heater contamination.

In Halifax, Nova Scotia, *Legionella* spp. were detected in water samples from 6 (8%) of 74 houses and 4 (25%) of 16 apartments (Marrie *et al.* 1994). Stout *et al.* (1992) found *Legionella* spp. in 14 (6%) of 218 homes surveyed. A positive detection was associated with lower hot water tank temperatures. None of the individuals living in these positive homes showed elevated legionella antibody levels. Zacheus and Martikainen (1994) found *Legionella* spp. in 30% of hot water distribution systems in 67 Finnish apartment buildings. Higher isolation rates were seen in those hot water systems using cold water processed in surface water plants than in those associated with groundwater. The authors suggested that this may be because of higher organic content in the former systems.

Perhaps because of the risk to immunocompromised patients, there has been much interest in the presence of *Legionella* spp. in hospital waters. Using both culture and PCR, Maiwald *et al.* (1994) found 75 (96%) of 78 hospital potable water samples to be positive. In a study of Nova Scotia hospitals, Marrie *et al.* (1994) reported that *Legionella* spp. were more likely to colonize the systems of older and larger (>50 beds) hospitals and those with total system recirculation.

Legionella spp. colonization of biofilms in water supply systems may be the reservoir for recolonization of water (Walker *et al.* 1993). This study also showed that copper piping is less likely than polyethylene to support the growth of *Legionella* spp. in biofilms.

EPIDEMIOLOGY

The first outbreak in Philadelphia during July 1976 affected 182 and killed 29 (Fraser *et al.* 1977). In many ways this outbreak was typical of many subsequent outbreaks. The disease tended to affect older smokers. The only other risk factor found in the case-control study was time spent in or just outside a particular hotel lobby. Based on this evidence, the authors suggested an airborne route of infection. In retrospect, this outbreak would probably have been due to aerosol contamination from a wet cooling and air conditioning system.

Soon after the description of the Philadelphia outbreak and the causative organism, Glick *et al.* (1978) re-assessed earlier outbreaks of unknown cause by using the newly available serological tests for Legionnaires' disease on stored sera. They found that one explosive outbreak of acute febrile illness at a health centre in Pontiac, Michigan, was associated with seroconversion to positive antibodies to *Legionella* spp. The outbreak of Pontiac fever affected at least 144 people, although with no deaths. At the time the investigations implicated a defective air conditioning system, but the mechanism of illness was unknown.

These two early outbreaks were typical, in that many subsequent outbreaks were traced to infected aerosols generated by inadequately maintained wet air conditioning systems. In particular, cooling towers have been major culprits. However, this was not the complete picture, since many outbreaks have also been shown to be due to contaminated aerosol from potable water sources such as showers (e.g. Cordes *et al.* 1981; Stout *et al.* 1982; Best *et al.* 1983) or mechanical humidifiers (e.g. Moiraghi *et al.* 1987). These have been major problems in hospitals and have been the cause of outbreaks among immunosuppressed individuals. So far, the outbreaks described have been due to aerosol spread and so are probably best thought of as airborne rather than waterborne. As such, most outbreaks of Legionnaires' disease fall outside the scope of this book. Good recent reviews of Legionnaires' disease have been produced by Hoge and Breiman (1991) and Quigley (1996). Further discussion of airborne outbreaks can be found in these reviews. There is no person-to-person transmission.

One source of outbreaks that has not yet been discussed is spa-pools and whirlpools. Although the mechanism of infection is still most probably inhalation of aerosols, the fact that individuals have immersed themselves in the source of these aerosols makes these outbreaks, in my view, water-associated and therefore within the scope of this book. The remainder of this section describes some of these outbreaks.

Perhaps the first outbreak linked to spa-pool use was in Michigan in 1982 (Mangione *et al.* 1985). Within two days of attending a racquetball party, 14 of 23 women developed features of Pontiac fever. All of the 14 ill women had used a spa-pool in the women's changing area, while the other 9 women had not ($p < 10^{-5}$). None of the 24 men attending the party was ill either. The investigators were able to identify 23 women who had used the spa-pool one week either side of the implicated party. Only 1 of these 23 had a compatible illness. Twenty of these twenty-three were interviewed as spa-pool controls. Compared to these controls, cases were likely to have visited the facility less often ($p < 0.01$) and to have spent longer in the spa-pool ($p < 0.05$). In addition, cases were more likely to report that more other women were using the pool at the same time. *L. pneumophila* was isolated from both men's and women's spa-pools. The concentration in the women's pool was 20 times greater. On the evening of the affected party, the spa-pool had been in use for longer than would normally have been the case. The spa-pool used bromine disinfection.

Bornstein *et al.* (1989) reported an outbreak of five cases of Legionnaires' disease among patients and therapists at a natural hot spring spa in eastern France. Sampling of the spa water yielded high counts of *L. pneumophila*. The spa area was then thoroughly cleaned and a prospective epidemiological study commenced. Because of the 'therapeutic properties' of the spa, it could not be chlorinated. Blood samples were taken from therapists, patients, administrative staff and blood donors from the area. Samples were taken from first-time patients at the beginning of their treatment period, at the end and four weeks later. Therapists at the spa had higher antibodies to several *Legionella* spp. than did patients, administrative staff or blood donors from the area. Although there were no cases of Legionnaires' disease during the three-month period, geometric mean antibody titres against *L. pneumophila* serogroup 3 among first-time patients increased from 8.1 (equal to blood donors) to 23.7 over the three samples. This confirmed that, despite the absence of overt disease, many patients were experiencing sub-clinical infection.

Three cases of Legionnaires' diseases were associated with exposure to a spa-pool in Vermont (Vogt *et al.* 1987). *L. pneumophila* serogroup 1 was isolated from one patient and from four of six samples from the spa-pool. The clinical and environmental strains were of the same electrophoretic type.

A large outbreak of a Pontiac fever-like syndrome affected 170 of 187 people who had visited a hotel and leisure complex in Lochgoilhead on the west coast of Scotland early in 1988 (Goldberg *et al.* 1989). The syndrome was slightly different from classic Pontiac fever in that symptoms were more prolonged and there was also breathlessness. The authors called the illness Lochgoilhead fever. *L. micdadei* was isolated from the spa-pool water by co-cultivation with *Acanthmoebea polyphaga*, and several cases were shown to seroconvert to this species. The spa-pool was disinfected with bromine. Records for bromination of the spa-pool were not kept, and on the day of inspection bromine levels were unrecordable.

During January 1991, six students became ill while attending a Vermont resort (Thomas, Mundy and Tucker 1993). The index case had diagnosed Legionnaires' disease, while the other five recovered fairly rapidly and were diagnosed as having suffered from Pontiac fever. High-titre convalescent antibodies were demonstrated in all six individuals. The case of Legionnaires' disease occurred in a student with diabetes, showing that the host is probably more important than the pathogen in determining whether an individual suffers from Legionnaires' disease or Pontiac fever. The authors considered a hot tub, the only common source exposure for all six, as being the likely cause of the outbreak. However, the tub had been emptied and disinfected before it could be sampled.

23   Leptospirosis

In the late 1980s there was a considerable flurry of interest in the UK popular press over the risks of leptospirosis. This interest led to unsubstantiated claims about the risks of the disease and the threats to human health of a supposed explosion in the rat population. Leptospirosis remains a feared disease, probably because of its mortality rate and its predilection for children and young adults.

Leptospirosis is a zoonosis and humans are usually infected by direct contact with animal urine or with waters contaminated with animal urine.

MICROBIOLOGY

Leptospira is one of two genera that are members of the family Leptospiraceae. They are flexible, regularly helical and motile organisms. They vary from 6–20 μm in length. They are obligate aerobes.

Currently three species are accepted: *L. interrogans*, *L. biflexa* and *L. parva*. *L. biflexa* and *L. parva* are non-pathogenic saprophytes and will not be discussed further. Within the pathogenic species *L. interrogans*, there are 22 serogroups and over 200 serotypes. (For the purposes of brevity, in this chapter these serotypes are written as though they are species names, i.e. *L. australis* rather than *L. interrogans* serotype *australis*.)

Some authors have proposed that *L. interrogans* be redefined into seven new species: *L. borgpetersenii*, *L. interrogans*, *L. meyeri*, *L. noguchii*, *L. santarosei*, *L. volbachii* and *L. weilii*.

PATHOGENESIS

Leptospires gain access to the bloodstream, either through intact mucous membrane, conjunctivae or damaged skin. Bacteraemia then carries the organisms to sites throughout the body including the liver, kidneys, CSF and eye. Multiplication at these sites is then responsible for end-stage disease. After infection many humans and animals can continue to excrete leptospires in the urine for some considerable time, so contaminating the environment and permitting further spread.

CLINICAL FEATURES

The incubation period is usually between 7 and 12 days, although this can range from 2 to 20 days.

The clinical presentation of infection depends in part on the infecting serotype. Nevertheless, sub-clinical infections are common during infection with all serotypes.

The illness has two stages: a septicaemic stage and an immune stage. The septicaemic stage presents as a non-specific flu-like illness, which lasts for three to seven days. There may be sudden onset of high fever, prostration, rigors and muscle pains. Headache and photophobia may suggest a meningitis, and vomiting and abdominal pain may suggest an acute abdominal emergency. There may also be respiratory symptoms. In severe cases thrombocytopenia may develop, leading to haemorrhage into the skin or from body cavities. Jaundice may develop at this stage. At the end of this period the temperature settles. Death is uncommon during this first stage.

About three days or so after resolution of the fever associated with the first stage, antibody levels are detected in the serum. There may then be a marked deterioration in clinical symptoms. The most common features are muscle tenderness, rash, conjunctival suffusion, hepatosplenomegaly and adenopathy. There may be a lymphocytic meningitis and patients may develop confusion and delirium. In those patients with jaundice it may deepen at this stage. Features of respiratory, renal and cardiac damage may be seen. Death occurs in 10–20% of patients during this stage. Recovery is seen from about three weeks, although leptospires may be found in the urine of untreated patients for up to 40 days. Complete recovery is the rule.

DIAGNOSIS

Diagnosis early in the course of the disease is rarely helped by laboratory investigations and must rely on clinical features and a history of water contact. Occasionally leptospires can be seen in blood or freshly voided urine but detection by these methods is of poor sensitivity and false positive results are not unknown.

The diagnosis is confirmed later in the course of illness by serology. Seroagglutination tests become positive about 6–12 days after the onset of symptoms. ELISA tests to detect both IgG and IgM antibodies are now the preferred diagnostic tool.

TREATMENT

Most cases recover spontaneously even without antibiotic therapy. Nevertheless, antibiotics are usually given when the diagnosis is suspected. Benzylpenicillin is the drug of choice, although tetracycline, sulphonamides and erythromycin also have some effect. Where illness is more severe, supportive therapies such as blood transfusion and renal dialysis may be needed.

ENVIRONMENTAL DETECTION

The isolation of leptospires from water samples is a time-consuming process. Larger bacterial contaminants are first removed by filtration and the sample is then cultured in selective liquid medium containing 5-fluorouracil at 30 °C for up to three months (Fewtrell et al. 1994). The medium is examined by dark-ground microscopy each week. Once the concentration of leptospires reaches about 10^6 spirochaetes per millilitre the stain can be tested for virulence. However, isolation of leptospires from water rarely gives any worthwhile information as non-pathogenic leptospires are common and the distribution of both pathogenic and non-pathogenic strains in waters is patchy.

ECOLOGY

As already mentioned, leptospires are zoonotic organisms that are excreted in the urine of infected animals. The distribution of pathogenic strains in the environment reflects the likelihood of contamination by urine of infected animals. In favourable conditions, leptospires can survive for several days in freshwater (Fewtrell et al. 1994). Survival is best at low temperatures (5–6 °C), neutral or slightly alkaline pH and in stagnant rather than running waters. Leptospires can survive in diluted cow's urine for up to 35 days and urine-saturated soil for six months.

EPIDEMIOLOGY

Infection by leptospirosis depends on direct contact with urine of an infected animal. The various serotypes tend to prefer particular animal groups and the dominant serotype in any country tends to differ. For example, in the UK the dominant serotypes are L. icterohaemorrhagiae, which tends to be carried by rats, and L. hardjo, which is carried by cattle. Consequently, L. icterohaemorrhagiae infection in the UK was traditionally associated with sewer workers, but as a result of improved health education and protective clothing of these workers it is now more likely to be seen in people who have recreational water contact. From 1980 to 1989 there were 178 reported L. icterohaemorrhagiae infections in the UK, of which 57 were water-related, and only 8 were in sewage workers. Of 241 infections by L. hardjo in the same period, 191 were in farmers or were farm-related. In the US the most important serotype is

L. canicola, which is associated with dogs. In recent years many serotypes have all but disappeared from some countries. Up to 1970, *L. pomona*, a pig-associated serotype, was the main strain in Switzerland, but it has now disappeared.

Drinking water outbreaks

I was only able to find one reported outbreak of leptospirosis associated with drinking water. This outbreak was identified in a small town in central Italy following the death of a 38-year-old male in July 1984 (Cacciapuoti *et al.* 1987). Over the next few weeks there were two more deaths. A total of 33 serologically confirmed (antibody > 1:1000, *L. australis*) cases, of whom one died, were identified. In addition, there were 24 unconfirmed cases of fever, of whom two died. In a case-control study of 18 confirmed cases and 36 age-, sex- and neighbourhood-matched controls, the only significant finding was drinking water from a local fountain ($p < 0.001$). Microbiological examination of water from this fountain found 140 faecal coliforms per 100 ml. During inspection of the water system to this fountain, a previously unknown additional reservoir was discovered. In this reservoir was a dead hedgehog. Eighteen serologically positive patients from this outbreak were followed up for five years (Lupidi *et al.* 1991). It was found that, in some individuals, peak antibody titres developed over a period of some months. Antibody was still detectable after 54 months in 2 of 15 cases.

Outbreaks associated with water contact

During June and August 1964, 61 cases of leptospirosis occurred in teenagers in southeastern Washington (Nelson *et al.* 1973). Serological investigations showed this outbreak to be due to *L. pamona*. All 61 serologically positive cases, 53 males and 8 females, gave a history of swimming at a certain point of a local irrigation canal. Analysis of questionnaire data from the five nearest schools showed that 16% of male students and 4.3% of female students reported swimming in the canal at this point. Inspection of the canal found a herd of 300 cattle, which had access to the water upstream of the suspect area. *L. pamona* was isolated from the canal near the cattle herd. Of 25 serum samples collected from cattle in the herd, 19 had antibodies against *L. pamona*.

Seven cases of leptospirosis were diagnosed in Stewart County, Tennessee during the first ten days of August 1975 (Anderson *et al.* 1978). Serological investigation showed antibodies to *L. grippotyphosa* in all seven. All cases were between 11 and 16 years old and all gave a history of swimming in a local creek. A further ten patients were identified with a similar illness but for whom serological investigations were negative. A case-control study of 16 proven and compatible illnesses identified swimming in the suspect creek as the only risk factor ($p = 0.005$). No leptospires were isolated from water samples. Serological examination of dogs belonging to affected cases was negative. Interviews with farmers identified no illness in local cattle. A serological study of five cattle herds in the area found only one cow to be positive for *L. grippotyphosa*. This cow was part of a herd that pastured in the vicinity of the swimming area, which also had direct access to the water.

The death of a worker on a trout farm in the UK from leptospirosis in 1980 stimulated an investigation of the farm (Robertson *et al.* 1981). Of eight other workers, four had a flu-like illness during the previous month, one of whom also had jaundice. Serological examinations showed that the second worker with jaundice had high titre antibody levels to *L. icterohaemorrhagiae*, while the remaining three had low-level antibodies. One of the four healthy workers also had low-level antibodies. Inspection of the farm found many rat holes along the banks of the ponds and dead trout floating near the edge. The shed where the trout food was stored was not rat-proofed and the food sacks were torn and their contents spilled on the floor. It was not clear whether the workers had been infected while handling food contaminated with rat urine or from contact with infected water while working in the pools.

The semi-tropical island of Okinawa, Japan, was the location for an outbreak affecting US military personnel during September 1987 (Corwin *et al.* 1990). As defined by a serological result of ≥ 200, there were 22 infected individuals, of whom 9 were symptomatic. Descriptive epidemiological studies suggested two separate clusters of illness. In the first cluster, seven laboratory-confirmed cases were identified among 13 individuals (53.8%) who had been swimming at a place called Aha Falls. All of the infected individuals in this group admitted to swallowing water, compared to only one of the six unaffected individuals ($p < 0.01$). In the second cluster, 15 of 82 (18.3%) who participated in combat training in a particular training area were infected, though only four were symptomatic. Again, there was a significant association between infection and swallowing water ($p < 0.05$). In neither cluster was simple immersion in water a risk factor.

During the summer of 1987, eight individuals were identified with flu-like illness and serological evidence of leptospirosis on the island of Kauai, Hawaii (Katz, Manea and Sasaki 1991). Six were shown by serology to have an *L. australis* infection, one an *L. bataviae* and one an *L. fort bragg* infection. All eight had been swimming in a local river. A few months before the human outbreak there had been several spontaneous abortions in cattle pastured adjacent to the swimming area. However, serological examination of the herd found eight with antibodies to *L. hardjo* and only one to *L. bataviae*. Therefore the link to this herd must be tenuous for most cases.

Early in July 1991 five boys from a small town in rural Illinois developed serologically confirmed leptospirosis due to *L. grippotyphosa* (Jackson *et al.* 1993). All five boys had been swimming in a particular location, compared to only 14 of 50 well children of similar ages ($p < 0.01$). Analytical epidemiology was unable to identify any other risk factors such as swallowing water during swimming. *L. grippotyphosa* was isolated from water samples taken from the suspect swimming area and 4 of 14 cattle tested in the area were serologically positive for *L. grippotyphosa*.

Prospective epidemiological studies

Caldas and Sampaio (1979) reported a sero-epidemiological study of 133 patients admitted to the infectious disease hospital in Salvador, Brazil. The fatality rate was 7.5%. Most cases occurred in months with the highest rainfall. The most likely sources of infection were suggested, in decreasing order of significance, as sewage, rats, water, dogs, mud and garbage.

To investigate the role that occupational factors could play in the risk of leptospirosis, Chan *et al.* (1987) investigated sera from 80 sewer and 120 public cleansing workers in Singapore. The sewer workers included sewer and sewage treatment works maintenance staff. The public cleansing workers included refuse collection workers and street and market cleaners. Sera from 100 controls were also examined. The incidence of infection as measured by a titre of >1:25 was 50.0% in public cleansing workers, 38.8% in sewer workers and 30.0% in controls. High antibody titres (>1:100) were found in 20.8% of public cleansing workers, 15.0% of sewer workers and 3.0% of controls. The subgroup with the highest rate was the market cleaners, perhaps suggesting greater contact with areas with high rat populations, because of discarded food.

A serological survey for leptospiral antibodies between 1980 and 1983 was done on 500 Barbadian and 500 Trinidadian schoolchildren aged 7–14 years (Everard, Hayes and Edwards 1989). The children were a random selection from various urban and rural schools. Blood samples were taken three times at approximately yearly intervals. At the initial survey 9.5% of the Trinidadian and 12.5% of the Barbadian children were positive for leptospire antibodies. The only risk factors for initial seropositivity was father's occupation in Trinidad. Incidence was highest in the children of labourers and agricultural workers ($p < 0.05$). In Trinidad there were 14 and in Barbados there were 3 seroconversions over the period of the study. The average annual incidence rates of seroconversion were 2.2, 4.9 and 13.3 per 100 000 in the 5–9, 10–14 and 15–19 age groups, respectively. Children living in a house without a tap ($p = 0.001$) and having livestock in the yard ($p = 0.01$) were independently associated with increased risk of seroconversion.

Another sero-epidemiological survey, this time in France, was reported by Andre-Fontaine, Peslerbe and Ganiere (1992). They studied sera from 26 young people involved in watersports such as canoeing and 58 individuals who worked on one of two local waterways. Using a titre of 1:40 as the positive cut-off point for the serological test, they found that 29% of the maintenance staff and 8% of the sports people were positive, although this was not statistically significant.

Sasaki *et al.* (1993) described an active surveillance programme designed to determine morbidity and risk factors in Hawaii. The study took place over two years, 1988 and 1989. The study covered Big Island and Kauai. On Big Island alone there were 20 serologically proven cases, giving an incidence rate of 128 cases per 100 000 person-years. There were two deaths. An additional 13 cases were identified from Kauai. All 33 cases were enrolled in a case-control study with 77 controls who presented with similar symptoms but in whom leptospirosis was excluded on the basis of serological tests. The majority (96%) of individuals in the case-control study were males. Household use of rain-water catchment systems ($p = 0.003$), presence of skin cuts during the incubation period ($p = 0.008$), contact with animal tissues ($p = 0.005$) and contact with cattle ($p = 0.05$) and cattle urine ($p = 0.03$) were all associated with an increased risk of leptospirosis. There was no significant association between leptospirosis and swimming in, or other contact with, fresh waters.

COMMENTS

Although generally causing only mild illness, some leptospires, especially *L. icterohaemorrhagiae*, can cause fatal disease. Furthermore, antibiotics are not always effective. Nevertheless, the risk of illness must be kept in proportion. Between 1981 and 1992 there were only 67 cases, with a mortality of 10–15%, of *L. icterohaemorrhagiae* infection associated with watersports and immersion in the UK. The British Canoe Union has estimated the risk of a canoeist dying of leptospirosis to be 1:330 000.

As with many diseases, prevention is better than cure. Individuals with occupational exposure to potentially infected waters should be educated about the risks and given appropriate protective clothing. Groups interested in water recreational activities should also be educated and advised about appropriate waters for their sports.

24   Mycobacterial Disease

Two mycobacterial diseases have had a profound effect on human history. The first, tuberculosis, was once described as the Captain of the Men of Death to reflect its importance as the leading cause of death in previous centuries. The other, leprosy, had once of the worst social stigmas associated with any disease. Fortunately, I can find no evidence that either is waterborne. Those *Mycobacteria* spp. that have been implicated in waterborne transmission are generally known as atypical mycobacteria or mycobacteria other than tuberculosis (MOTT).

Mycobacteria associated with water present an interesting spectrum of disease. Some, such as *M. ulcerans*, are pathogenic in previously healthy individuals; others, such as *M. avium*, usually cause disease only in compromised individuals, especially those with AIDS; and some, like *M. kansasii* rarely cause disease even when isolated in clinical specimens. The latter group is still potentially dangerous when it confuses diagnosis and leads to people being treated with weeks or months of unnecessary anti-tuberculous therapy.

MICROBIOLOGY

Mycobacteria are aerobic or microaerophilic, straight or slightly curved bacilli. They are acid-fast on staining with the Ziehl–Neelsen method. They differ from other bacteria by having a thick, complex cell wall containing mycolic acid. Many species grow only very slowly.

There are some 50 species described. These are usually speciated by physiological and biochemical differences, such as speed of growth, optimal temperature for growth and whether pigment is produced in the light, in the dark or not at all. Table 24.1 shows some characteristics of species that have been associated with waterborne spread.

PATHOGENESIS

The pathogenesis of atypical mycobacterial disease depends on the infecting agent and the site of infection. The two infections that are primary skin diseases (*M. marinum* and *M. ulcerans*) follow inoculation of the bacterium

Table 24.1 Characteristics of *M. tuberculosis* and some mycobacteria associated with waterborne spread. Adapted from Collins, Lyne and Grange (1995)

Species	Pigment[a]	Growth at (°C):					Rate of growth[b]
		20	25	33	42	45	
M. tuberculosis	N	−	−	+	−	−	S
M. avium	N	V	+	+	+	V	S
M. fortuitum	N	+	+	+	V	−	R
M. gordonae	S	+	+	+	−	−	S
M. marinum	P	+	+	+	−	−	R
M. scrofulaceum	S	V	+	+	+	−	S
M. terrae	N	V	+	+	−	−	S
M. ulcerans	V	−	−	+	−	−	S
M. xenopi	V	−	−	−	+	+	S

V, variable.
[a] N, no pigment; P, photochromogen; S, scotochromogen.
[b] R, rapid; S slow.

into the skin. Other infections probably follow from inhalation. Virulence factors are poorly understood for the mycobacteria. However, the robust nature of these organisms, largely due to their thick wall and capsule, and their resistance to many natural defence mechanisms must play a significant role in disease causation.

CLINICAL FEATURES

The clinical features of the various mycobacteria are very varied. The two main diseases associated with this genus are tuberculosis and leprosy. Both are chronic diseases that continue to cause considerable suffering worldwide. The presentation of each can also vary markedly from one patient to another. Fortunately, neither appears to be transmitted by water. Those interested in the clinical features of mycobacterial disease would be well advised to consult a more detailed description. I will only give a thumbnail sketch of the clinical features associated with the mycobacteria whose epidemiology is discussed later in the chapter.

The clinical presentation of *M. avium* is often vague. In non-AIDS patients symptoms include cough, sputum production, weight loss, fever and haemoptysis. Chest radiographic appearance may be similar to tuberculosis. AIDS patients may suffer from similar symptoms but may also develop disseminated disease. In disseminated disease, weight loss and fever are more severe and the patient may complain of drenching night sweats. There may be also diarrhoea, malaise, anorexia and anaemia. *M. xenopi* can also produce chest disease similar to tuberculosis, although most infections are asymptomatic.

M. fortuitum has been implicated in the causation of a wide variety of clinical syndromes affecting several body systems. The outbreaks discussed below were associated with both respiratory disease and wound infections.

M. marinum infection usually follows injury in association with contact with water from aquaria, swimming pools or other sources. The incubation period is two to three weeks. The infection presents initially as a small papule, which gradually enlarges and develops a blue-purple colour. The papule may suppurate or ulcerate. Dissemination has been reported but is uncommon. *M. ulcerans* causes extensive, chronic and relatively painless ulcers. The ulcer usually develops over about six weeks.

DIAGNOSIS

Diagnosis may be suggested by seeing acid-fast bacilli in sputum or during the histological examination of biopsy specimens. Diagnosis is confirmed by culture on appropriate media such as Lowenstein–Jensen solid medium or in Kirchner's liquid medium. However, growth may be slow and slopes should be incubated at 37 °C for at least eight weeks. Several of the atypical bacteria grow better at 30 °C and culture should be performed at both these temperatures if *M. marinum* or *M. ulcerans* is suspected.

A useful adjunct to diagnosis is skin testing with purified protein derivatives of various species.

TREATMENT

There are a variety of anti-tuberculous drugs available which are effective against some, but not all, of the waterborne mycobacterial species. However, treatment may need to be prolonged for as much as two years. There is also a high failure rate. Surgical excision may be necessary for some cases.

ENVIRONMENTAL DETECTION

For culture for mycobacteria in water samples, 1–10 l of water is filtered through a membrane filter with a 3 μm pore size (Kubalek and Komenda 1995). The filter is then shaken in sterile phosphate-buffered saline to resuspend any organisms. The saline is then centrifuged to concentrate the mycobacteria. The deposit may be treated with NaOH to kill other bacteria and is then cultured onto Lowenstein–Jensen slopes as for clinical specimens.

Alugupalli *et al.* (1992) described a gas chromatography–mass spectrometry method for detecting *M. xenopi* in drinking water. The method was rapid, but not as sensitive as culture.

ECOLOGY

Various mycobacteria are widely distributed in both natural and treated waters. Wallace (1987) reviewed the available literature up to that point. Studies of the isolation of mycobacteria from surface waters include a study of 100 surface waters (river and canal) and tap-waters sampled in Bangkok (Imwidthaya *et al.* 1989). The authors isolated *M. fortuitum* on 18 occasions and *M. chelonei* once. They also isolated *M. fortuitum* 57 times from 100 soil samples, *M. chelonei* twice and *M. gordonae* once. The were unable to isolate mycobacteria from any of 30 swimming pools. Sabater and Zaragoza (1993) reported on the identification of 15 strains of *M. gordonae* and 10 strains of *M. avium* isolated from surface waters in Spain. Von Reyn *et al.* (1993) reported on a study comparing the isolation of *M. avium* from surface and mains water at two locations in the USA, Finland, Zaire and Kenya. In New Hampshire, USA, *M. avium* was isolated from 33% of environmental samples. The rate for Boston was 38%, for Finland 37%, for Zaire 33% and for Kenya 12%.

Kirschner, Parker and Falkinham (1992) studied the isolation of MOTT from soil and water samples taken from four sites in the USA. Two sites were acid swamps and two were freshwater sites. MOTT were isolated more frequently from the acid swamp environments. Isolation rates were also higher in warmer temperatures.

In a study of surface waters in Finland, *M. avium–intracellulare–scrofulaceum* complex were isolated from 40% of stream-water samples at concentrations of between 50 and 1400 CFU/l (Katila *et al.* 1995). *M. malmoense* was isolated from two samples.

Eaton *et al.* (1995) cultured *M. avium* from three of seven (43%) water and three of seven soil samples collected in Kampala, Uganda. The average number of colony forming units was 3.3/ml for water and 7825/g for soil. The strains isolated were similar to strains isolated from AIDS patients in Europe, despite the previous findings that *M. avium* does not appear to infect AIDS patients in Uganda (Morrissey *et al.* 1992).

Several studies have reported on the isolation of *Mycobacteria* spp. from tap-water. For example, Imwidthaya *et al.* (1989) isolated *M. gordonae* from 3 of 30 samples of Bangkok tap-water. Du Moulin *et al.* (1988) cultured water from hot and cold taps on two temporarily vacant floors in a hospital. *M. avium* was cultured from 11 of 16 hot and 3 of 18 cold water samples. Counts in hot water samples were as high as 500 CFU/100 ml. The hot water taps had an average temperature of 55 °C. In their study of isolation rates in several countries, Von Reyn *et al.* (1993) reported isolating *M. avium* in 17% of mains water samples from New Hampshire, 25% from Boston, 45% from Finland, 20% from Zaire and 0% from Kenya.

Peters *et al.* (1995) cultured hot and cold tap samples from two hospitals and four homes in Berlin. Of 118 samples, 42.4% grew *Mycobacteria* spp.

Over half, 33 of 64 isolates, were *M. gordonae*. Also isolated were *M. chelonae* (9), *M. gastri* (6), unnamed rapid growing mycobacteria (6), *M. kansasii* (2), *M. fortuitum* (2), *M. avium* (2), *M. flavescens* (2), *M. malmoense* (1) and *M. xenopi* (1).

Yajko *et al.* (1995) studied the home environments of 290 patients with HIV infection in San Francisco. *M. avium* was isolated from just one (0.19%) water and one (0.25%) food sample. By contrast, *M. avium* was isolated from 27% of soil samples taken from patients' potted plants. Several of the soil samples matched types of *M. avium* isolated from patients themselves.

At least in the Czech Republic, there is a seasonal variation in the colonization of mycobacteria in potable water systems (Kubalek and Komenda 1995; Kubalek, Komenda and Mysak 1995). They demonstrated that water samples were more likely to yield rapid growing *Mycobacteria* spp. in the spring than in the autumn ($p < 0.05$).

An important study by Schulze-Robbecke, Janning and Fischeder (1992) found that 90% of 50 biofilm samples were positive for *Mycobacteria* spp. These biofilm samples had been collected from water treatment plants, domestic water supply systems and aquaria. Counts were quite high, up to 5.6 $\times$ 10^6 CFU/cm^2, and were higher on plastic and rubber materials than on copper and glass.

The aquatic mycobacteria are highly resistant to disinfectants used in water treatment (Carson *et al.* 1978; Pelletier, du Moulin and Stottmeier 1988). Although the resistance varies, many are also relatively resistant to high temperatures (Schulze-Robbecke and Buchholtz 1992). In particular, two significant pathogens, *M. avium* and *M. xenopi*, are more thermoresistant than *Legionella pneumophila*.

EPIDEMIOLOGY

Tuberculosis is spread from person to person or via contamination of the environment, although waterborne spread has not been recorded to my knowledge. Several of the other species of mycobacteria have been associated with waterborne spread. The published literature on waterborne mycobacterial disease is grouped by the implicated species.

M. avium complex

From 1972 to 1983 the isolation of *M. avium* complex increased fivefold in Massachusetts (du Moulin *et al.* 1985). In 1972 *M. avium* was isolated from 0.19% samples and in 1983 from 0.91% of samples. The incidence rate in various communities increased with the size of the community. Independent of community size, incidence rates were higher in those communities that received their water supplies from a particular company (3.93 versus 2.12

cases per 100 000, p < 0.001). This company's water was taken from a series of watersheds and then transported up to 65 miles through an ageing distribution system. *M. avium* was isolated from this supply.

Horsburgh *et al.* (1994) reported a case-control study of *M. avium* infections in 83 patients with HIV disease and 177 HIV-positive but *M. avium*-negative controls. All patients were adults who attended the San Francisco General Hospital. Among other possible risk factors, the authors asked about drinking home tap-water, filtered water, bottled water and untreated water. They also enquired about swimming, daily showering, baths, visits to the beach, use of hot tubs, spas or whirlpools and recent plumbing repairs. In the final multivariate model, having a positive *M. avium* blood culture was positively associated with having a low CD4+ count (OR 3.58, CI 1.71–7.49) and eating hard cheese (OR 5.63, CI 1.58–20.1) and negatively associated with daily showering (OR 0.58, CI 0.28–0.88). Risk factors for having *M. avium* in sputum included consumption of raw shellfish (OR 7.28, CI 1.63–32.6) and intravenous drug use (OR 3.72, CI 1.32–10.5). Daily showering (OR 0.27, CI 0.09–0.79) and having a cat (OR 0.27, CI 0.09–0.85) were negatively associated with the risk of sputum carriage. None of the other water risk factors was associated with risk in either univariate or multivariate models.

In another American study, von Reyn *et al.* (1994) studied multiple isolates of *M. avium* from 36 patients with HIV infection and CD4 counts of less than $200/\mu l$. Strains were characterized by pulse field gel electrophoresis. Of the 36 patients, 29 (81%) were infected with one or more strain of *M. avium*. Of 25 patients from whom more than one isolate was available, 5 (20%) carried more than one distinct strain. *M. avium* was also isolated from 10 (30%) of 33 water samples in one study and from hot water samples at the two main hospitals. Four strain groups were identified. Group 1 strains were isolated from three patients at hospital A with symptomatic disseminated *M. avium* infection. Group 1 strains were also isolated from two water samples from hospital A, but not from the patients' homes. There were two patients with group 2 strains and both had been treated at hospital B. Group 2 strains were isolated from hospital B on three separate occasions. Group 3 strains were isolated from two patients but not from environmental samples. Group 4 strains were isolated from one patient and a river, although no information was available about possible contacts with the river. The isolation of group 1 and 2 strains from patients and from water from the hospitals where they were treated but not from other sites is strong circumstantial evidence of waterborne spread.

M. fortuitum

Burns *et al.* (1991) described an outbreak of *M. fortuitum* infections on a alcoholism rehabilitation unit between August 1989 and January 1990. A total of 16 patients were identified. In a case-control study cases were more likely to report having chronic bronchitis (OR 6.6, CI 1.5–28.6), to have ever used shower number 2 (OR 5.6, CI 1.2–25.8) and to have eaten ice on the ward (OR 6.6, CI 1.5–28.3). The ice-making machine was removed from the ward early in the outbreak because the nursing supervisor had noted a brown scum on several of its components. *M. fortuitum* was isolated from one of the showers, a hot tap on an adjacent ward that used the same feed as the showers and an evaporator on an ice machine. However, typing of both human and environmental strains by pulsed field gel electrophoresis showed that only the isolate from the tap was the same type as the clinical isolates.

Using DNA methods to type strains from four nosocomial outbreaks, Hector *et al.* (1992) showed that environmental strains from two outbreaks were found that were identical to one or more outbreak strains. The first was an outbreak of sternal wound infections in Texas (Kuritsky *et al.* 1983). The same strain was isolated from both clinical samples and several water samples taken from the hospital, including municipal water coming into the hospital, water from a cold-water tap in the operating room, water used to cool cardioplegia solution in the operating room and water in an ice machine. The second outbreak was that described above, of 20 respiratory infections (Burns *et al.* 1991).

M. gordonae

Panwalker and Fuhse (1986) reported a marked increase in the isolation of *M. gordonae* from clinical specimens from a single hospital. From July 1980 to June 1981 they isolated this organism on 32 occasions compared to only 7 isolates in the previous 54 months. Few, if any, patients exhibited a compatible disease. Extensive environmental sampling implicated ice machines as the source. Improved maintenance and cleaning of the ice machines led to a marked reduction in the isolation of *M. gordonae* from clinical samples.

M. marinum

Most infections with *M. marinum* are associated with water contact, usually swimming pools or aquaria (Collins, Lyne and Grange 1985). Although there have been outbreaks of swimming pool granuloma due to *M. marinum*, most cases from aquaria and other sources are sporadic. Iredell, Whitby and Blacklock (1992) reported on all cases of *M. marinum* infection that presented in Queensland, Australia, during the 20 years from 1971 to 1990. They identified 29 patients from whom *M. marinum* had been isolated. There were three times as many cases in males as in females. Of 25 patients with sufficient information, 5 (20%) had contact with fish tanks and 9 with marine or surface water or fish.

M. scrofulaceum

One study set out to investigate the epidemiology of MOTT by skin testing of military recruits in Greece (Dascalopoulos, Loukas and Constantopoulos 1995). Initially, 508 recruits were tested with five sensitins (*M. tuberculosis*, *M. scrofulaceum*, *M. intracellulare*, *M. avium* and *M. kansasii*). Of these 508, 94 (18.5%) had a reaction to one or more sensitin. Of the non-tuberculosis sensitins, the commonest positive reaction was seen for *M. scrofulaceum*, so further testing was restricted to *M. tuberculosis* and *M. scrofulaceum*. In the subsequent study of 17 403 recruits, 7.0% were considered to have been previously infected with MOTT alone, 8.9% with tuberculosis and 3.8% with both. The prevalence of past tuberculosis did not differ much between areas of Greece. However, MOTT positivity was commoner on islands and near the sea when compared to mountainous areas (7.05 versus 4.08, *p* < 0.001). Furthermore, in non-mountainous inland areas, MOTT prevalence was higher near big rivers.

M. terrae

Lockwood *et al.* (1989) reported a sudden increase of isolations of *M. terrae* from clinical samples taken from patients at a single hospital in 1986. Altogether, they identified 163 positive samples from 131 patients; no patient appeared to suffer from disease related to this organism. The authors were able to isolate *M. terrae* from water taken from several sites in the water distribution system within the hospital. Hyperchlorination of the water supply and advice on avoiding contact with water when taking samples terminated this pseudo-outbreak.

M. ulcerans

M. ulcerans infections are essentially restricted to tropical countries. They have been reported from Australia, several African countries, Central and South America, New Guinea, Malaysia and Sumatra (Barker 1973; Hayman 1991). As early as 1973, it was realized that the infection was more common in those areas near major rivers or swamps (Barker 1973). Evidence during investigations of an outbreak in the Kinyara refugee settlement, Uganda, found no evidence of person to person transmission (Uganda Buruli Group 1971). The Kinyara refugee settlement was within four miles of the Nile and the infection rate in women was higher in those living closer to the river, even though few of the refugees visited the river.

Barker and Carswell (1973) reported a study of the prevalence of Buruli ulcers in tsetse fly control workers in Uganda. The tsetse control division employed 170 men, who lived with their families in camps scattered along the west bank of the River Nile. During the study 47 cases of Buruli ulcer were identified in 170 families. Compared to those families whose source of water was boreholes, the attack rate was higher in those taking water from seasonal swamps (RR 4.2, CI 1.4–12.2) and even higher in those taking water from permanent swamps (RR 8.8, CI 3.3–23.6).

Oluwasanmi et al. (1976) reported on 24 cases of M. ulcerans infection in Ibadan, Nigeria. Fourteen cases were in people who lived or worked at the University of Ibadan. It was noted that although the university had been in existence for some 25 years, cases of Buruli ulcer only started to appear in university people when a stream running through the university grounds was dammed to create a fish pond. Cases were more common in people who visited or lived near this pond.

Based on his experience of working in Bairnsdale, Australia, Hayman (1991) has proposed a mechanism for the epidemiology of M. ulcerans infections. He noted that the number of cases of infection during the 1980s was much greater than in previous decades after 1950. The increase in cases followed two years after severe flooding of local rainforest. Basically, he suggested that the normal habitat of M. ulcerans is certain plants in rainforest. However, following disruption of the forest by fire or flood, the organism is washed into streams and lakes, where it multiplies. Dispersal from this aquatic environment either back into the forest or to infect man is by aerosol spread.

Following reports of an increasing incidence of Buruli ulcer in West Africa, Marston et al. (1995) investigated the epidemiology of the disease in a rural area of the Cote d'Ivoire. The authors identified 312 patients with active or healed ulcers and were told of 14 others who had died. Most of the lesions were situated on the legs or arms (92%). In the villages surveyed the prevalence ranged from 0 to 16%, with the incidence higher in those villages nearer to the Lobo River. In a multivariate analysis of a case-control study with 46 cases and 90 controls, disease was associated with living closer to the river (for every 10 minutes walk closer to the river OR 1.52, CI 1.01–2.28) and negatively associated with wearing long trousers (OR 0.20, CI 0.06–0.62).

M. xenopi

During the years 1980–1983, M. xenopi was isolated from 37 patients in northern Bohemia, Czechoslovakia (Horák, Poláková and Králová 1986). Thirty of these patients lived in the regional town. Only 7 of the 37 patients had pulmonary disease, and sputum culture was repeatedly positive in 5 of these 7. The authors reported isolating M. xenopi from tap-water from the homes of five of nine patients and one of two controls.

During a 12-year (1978–1989) survey of the isolation of M. xenopi in Israel, it was noted that most strains came from patients attending a single hospital (Lavy, Rusu and Mates 1992). Subsequent investigations identified the organism in the hot water system of the hospital.

Another study from the Czech Republic looked at 21 excreters of *M. xenopi* identified in Prague during 1990 (Šlosárek, Kubín and Jarešová 1993). In 13 cases, culture was positive on repeat occasions, and all of these cases had severe respiratory disease. Water samples from the flats of 11 of these people were positive for *M. xenopi*, as were samples from 5 of 17 adjoining flats. *M. xenopi* was not isolated from the distribution network.

An Indiana general hospital, which had previously never submitted a culture of *M. xenopi* for identification, submitted 13 strains over a 13-month period starting in June 1990 (Sniadack *et al.* 1993). Initial microscopy was negative on all positive specimens and no patient was though to be suffering from disease related to *M. xenopi*. In a case-control study it was shown that specimens collected in a non-sterile manner were more likely to be positive (3.1% versus 0%, OR ∞, $p = 0.003$). *M. xenopi* was isolated from tap-water, and all positives were though to be related to specimen collection being contaminated by tap-water. For example, bronchoscopes were rinsed in tap-water after disinfection, patients gargled with tap-water before giving a sputum sample and bed pans were rinsed in tap-water before use. This pseudo-outbreak is an important reminder that correct specimen collection is extremely important in microbiology. Five of these patients received anti-tuberculous therapy for between one and six months – a costly and potentially toxic treatment regime for a disease that was not present.

25 Tularaemia

Tularaemia is the disease associated with infection by the bacterial pathogen *Francisella tularensis*. The infection occurs in many parts of the Northern Hemisphere. It is a zoonotic infection of rodents and birds, and has been given several exotic names, such as rabbit fever, deer fly fever and water-rat trappers's disease.

MICROBIOLOGY

The causative organism, *F. tularensis*, is a small, Gram-negative, aerobic, pleomorphic coccobacillus. The organism requires cysteine for growth.

At various times *F. tularensis* has been classified as a *Pasteurella* and a *Brucella* organism. There are two species in the genus, *F. tularensis* and *F. philomiragia*. There are two biogroups of *F. tularensis*, *F. tularensis* biogroup *tularensis* and a low virulence biogroup *F. tularensis* biogroup *novicida*. There are also two biotypes of *F. tularensis* biogroup *tularensis*, the more virulent American biotype A or *nearctica* and the less virulent American, European and Asian biotype B or *holarctica*. These two biotypes are indistinguishable by serology.

PATHOGENESIS

F. tularensis is a highly virulent pathogen. The exact infectious dose varies according to the route of infection. If infection is through a skin abrasion or by inhalation, it is about 10–50 organisms. Following ingestion the infectious dose is up to 10^8 organisms.

Initially, organisms reproduce at the site of entry for three to five days. From here there is spread to regional lymph nodes, followed by bacteraemia. Disseminated infection can affect several organs, causing focal necrotic lesions and granulomas. Humeral immunity is insufficient and recovery depends on the development of cellular immunity.

CLINICAL FEATURES

Clinical features, at least in the early stages, depend on the portal of entry. The incubation period is usually two to five days, although it can range from less than a day up to three weeks.

Clinical disease can be either of the cutaneous-lymphatic type where a nodular, suppurative or ulcerative lesion develops at the site of entry. Local lymph nodes are often considerably enlarged and very tender. There may be obvious lymphangitis between the primary lesion and the lymph nodes. In the typhoidal presentation the main feature is high fever with occasional pneumonitis. However, these two main forms of presentation overlap considerably. Sometimes the primary lesion is not obvious even though regional lymph nodes are affected. At other times, the lymphatic type progresses to typhoid disease. Untreated, the mortality is up to 15%.

DIAGNOSIS

F. tularensis is extremely infectious in the laboratory and great care must be taken when handling the organism. The pathogen may be cultured from the skin lesion and from lymph nodes, but it does not tend to grow in blood cultures. Preferred culture media include glucose cysteine blood agar, modified Thayer–Martin medium and inspissated egg yolk medium. If the diagnosis is under consideration then samples such be cultured on more than one type of medium.

Histological examination of tissue with fluorescent antibody staining may also demonstrate the organism. Diagnosis can be confirmed by sero-agglutination tests or enzyme-linked immunosorbent assay.

TREATMENT

The treatment of choice is one of the aminoglycosides such as streptomycin or gentamicin.

ENVIRONMENTAL DETECTION

Primary isolation of *F. tularensis* from water samples probably requires preliminary passage in laboratory animals followed by culture as for human diagnosis.

ECOLOGY

The distribution of the infection seems to be restricted to the Northern Hemisphere, being most frequent between 30° and 71° latitude. Its main reservoirs are animals such as hares, rabbits and rodents (voles, squirrels and beavers). The environment may be contaminated by these animals.

EPIDEMIOLOGY

Transmission of infection to humans usually follows direct contact with infected animal tissues or by biting insects. Infection may also be airborne or by contact with water or by animal bite. In the latter case, this may be as a result of a carnivore such as a cat taking the infection onto its teeth. It is not surprising, therefore, that most infections occur in hunters and others working with wild animals or in residents of, or tourists to, affected rural areas.

Although there are reports in the 1970–1995 literature of individual cases where a waterborne source was suspected, I have only been able to find two reports of waterborne outbreaks. Both occurred in Italy. The first outbreak affected 49 individuals in or around the small medieval town of Sansepolcro during March to May 1982 (Greco *et al.* 1987). The distribution of cases was significantly more common in those areas taking their drinking water from just one of the two water systems supplying the town (RR 53.2, CI 12.9–219.0). The implicated supply system was in a poor state of repair and unchlorinated. It was said to be preferred by those residents who liked 'natural spring water'. An inspection found it to be uncovered and surrounded by animal prints. A sick hare captured in the area was found to be infected with *F. tularensis*.

The second waterborne outbreak occurred in the Ligurian Apennines (Mignani *et al.* 1988). The authors identified four cases in patients from the same mountain area during April and May 1988. A subsequent serological survey of 160 other individuals from the same area identified a total of 20 sero-positive individuals. Nine of these twenty reported recent compatible symptoms. All affected individuals got their water from the same aqueduct, while all of the houses with all sero-negative individuals got their water from other aqueducts. Furthermore, the risk of infection was greater in those houses nearer the source of the aqueduct.

26   Helicobacter Infections

The decision to include a chapter on *Helicobacter pylori* in this book was taken just as I was finishing writing the first draft. The reason was the publication of two papers in 1996 that considerably strengthened the water-borne hypothesis, at least for some communities. Like so many of the pathogens described in this book, *H. pylori* is a newly described agent. It was only in the early 1980s when its pathogenic role was first suggested (Marshall and Warren 1984). Indeed, the history of its discovery and the gradual and begrudging acceptance of its role in gastric ulceration is one of the better medical stories of recent times. It is now accepted as a major cause of peptic ulcer disease and, increasingly, as a major factor in the aetiology of gastric cancer.

MICROBIOLOGY

H. pylori are small microaerophilic, Gram-negative bacilli. In the stomach they are spiral organisms but on agar culture they are usually only singly curved. On exposure to air for one to two hours, the cells become coccal and can no longer be cultured. This coccal form is still metabolically active.

   When it was first described, the species was placed in the genus *Campylobacter*, although in 1989 it was given its own genus. Several other *Helicobacter* spp. have now been described. Most are inhabitants of the stomachs of other mammals.

PATHOGENESIS

The pathogenesis of human disease is still not fully understood. An important virulence characteristic is the ability of *H. pylori* to survive gastric acidity. Indeed, if gastric pH rises as a result of gastritis, then *H. pylori* is replaced by other, less acid tolerant organisms. Motility and urease activity appear important, the first to allow movement in the mucous layer and urease to produce ammonium ions to help buffer gastric acid. The mechanism of tissue damage is not clear.

CLINICAL FEATURES

Acute infection presents as nausea and abdominal pain, which last for between 3 and 14 days. Gastritis develops and hypochlorhydria may persist for up to a year. In most patients infection persists for several years or more. Although most chronically infected individuals will be asymptomatic, almost all will have histological evidence of chronic superficial gastritis. *H. pylori* is, however, more common in patients with non-ulcer dyspepsia than in controls.

The most common chronic disease associated with *H. pylori* infection is duodenal ulceration. Almost all patients with duodenal ulcer will have an infection by *H. pylori*. Because of other causes such as non-steroidal anti-inflammatory drugs, the proportion of cases of gastric ulcer associated with *H. pylori* is somewhat less (50–80). However, infection with *H. pylori* increases the risk of gastric or duodenal ulceration by about 50 fold.

H. pylori is one of the stronger candidates for a carcinogenic bacterium. Gastric lymphoma is strongly associated with *H. pylori* infection, and cure of the bacterium may lead to improvement in the histological appearance of the tumour. There is also an increasingly firm body of evidence suggesting that *H. pylori* predisposes to gastric carcinoma.

DIAGNOSIS

Diagnosis can be confirmed by endoscopy followed by microscopy or culture of biopsy material onto appropriate selective media. Other less invasive tests include a serological blood test, athough this remains positive for a long time after eradication of infection. A urease breath test using radiolabelled carbon meals is also available.

TREATMENT

At present, the preferred treatment seems to be a combination of amoxycillin plus metronidazole plus bismuth for about one month.

ENVIRONMENTAL DETECTION

Enroth and Engstrand (1995) have described a two-stage method for the detection of *H. pylori* in water samples. Initially the organism is concentrated by immunomagnetic separation and then detected by PCR. For three-day-old cultures they could detect 100 bacteria per millilitre. However, as the culture aged, the sensitivity declined, presumably due to changing antigenicity of the coccal form.

ECOLOGY

There is still a considerable amount not known about the ecology of *H. pylori*. However, at present, it would appear that man is the main host and environmental contamination derives from infected humans. Using the PCR technique already mentioned, Hulten *et al.* (1996) reported identifying *H. pylori* in 24 of 48 drinking water samples from various new towns near Lima, Peru.

The spiral form of *H. pylori* remains culturable for at least 10 days in river water at 4 °C and the coccal form for at least a year (Shahamat *et al.* 1989a, b). Furthermore, *H. pylori* can remain viable under a wide range of environmental conditions (West, Millar and Tompkins 1992).

EPIDEMIOLOGY

While the full epidemiology of *H. pylori* infection is still to be elucidated, it would appear that direct and indirect person to person spread are the likeliest routes of transmission. Goodman and Correa (1995) have published a comprehensive review of the literature on the transmission of *H. pylori*. There have now been several studies investigating the role of waterborne transmission.

The first study to report an association between water and *H. pylori* infection was done in Peru (Klein *et al.* 1991). They used the urea breath test in 407 children from Lima aged between 2 months and 12 years. The prevalence of infection for the whole group was 48%. Prevalence increased with age. Infection was negatively associated with high family income ($p = 0.001$). Children who lived in homes with an external source of water were more likely to be positive (OR 3.1, $p = 0.001$). Among the high-income group, those using municipal water were much more likely to be positive than those using private well supplies (37% versus 4%, OR 11.4, $p = 0.02$). This difference was not seen in the low-income group. The authors concluded that transmission was associated with poor hygiene or, in good hygiene homes, with consumption of municipal water supplies.

In a sero-epidemiological study of 245 healthy children in Arkansas, no association was found with drinking water source (Fiedorek *et al.* 1991). The authors did, however, note an inverse relationship with family income.

A large cross-sectional study from southern China was published the following year (Mitchell *et al.* 1992). Diagnosis was based on serological testing. The overall prevalence was 44.2%. The prevalence in all age groups was higher in the city (52.4%) compared with the rural provinces (38.6%, $p < 0.05$). In the univariate analysis there was a significant association with drinking city water, but water source was completely linked to place of residence and was found not to be significant in the multivariate model. This may be explained by the finding that most people reported boiling their drinking water. It is not clear to me why the authors decided that drinking water was a proxy for place of residence and not vice versa.

A serological survey of 823 people, mostly adult residents of Taiwan, found no association between infection and drinking water source (Teh *et al.* 1994). A similar survey of 252 Korean children (Malaty *et al.* 1996) found a significant negative association between *H. pylori* infection and social class but no association with source of water supply.

Goodman *et al.* (1996) reported a survey, using the breath test to diagnose *H. pylori* infection, of 684 children in an Andean rural community. They correlated infection with a large number of social, economic and behavioural factors and used logistic regression modelling to analyse the data. In the model adjusted for background variables they found evidence for person to person transmission because infection was commoner in children whose mothers rarely used soap (OR 2.7, CI 1.1–6.6). They also found that infection was commoner in children who reported swimming in rivers or streams (OR 3.3, CI 1.2–9.4), swimming in swimming pools (OR 3.6, CI 1.5–8.5) and drinking from a stream at some time (OR 2.8, CI 1.2–6.8).

Although still open to further study, the evidence in favour of waterborne transmission in some developing communities now appears strong. The challenge remains to attempt an estimate of the relative importance of waterborne as opposed to other forms of transmission in both developed and developing countries. It may be that in some communities waterborne *H. pylori* infection is a significant cause of infection and, indeed, gastric carcinoma.

27 Viral Hepatitis

Viral hepatitis is an inflammation of the liver caused by one of several very different viruses (Table 27.1). Two of these viruses, hepatitis A and hepatitis E, have been regularly associated with waterborne outbreaks of disease. Hepatitis E appears to be exclusively spread by drinking water, and outbreaks of this pathogen demonstrate many of the problems associated with providing safe water supplies in tropical countries.

VIROLOGY

Many viruses cause a hepatitis as part of their clinical presentation. However, most authors tend to lump together just a few that have hepatitis as their main clinical feature (Zuckerman and Harrison 1995). These are denoted by a letter of the alphabet. Currently five viruses have been named, hepatitis A to E, although particles of a possible hepatitis F have also been described. Of the alphabet of viral hepatitis, only those illnesses causing infectious hepatitis (hepatitis A, hepatitis E and probably some other forms of non-A, non-B hepatitis) are associated with waterborne transmission. Consequently, further discussion is restricted to these infections.

Hepatitis A virus (HAV) is a small, positive sense, single-strand RNA virus, about 7.5 kb in length. It is now classified as belonging to the family Picornaviridae. The virus particle is spherical, 27–28 nm in diameter and has no envelope. The capsid consists of three major polypeptides, VP1, VP2 and VP3. Compared to many viruses it is relatively resistant to heat and chemical disinfectants, including chlorine. Humans are considered to be the only natural host for HAV. Although not culturable in many cell lines, it can be grown in cell cultures of primate liver cells.

Hepatitis E virus (HEV) is a small, 30 nm, single-strand RNA virus about 7.2 kb in length. HEV was thought to belong to the Calicivirus group, although recent studies have shown it to be quite distinct from Norwalk virus, another Calicivirus. It is though that humans are the only natural host, although chimpanzees and other species of monkey are susceptible to infection.

Table 27.1 Agents causing viral hepatitis

Virus	Virus family	Nucleic acid	Incubation period	Mode of infection
Hepatitis A (HAV)	Picornavirus	ssRNA	2–4 weeks	Faecal–oral
Hepatitis B (HBV)	Hepadnavirus	dsDNA	1–3 months	Parenteral/sexual
Hepatitis C (HCV)	Togavirus	ssRNA	2 months	Parenteral
Hepatitis D (HDV)	Very small	ssRNA	2–12 weeks	Parenteral
Hepatitis E (HEV)	Calicivirus	ssRNA	6–8 weeks	Faecal–oral

PATHOGENESIS

Both viruses are acquired orally. The virus passes through the stomach, where it replicates in the lower intestine before being carried to the liver, where most replication occurs. Virus is shed from the liver in the bile, from which it contaminates the faeces. Liver damage occurs at the point when circulating antibody appears in the blood.

CLINICAL FEATURES

The incubation period of hepatitis A is 15–45 days. Generally the disease is benign and many cases of infection are sub-clinical. Initial symptoms are non-specific, and include malaise, lassitude, myalgia, arthralgia and fever. Many individuals with this early illness will not even seek medical attention. Probably less than a quarter of cases become jaundiced. In those patients who develop jaundice, this develops 2–7 days after the development of the prodromal illness. Often the first feature noticed by the patient is darkening of the urine, soon followed by pale or clay-coloured stools. Sometimes severe itching can accompany the jaundice. On examination the patient may be jaundiced, most obviously noted in the whites of the eyes. The liver is also often enlarged. Rising plasma transaminases is an early feature. Complications include prolonged cholestasis, at times lasting for months, and relapsing disease. Fulminant hepatitis and fatality are rare complications; even in hospitalized patients they may only be present in 1 per 1000 cases. The patient probably remains infectious for up to 7 days after the onset of jaundice. Unlike hepatitis B and C, there is no chronic infection.

Hepatitis E has broadly similar clinical features to hepatitis A. However, the incubation period is longer – 4–8 weeks – and the disease can last somewhat longer as well. Progression to fatal fulminant hepatitis is commoner than in any other viral hepatitis, at 1–2% of cases. This may be even higher in pregnant women.

DIAGNOSIS

The diagnosis for both hepatitis A and E is by the detection of specific IgM antibodies in serum or by the demonstration of a rise in IgG antibodies.

TREATMENT

Most cases of hepatitis A and E only require non-specific supportive treatment of rest and analgesics. Itching can be controlled by antipruritic drugs. Prolonged severe cholestasis responds to steroids.

ENVIRONMENTAL DETECTION

The initial steps in the identification of hepatitis viruses in water are the same as for most viruses. This follows a two-step approach, concentration and detection. The method is reviewed in more detail elsewhere and is only outlined here (Fewtrell et al. 1994; Sellwood and Wyn-Jones 1996).

For river and sea water 10 l samples are filtered through cellulose nitrate disc membranes or fibreglass cartridges. In treated water virus concentrations are expected to be much lower, so larger volumes, 100 l, need to be filtered using large-scale fibreglass cartridges. Viruses adsorbed onto the filters are then released into a proteinaceous solution at high pH. Lowering the pH of this solution will then allow floc formation, to which the virus particles are adsorbed. This floc is then centrifuged down and finally resuspended in 5–10 ml of buffer.

Once the final concentration has been made, the virus has to be detected. Detection of hepatitis A can be by tissue culture, although it grows only in certain cell lines such as FRhMK-4 and then only very slowly, requiring several weeks (Pana et al. 1987; Sellwood and Wyn-Jones 1996). More rapid detection methods include DNA and RNA probes (Jiang et al. 1986; Metcalf and Jiang 1988; Shieh et al. 1991), an ELISA test (Nasser and Metcalf 1987) and, more recently, the polymerase chain reaction (PCR) (Morace et al. 1993; Monceyron and Grinde 1994; Tsai et al. 1994). A PCR has also been developed for hepatitis E (Jothikumar et al. 1993).

Jehl-Pietri et al. (1993) compared immune electron microscopy (IEM), radioimmunoassay (RIA) and molecular hybridization (MH) using a cDNA probe to detect HAV in raw and treated sewage. HAV was detected in 3 of 13 raw and 8 of 13 treated samples by MH. No sample was positive by RIA, and six effluent but no affluent samples were positive by IEM. Two samples found to be positive by IEM were negative by MH. MH was found to be far more sensitive than either IEM or RIA.

In a study of HAV in river waters, Morace *et al.* (1993) found 15.3% positive by ELISA, 23% by cell culture, 38.4% by DNA hybridization and 67% by PCR.

Monceyron and Grinde (1994) developed a method for the detection of HAV using immunomagnetic separation (using metal balls coated with anti-HAV antibody to bind HAV virus followed by their separation from the sample by magnetic extraction), followed by PCR. The authors suggested that this method was particularly suited for use in polluted river and sea waters.

ECOLOGY

It is believed that both hepatitis A and E viruses are essentially restricted to human hosts. As with all viruses, they only replicate in their host, so water-borne transmission of viral hepatitis must be preceded by faecal contamination. Therefore, the ecology of these viruses in the environment must mirror that of the distribution of human faecal contamination. Indeed, any surface water that is subject to faecal or sewage contamination will be at risk of contamination by HAV or HEV virus from time to time, depending on the prevalence of the diseases in local human populations. For example, Morace *et al.* (1993) reported that 67% of river samples were positive for HAV by PCR. HAV was not detected in seawater off Bondi beach (Kueh and Grohmann 1989). However, one must be careful not to take these contamination rates as too reliable. Differences in detection rates between studies are as likely to be due to differences in sensitivity of the detection methods as to the real concentration of virus in water.

EPIDEMIOLOGY OF HEPATITIS A

Hepatitis A is common throughout the world, is very infectious and can spread in a variety of ways. Direct person to person transmission by the faecal–oral route is probably the commonest, especially in children. This route of transmission is probably the cause of most of the school-based outbreaks described in the UK and elsewhere. Person to person transmission between homosexuals has also been described. Foodborne outbreaks are also common. In such outbreaks the source of the infection is usually an infected food-handler who was incubating the disease. However, outbreaks associated with raw or undercooked shellfish, harvested from polluted waters, have also been described. Hepatitis A is most common in tropical and subtropical countries, and travellers to these areas are at particular risk.

Outbreaks associated with drinking water

During November and December 1966, approximately 375 inhabitants of Olivet, France developed hepatitis out of a population of a little under 10 000 (Gavan and Nutt 1970). At that time a US army facility was located nearby and 52 cases of hepatitis occurred in US army personnel. Of these 52 cases, 40 lived in Olivet (an attack rate of 0.03%). Only 12 cases were identified in individuals not resident in Olivet (attack rate of 0.0017%). The authors estimated an attack rate of 0.41% among French residents of Olivet. It was noted that the outbreak of hepatitis among French residents was almost entirely restricted to residents of Olivet. Furthermore, a month before the outbreak of hepatitis there had been an outbreak of gastroenteritis among the French residents. A review of both French and American army records of water examination showed that between 3 and 10 October, residual chlorine levels were absent on more than one occasion. Also during that period microbiological analysis of drinking water revealed heavy faecal contamination; *Escherichia coli*, *Streptococcus faecalis* and *Clostridium perfringens* were all detected. The source of the faecal contamination was not discovered, although major works on the distribution system were undertaken during early October.

Circumstantial evidence suggested that an outbreak of infectious hepatitis during July and August 1969 in a Sydney residential school for the intellectually handicapped was waterborne (Rennie 1970). One staff member and 12 residents were affected. It was noted that the water supply came from two sources; rain-water collected from the roof and untreated water from a nearby creek. Although the rain-water was supposed to be for drinking, the taps from both sources were situated close together and it was suggested that many of the residents would have been unable to distinguish between them.

The Holy Cross College football team outbreak of hepatitis during September and October 1969 is interesting in that an unusual chain of events led up to the outbreak (Morse *et al.* 1972). The attack rate was very high – 93%. Of 97 athletes using the sports facilities between 26 and 31 August, 32 developed jaundice, 22 developed an anicteric illness and 36 developed asymptomatic hepatitis as measured by liver enzymes. Non-athletes using the same dining facilities were not affected, nor were athletes starting the following week. The water supply to the practice area was from the municipal system and it was used for both drinking and irrigation. The drinking tap was at the lowest point of the supply pipe, which also supplied underground irrigation systems. The field drainage systems ran close to the water supply pipe. Although the pressure in the pipe was normally sufficient to prevent field water from entering the pipe, it was discovered that pressure was very sensitive to increased use further up the supply network. If two fire hydrants were opened just before the playing fields, negative pressure developed in the pipe, such that surface water could siphon into the drinking water supply.

Furthermore, a family who lived in condemned property adjacent to the playing fields experienced an outbreak of hepatitis during August. The children apparently enjoyed playing in water that accumulated around the field irrigation system. Finally, on the morning of 29 August a fire broke out in a building two miles away from the college, but along the course of the main water supply line. Thus, the outbreak was solved: infected children playing in surface water by a poorly designed drinking water supply and irrigation system that allowed siphoning of infected water into the pipe when the demands of a fire reduced pressure in the pipe.

An outbreak of hepatitis A affected 49 children and 1 adult in a rural elementary school in Alabama during October and November 1972 (Baer, Walker and Yager, 1977). An epidemiological study found a significant association with illness and drinking school water ($p = 0.047$). The school water supply was from small springs situated 125 yards downhill of the school. The spring water came primarily from surface seepage and it was noted that some of this subsurface water came from septic tanks further uphill. Thirty days before the outbreak occurred there had been heavy rainfall. Although normally chlorinated, the school supply was probably unchlorinated at that time.

Sixteen cases of hepatitis A occurred among staff at a research centre on Fundao Island, Rio de Janeiro, Brazil, during March and April 1980 (Sutmoller *et al.* 1982). Although no analytical epidemiological study was done, the authors concluded that the outbreak was waterborne, as several water samples found no residual chlorine and high coliform and faecal coliform counts. No reason for the faecal pollution was identified. However, about a month before the outbreak the water supply to the plant was interrupted.

An outbreak in Lancaster County, Pennsylvania, between August and October 1980 affected 49 people (Bowen and McCarthy 1983). Eleven of these people worked at a hardware store and all other cases had contact with the store or the home of the store's owner, who lived next door. In a cohort study, drinking water from either the store's water fountain or in the owner's home was highly associated with illness ($p < 0.001$). No other risk factor was identified. The water supply for both the store and the owner's home came from a 61 m well drilled through limestone and dolomite rocks. The septic tank from the store was situated about 30 m from the well. However, the exact route of contamination was not discovered. Dye placed in this toilet did not appear in the well-water.

In November 1982 there was a marked increase in the incidence of hepatitis A infection in Meade County, Kentucky (Bergeisen, Hinds and Skaggs 1985). It was noted that the local physicians had been aware of the increase for some time but 'never had the time to report them'. In a case-control study the risk factor was found to be consumption of water from Buttermilk Falls. Furthermore, there was found to be a dose–response relationship between hepatitis and drinking unboiled Buttermilk Falls water ($p = 2 \times 10^{-5}$). The local rock in Meade County was limestone. There is little surface runoff, as most rain-water percolates down through sinkholes into fractures in the limestone rock. These sinkholes are frequently used for dumping human and animal wastes. The porous nature of the rock would also permit contamination from septic tanks and other sources of faecal pollution. Buttermilk Falls is one of several springs draining water from this aquifer. The water was usually collected by trucks and distributed untreated to people's homes. Microbiological analysis revealed more than 400 faecal coliforms per millilitre (40 000 faecal coliforms per 100 ml). Fluorescein dye flushed into a patient's septic tank appeared two weeks later in water from Buttermilk Falls.

An outbreak of hepatitis A affected 16 residents and 11 visitors at a trailer park in north Georgia, USA, between July and October 1982 (Bloch *et al.* 1990). The index case developed his illness four weeks before other cases. The water supply was from a common well and sewage was to individual septic tanks for each trailer. Faecal coliforms were detected in several drinking water samples and hepatitis A Ag detected in groundwater samples. However, the route of contamination of the groundwater was not identified by dye tests. The outbreak abated four weeks after a boil water notice was issued.

Between September 1988 and January 1989 an outbreak of hepatitis A in central Italy was linked to a single brand of bottled mineral water (Stroffolini *et al.* 1990). A total of 47 cases were identified, of whom the majority were males. In a case-control study of 41 cases, the consumption of raw mussels while on holiday at various places on the coast (OR 6.6, CI 2.3–19.2) was implicated. However, only 41% of cases had eaten raw mussels so other factors must have been important. Consumption of a single brand of bottled mineral water was reported by 63% of cases and 41% of controls (OR 2.5, CI 1.1–5.4). Supporting the observation of a link with bottled mineral water was the finding of coliform bacteria in September but not in subsequent months.

An outbreak of hepatitis A in a rural district of Saudi Arabia affected 23 children and adolescents during a thirty-day period (Al-Majed *et al.* 1990). The authors suggested that this was a waterborne outbreak, based on the abrupt onset of the epidemic. The water supply to the village was from three wells situated about 3 km distant and delivered by truck. It was thought that the source of the infection was probably a water worker.

During April and May 1987, 13 cases of hepatitis A infection, of whom only 6 were symptomatic, occurred in a school and college in Rome (Divizia *et al.* 1993). The index case in the outbreak was probably a sister at the college who had been ill in March. Although no analytical epidemiology was done, hepatitis A virus was cultured from concentrated well-water samples and a polymerase chain reaction test was positive on an unconcentrated sample.

Outbreaks associated with recreational water contact

Bryan *et al.* (1974) reported an outbreak of hepatitis A that affected 14 members of a Boy Scout troop during September 1969. Between 14 and 17 August (28 days before the outbreak), 25 boys and 5 adults had camped on an island in a lake in South Carolina. All 14 cases had attended the camp. A cohort study of all 30 members of the camp showed a significant association with drinking lake water, either deliberately or accidentally while swimming ($p = 0.007$).

Hepatitis A infection affected 26 individuals in Salishan, a relatively deprived area of Washington, during 1974 (Chapman 1976). It was noted that many of the affected children played in a small stream that ran through the housing development. Indeed, the geographical distribution of cases followed the length of this stream. Microbiological examination of this stream water found evidence of faecal pollution, which was shown to be due to failing septic tanks.

Of 822 campers who attended a campsite in Louisiana during one weekend in August 1989, 20 developed hepatitis A the following month (Mahoney *et al.* 1992). The highest attack rate was in children aged 5–9 years. In a case-control study, cases were more likely to report drinking the campsite's water (16 of 19 cases versus 17 of 35 controls; OR 5.7, CI 1.2–34.5) and particularly drinking from the site's only water fountain (OR 13.8, CI 2.7–88.0). However, all 19 cases swam in one of the public pools on the Saturday afternoon compared to only 15 of 26 controls (OR undefined, lower CI 3.3). Other swimming-associated risk factors were swimming for more than one hour (OR undefined, lower CI 1.6), putting the head under water (OR undefined, lower CI 0.7), swallowing water (OR 3.8, CI 0.8–19.6) and spitting water (OR 2.4, CI 0.5–13.2). Because of the stronger association with swimming and swimming-associated factors, and doubts about recall bias on drinking water, the investigators concluded that the most probable explanation was the swimming pool. The particular Saturday afternoon when infection had occurred was rather hot and the pool was busy, so putting particular load on the chlorination systems. It was also noted that the plumbing in the most likely pool was potentially subject to contamination from the sewer.

Prospective studies of faecal pollution of water supply incidents

As discussed above, many waterborne outbreaks of viral hepatitis have followed faecal contamination of the water supply. Several studies have attempted to quantify the risk of hepatitis following such incidents by prospectively attempting to identify cases. In June and July 1975, massive faecal contamination of the water supply in Crater National Park, Oregon, followed an obstructed sewage pipe (Rosenberg, Koplan and Pollard 1980). An estimated 100 000 people had visited the park during the time that the drinking water had been contaminated. More than 2000 people who had drunk the park water developed gastroenteritis due to enterotoxigenic *E. coli*. It was known that two people had used the park toilets while incubating non-B hepatitis. Immunuglobulin was given to all park staff and many visitors. None of 320 park staff interviewed had symptoms of hepatitis. Twenty of 3997 people who had stayed overnight in the park and returned a questionnaire claimed to have had hepatitis, although follow-up telephone contact showed that 15 of these 20 had confused gastroenteritis with hepatitis. All five cases had drunk the water and none of them had received immunoglobulin. However, the relationship between drinking water and developing hepatitis did not achieve statistical significance ($p = 0.15$). The authors pointed out that the attack rate among those respondents who had drunk water and had not received immunoglobulin was about nine times higher than would be expected from national reporting, supporting the hypothesis of a waterborne outbreak. Receiving immunoglobulin was found to be protective ($p = 0.06$). Nevertheless, the authors concluded that the cost of administering immunoglobulin was greatly in excess of the cost benefit of reduced illness.

During October 1991 the water supply to almost 6000 residents of a town in the Republic of Ireland became contaminated with sewage (Thornton *et al.* 1995). A large outbreak of gastroenteritis followed this incident. To identify whether the incident would cause an increase in the incidence of hepatitis A, two sero-epidemiological surveys were conducted in the town using saliva antibody tests. Two hundred households were randomly chosen and asked to participate, half of which were in the affected area. The first study was conducted three weeks after the contamination episode and the second six weeks later. In the first study 495 samples were analysed of which 213 (43%) were immune and three showed evidence of recent infection. In the second survey a further three samples were indicative of recent infection. Thus six cases of hepatitis A were identified, four of whom lived in the affected area, although only one probably drank the polluted water. There were no formal notifications of hepatitis A during the period. The study gave no evidence of increased hepatitis A infection secondary to the pollution incident.

Other epidemiological studies of sporadic disease

Hoffman, Crusberg and Savilonis (1979) analysed the geographical distribution of infectious hepatitis cases occurring in Worcester, Massachusetts, between the years 1968 and 1972. During 1970 there had been a large epidemic affecting almost 500 people. The authors then correlated the distribution of cases with what was known of the water distribution and sewage collection systems. Factors that were correlated with the incidence of hepatitis in the various census tracts were the percentage of the population with combined sewers (taking foul waste and street runoff) ($p < 0.0005$) and with pre-1915 pipes ($p < 0.0005$). The percentage of people in the census tract with post-1940 pipes was found to be protective ($p = 0.0025$). Social factors such as the percentage of families below the poverty line were also found to be strongly significant ($p < 0.0005$).

Tsega et al. (1986) studied the distribution of antibody to hepatitis A among 500 individuals from five different regions of Ethiopia. Antibody to hepatitis A virus was present in 84.4%. No association was demonstrated between HAV positivity and type of water consumption or mode of excreta disposal.

In a study of 109 individuals who took military diving courses in 1991 and 1992 in France and 49 non-diving controls, serological examination for hepatitis A was done at the start and repeated throughout (Garin et al. 1994). No diver or control seroconverted to hepatitis A during the course. Furthermore, the seropositivity rates were the same in both groups, suggesting that diving was not a risk factor.

Lagarde et al. (1995) investigated serological markers for hepatitis A in 936 French military recruits from October 1992 to June 1993. The overall prevalence of antibody was 16.3%, having fallen from 48.0% in 1979. In a multivariate logistic regression model, the factors associated with past infection were: belonging to the lower classes (as defined by father's occupation) (OR 2.00, CI 1.35–3.03), having two or more siblings (OR 2.25, CI 1.48–3.44), having a history of jaundice (OR 2.27, CI 1.19–4.33), having travelled overseas (OR 2.26, CI 1.38–3.70) and drinking tap-water (OR 1.56, CI 1.03–2.35). To investigate the role of tap-water further, 211 recruits who drank tap-water were asked about chlorine taste in their drinking water. Of 79 reporting a chlorine taste 11 (13.9%) were antibody positive compared to 26 (19.7%) of 132 who did not report a chlorine taste ($p < 0.06$).

EPIDEMIOLOGY OF NON-A, NON-B HEPATITIS (HEPATITIS E)

Hepatitis E is less common than hepatitis A and is restricted to tropical and subtropical countries. This infection also appears to be less infectious, since secondary cases are much less common than is reported for hepatitis A. Indeed, it would appear that waterborne transmission is the predominant route for hepatitis E.

Outbreaks associated with drinking water

A large outbreak of non-A, non-B hepatitis affected at least 275 people living in the Kashmir valley over a six-month period from November 1978 to April 1979 (Khuroo 1980). The attack rate over the six months was 1.65%. One patient died with fulminant hepatitis. There were 15 villages in the area under investigation, of which only 4 had a piped water supply. In the remaining 11 villages people took their water from the local streams. Only 6 of 275 cases identified lived in a village with a piped supply (χ^2 = 26.4, p < 0.001). Coliform counts in the stream were high in all samples tested. It was noted that in the majority of homes only a single case occurred, suggesting a low rate of secondary infection.

Another outbreak of non-A, non-B hepatitis in India affected students living in a hostel in Madhya Pradesh during 1980 (Chakraborty *et al.* 1982). Between July and September 38 of 153 students developed hepatitis. The attack rate was higher among boarders (40.0%) compared with day students (5.9%) (p < 0.001) and was higher in the right wing of the hostel (60.5%) compared with the left wing (24.1%) (p < 0.01). The water supply to the college was from a dug well. Chlorination was only intermittent. It was noted that the water supply pipes were rusted in many places and that a septic tank had overflowed into low-lying ground through which the water supply pipe to the right wing passed.

Nouasria *et al.* (1984) reported a small outbreak of non-A, non-B hepatitis during September 1983 in Constantine, Algeria. Six of 36 residents in one building developed jaundice over a two-week period. A plumbing cross-connection between toilets and the drinking water supply had been made 28 days before the first case and had not been rectified for two weeks. Very high coliform counts (1400 per 100 ml) were found in the drinking water in the affected building.

Between January and March 1980, 226 cases of non-A, non-B hepatitis were identified in a Calcutta slum (Pain, Chakraborty and Choudry 1983). Water for the area came from eight filtered water standpoints and two open shallow dug wells, which were in close proximity to latrines. Bacteriological analysis of the well-water and tap showed them to be highly contaminated with coliforms. Most of the filtered water taps were 'submerged under highly contaminated sewage water'.

A large outbreak of non-A, non-B hepatitis affected at least 1200 people in Kolhapur City, Maharashtra State, India, between February and March 1981 (Sreenivasan *et al.* 1984). Three people died. The attack rate for symptomatic cases was 0.0034%. The attack rate in one ward of the city reached 0.0066%, which was three times higher than in any other ward. The water supply to the affected ward was different from that to the other areas of the city. This water was extracted from the Panchaganga River and treated by sedimentation, rapid sand filtration and chlorination. The geographical distribution of cases closely followed the water supply line. Water samples taken in January had shown high counts of *E. coli*. It was suggested that inadequate water monitoring had contributed to the outbreak.

From October 1980 to January 1981 there were 788 cases of non-A, non-B hepatitis notified in Medea, Algeria (Belabbes *et al.* 1985). Nine pregnant women were infected and all died. There were only two other deaths, in males who already had a debilitating disease. An epidemic of typhoid coincided with the increase in hepatitis cases. The waterborne nature of the outbreak was suggested by the geographical distribution of cases. The areas supplied with river water had the highest incidence (0.74%), those supplied by spring water the lowest (0.08%). Areas supplied with a mixture of the two had an intermediate incidence (0.23%). The river water was chlorinated before distribution. Six weeks before the outbreak there was a breakdown in the automatic chlorination system for several days. There was also a rupture of a main pipe in the town centre, allowing contamination of the river drinking water (now unchlorinated) by raw sewage.

A military unit in Pakistan suffered an outbreak of non-A, non-B hepatitis which affected 21 of 200 soldiers living in a single barracks (Quraishi et al. 1988). Water for drinking and cooking was taken from a tube well. The water supply pipe was found to be cracked. The septic tank was overflowing such that sewage was in contact with the cracked pipe.

An outbreak of non-A, non-B hepatitis affected 133 students and others at a college in Sargodha, Pakistan, in early 1987 (Iqbal et al. 1989). Inspection of the water supply to the affected college showed that it was extracted from a stream and passed to an underground reservoir. A sewage pipeline crossed the water pipe just before the reservoir. Samples of water from this tank found it to be heavily contaminated with coliforms, too frequent to count.

During December 1986 and January 1987 an outbreak of non-A, non-B hepatitis affected 61 people in a village of south Delhi (Panda et al. 1989). The village was next to an open, unlined sewer. Water used by the village came from hand-pumped groundwater or municipal water stored in underground reservoirs. Virus-like particles were identified in the stool of cases and were used to infect rhesus monkeys.

During the latter six months of 1985, an outbreak of non-A, non-B hepatitis affected 273 individuals in Maun, Botswana (Byskov et al. 1989). There were four deaths, including the death of a pregnant woman, and 47 admissions to hospital. In addition to these deaths four pregnant women lost their foetuses, either spontaneously or after induction. Among cases, 80% took their water entirely from standpipes, 8% entirely from the river and the rest a mixture. Inspection of the water distribution system found it to be in a poor state of repair and that chlorination was inadequately monitored. Furthermore, sewage disposal was poor, with local collections. About 11% of cases were in people who were water construction workers, which added further weight to the waterborne hypothesis.

Velazquez et al. (1990) described two outbreaks of non-A, non-B hepatitis in rural villages in Mexico during late 1986. The first outbreak started in June and affected 94 people (an attack rate of 5.4%). The second outbreak, which started in August, affected 129 people (attack rate 5.9%). Case-control studies were done in both villages. Factors associated with increased risk of disease in the first village were: cases noting visibly dirty water in the well (OR 36.3, CI 5.9–278.1) and contact with a hepatitis case (OR 7.4, CI 1.6–35.8). Protective factors were: having a protective wall for the well (OR 0.1, CI 0.03–0.54) and boiling drinking water (OR 0.2, CI 0.05–0.96). In the second village using stream water for drinking (OR 16.9, CI 2.1–98.1), using stream water for cooking or washing dishes (OR 12.6, CI 1.5–84.6) and contact with a hepatitis case (OR 3.6, CI 1.4–9.5) were all associated with an increased risk of infection.

Between February and April 1987, 125 patients with non-A, non-B hepatitis were admitted to hospital from one of two villages in Xinjang, China (Wang et al. 1990). Of these cases 90% had drunk water from pools. People from these villages who boiled their water did not develop the disease.

An outbreak of hepatitis E virus infection affected military personnel in northern Ethiopia between October 1988 and March 1989 (Tsega et al. 1991). During the outbreak over 750 personnel were seen in the military hospital, of whom 423 were hospitalized; there were no deaths. The authors pointed out that their information came from just one hospital in the area, which suggests a huge outbreak, especially when sub-clinical infections are taken into account. Examination of drinking water found evidence of faecal contamination, and the outbreak declined after general hygiene measures and health education were introduced.

Between July and October 1987 residents in an area of south Delhi complained on several occasions about a foul smell in their drinking water (Vrati et al. 1992). Microbiological analysis of this water revealed very high coliform counts. Investigations of the water supply found damage to both the water pipe and sewage pipe where they were running close to each other. Subsequently in November of that year there was an outbreak of hepatitis in the area of distribution of the affected supply; 43 individuals developed clinical hepatitis. Serological markers for hepatitis A and hepatitis B were negative. The authors were able to transmit the infection to rhesus monkeys by inoculating a cell-free concentrate of human faeces.

Perhaps the largest waterborne outbreak of hepatitis E to be described so far occurred in Kanpur, India, between December 1990 and April 1991 (Nail et al. 1992). After widespread reports of acute hepatitis in the city, the investigators undertook a systematic survey of a random sample of houses. The incidence of hepatitis with jaundice during the study period in this sample was 3.76%, suggesting that the true incidence of the disease was over 79 000. There were two peaks in incidence, in February and in April. The incidence of disease was higher in those wards that were supplied with a mixture of River Ganges and tube-well water compared to those supplied only with tube-well water ($p = 10^{-6}$). There was, furthermore, a gradient of increasing illness with the increased proportion of Ganges water supplied. Investigations of the water supply records suggested that the first peak of illness was associated with faecal contamination of the river water and the second peak with inadequate chlorination of a water reservoir. Aggarwal and Naik (1994) used this outbreak to determine the relative importance of waterborne and person to person transmission. The authors surveyed households at the peak of the epidemic and again a year later. Where second cases occurred in a family the time interval between first and second cases was recorded. Of 111 cases of hepatitis recorded, 81 were first or only cases and 22 occurred within two weeks of the index case. Thus, 103 (92.8%) of cases were not acquired from family members. The remaining eight cases occurred between 2 and 6 weeks after the index case, which could be either person to person or waterborne. It would appear that person to person spread in families plays, at best, a very minor role in the transmission of hepatitis E.

Another outbreak of non-A, non-B hepatitis in India affected at least 127 people in Rairangpur Town, Orissa, during December 1989 and January 1990 (Bora *et al.* 1993). There was one death. The drinking water for 9 of the 15 wards in the city was by an intermittent piped supply. The other wards relied on hand pumps and dug wells. The geographical distribution of cases followed the piped water supply (attack rate 1.9% compared to 0.5%). In a case-control study that matched for ward or residence, use of the piped supply was still highly associated with illness (OR 9.0, CI 4.2–19.3). Although the exact source of contamination of the water supply was not identified, it was noted that there had been a leakage of the main supply early in December.

An epidemic of non-A, non-B hepatitis commenced in December 1989 and reached a peak in March the following year in Rewa District, Madhya Pradesh (Risbud *et al.* 1992). During the first four months of 1990, 302 patients were admitted to the local hospital. Of hospitalized patients, the case fatality rates were 7.9% in males and 20.6% in females. A survey of the 2691 families in affected wards revealed another 517 cases. Inspection of the water supply system revealed 427 leaks, and at 903 places the supply crossed foul drainage. The team also visited surrounding rural areas and identified 82 cases, all of whom gave histories of daily visits to and water consumption in the main affected area.

Yet another outbreak of non-A, non-B hepatitis affected residents in a part of Delhi during February and March 1992 (Bandyopadhyay *et al.* 1993). The index case was a six-year-old girl who had acquired the infection elsewhere. Inspection of the water supply found sewage contamination around the water supply line.

Bile *et al.* (1994) studied the role of river- and well-water consumption in the transmission of hepatitis E during an outbreak in Somalia in 1988. In a survey of 142 villages 11 413 jaundiced cases were recorded out of a population of 245 312. There were 346 deaths. Antibodies to hepatitis E virus were detected in 128 of 145 sera examined. The attack rate was highest in the coastal area (9.6%) compared to the riverine (5.0%) and semi-arid (1.0%) areas. The fatality rates were the inverse of this: semi-arid 5.2%, riverine 3.0% and coastal 1.8%. The recorded attack rates and fatality rates for each village were also analysed according to their source of water. The attack rate was highest in those taking their water from rivers (6.0%) compared to wells (1.7%) and ponds (1.2%). The case fatality rate was much higher in people taking their water from wells (8.6%) than in those taking water from rivers (2.5%) or ponds (0.8%). There was also a higher incidence of disease following heavy rainfalls, after which the river level rose. Detailed study of a smaller number of villages found no evidence of person to person spread. The higher mortality rates in villages with well-water was explained by the increased dose of virus in contaminated well-water.

During March, April and May 1994 an outbreak of HEV disease affected 27 patients living in a relatively affluent apartment block in northwest Delhi (Singh *et al.* 1995b). The attack rate for residents in this block was 1.9%. Samples from the drinking water supply reservoir were of high quality, but high faecal coliform counts were detected in tap-water in the affected block. Although no exact point of contamination was identified, it was noted that many of the residents had installed booster pumps in their homes to increase water pressure at the tap. At times of relatively low pressure, this had the effect of causing negative pressures in the pipes.

Prospective epidemiological studies

A study of acute hepatitis among 261 children living in Cairo, Egypt, investigated the prevalence of serological markers for viral hepatitis (el-Zimaity *et al.* 1993). Acute hepatitis A (as indicated by IgM test results) was diagnosed in 85 (32.6%), hepatitis B in 19 (7.3%), mixed hepatitis A and B in 2 (0.8%) and hepatitis E in 58 (22.2%). No risk factors were identified other than for hepatitis E. Those with hepatitis E were more likely to take their water from a common village tap or well rather than an indoor tap ($p = 0.03$) and to use a pit rather than a flush toilet ($p = 0.0006$).

A prospective sero-epidemiological study of hepatitis E was done in South Africa in 1992 (Grabow *et al.* 1994). Blood samples were taken from 555 canoeists and 227 healthy medical students. Evidence of past infection was found in ten (1.8%) canoeists and six (2.6%) of the medical students. The increased incidence among students compared to canoeists was interesting given that they were generally younger and had no regular contact with sewage-polluted waters, unlike the canoeists. This study would suggest that canoeing was not a risk factor for hepatitis E infection.

Arif *et al.* (1994) conducted a sero-epidemiological study in two areas of Saudi Arabia. The two areas were Riyadh, an urban area, and Gizan, a rural area with primitive sewage disposal and an inferior water sanitation system. A total of 1418 people were included in the study. The prevalence of positive markers was higher in the rural area (14.9%) than in the urban area (8.36%).

Two years after an outbreak of hepatitis E infection in west Kalimantan, Indonesia, a follow-up study was done to investigate the subsequent epidemiology of the disease (Corwin *et al.* 1995). A cross-sectional survey of eleven villages included administration of a questionnaire and serological testing for HEV IgG in 127 households. Of the 127 households, 112 (88%) had at least one member positive. Use of river water for drinking was almost universal. However, if areas were grouped into high ($\geq$60%), medium and low (<40%) prevalence of hepatitis E virus infection, significant associations were found with use of river water for drinking and cooking ($p < 0.001$), bathing ($p < 0.0001$) and disposal of human excreta ($p < 0.001$). Boiling drinking water was found to be protective ($p = 0.02$).

28   Viral Gastroenteritis

Viral gastroenteritis is a very important cause of diarrhoeal disease, with between three and five billion cases each year and up to ten million deaths. A wide variety of viruses are responsible for causing gastroenteritis. Viral gastroenteritis seems to be on the increase, at least in the UK. While some of this increase may be due to better diagnosis and ascertainment, my own experience suggests that a large part of the reported increase is real.

VIROLOGY

Although many viruses can be identified in faeces by isolation in tissue culture, those viruses that are typically associated with epidemic gastroenteritis do not grow in routine cell cultures. They can, however, be seen by electron microscopy (EM). Indeed EM was for a long time the only diagnostic tool available and these viruses are often still known as fastidious viruses. Table 28.1 lists those fastidious viruses associated with gastroenteritis. The exact prevalence of each pathogen is not fully known, as the majority of illnesses are not accurately diagnosed. However, of the available reports of water-associated viral gastroenteritis, rotavirus and Norwalk or Norwalk-like viruses seem to account for the vast majority.

Rotaviruses are large-structured spherical viruses of about 70 nm diameter. Under the EM they appear to have a wheel pattern. Three antigenically different rotavirus types (A, B and C) have been associated with disease in humans. They are relatively resistant to many disinfectants other than chlorine to which they are quite sensitive (Figure 28.1a).

Norwalk viruses are small, single-stranded RNA viruses about 7.5 kb long. They are spherical and about 32 nm in diameter (Figure 28.1b).

PATHOGENESIS

Rotaviruses replicate in the villus epithelial cells of the small intestine and causes a loss of the absorptive cells. This may in part explain the cause of the diarrhoea due to reduced fluid absorption. Norwalk virus causes changes in

Table 28.1 Fastidious viruses associated with gastroenteritis

Virus	Nucleic acid	Shape	Size (nm)
Rotavirus	Double-stranded RNA	Circular	72
Small round virus (SRV), including Norwalk	Single-stranded RNA	Circular	30–35
Adenovirus	Double-stranded DNA	Icosahedral	75
Astrovirus	Single-stranded RNA	Circular	28
Calicivirus	Single-stranded RNA	Circular	33
Coronavirus	Single-stranded RNA	Enveloped	>100

the jejunum. Cell death does not appear to occur and the mechanism for the illness is unknown.

CLINICAL FEATURES

Rotavirus most commonly affects infants and young children. It has an incubation period of about 24 hours. The illness starts abruptly, with fever, vomiting and diarrhoea, which normally last 24–48 hours, although diarrhoea can last for up to five days.

The small round viruses such as Norwalk have a slightly shorter incubation period of a few hours to a day. The illness presents as vomiting and/or diarrhoea, which can have a very abrupt onset. Often affected individuals do not have time to get to the toilet to vomit. Illness last up to about 48 hours and recovery is complete, without sequelae.

DIAGNOSIS

For all these viral pathogens, EM of stool samples was the standard method for many years. Various commercial test kits are now available for rotavirus, based on latex agglutination, ELISA or polyacrylamide gel electrophoresis with silver staining (PAGE-SS). Tests for serum antibody exist for both rotavirus and Norwalk virus. Polymerase chain reaction tests are also becoming available.

TREATMENT

For all these pathogens management is based on fluid replacement and supportive care.

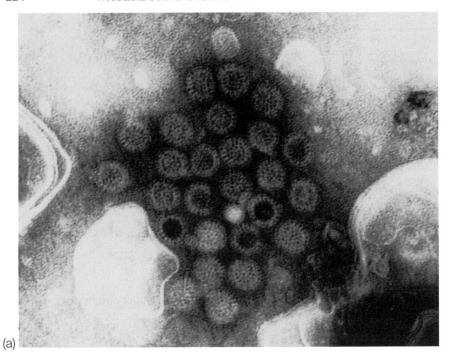

(a)

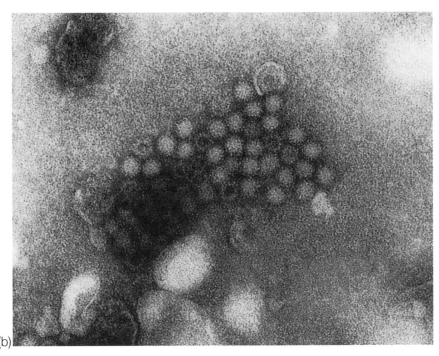

(b)

ENVIRONMENTAL DETECTION

The basic methodologies available for the detection of rotavirus and Norwalk virus in water and other environmental samples is as described in Chapter 27, on viral hepatitis. Rotavirus detection has been done with indirect immuno-fluorescence (Mehnert and Stewien 1993) and PCR (Jothikumar *et al.* 1995; Tsai *et al.* 1994).

ECOLOGY

As with the hepatitis viruses, viruses associated with human gastroenteritis replicate only in their human hosts. The distribution of viral gastroenteritis agents in the environment reflects the distribution of human faecal contamination. Rotavirus has been detected in 20.6% of sewage and 34.5% of creek water samples in the Sao Paulo area (Mehnert and Stewien 1993) and in 42% of drinking water sources in New Delhi (Jothikumar *et al.* 1995). Using somewhat older immunoassay-based methodology, Guttman-Bass, Tchorsh and Marva (1987) were unable to detect rotavirus in a one-year survey of Jerusalem.

EPIDEMIOLOGY

Viruses are the most commonly reported cause of acute gastroenteritis in any country. As viral replication occurs only in the human host, infection is acquired either directly from infected humans or indirectly through contaminated articles, food or water. Most of the viruses are very infectious and attack rates are often high. Many outbreaks are reported each year, especially in institutions. Person to person spread can be very rapid, mimicking a point source outbreak. Foodborne outbreaks occur when food has been handled by an infected food worker. Airborne spread, when a sufferer vomits, is probably common for Norwalk-like viruses. Waterborne outbreaks occur if the water supply or swimming area has been contaminated with human sewage. In all drinking water associated outbreaks the supply was unchlorinated.

Drinking water associated outbreaks

Perhaps the first well-documented outbreak of Norwalk virus gastroenteritis linked to drinking water occurred in a Washington State elementary school during May 1978 (Taylor, Gary and Greenberg 1981). Of 495 children and

---

Figure 28.1 (*opposite*) Electron micrographs of (a) a rotavirus and (b) a small round structured virus. Provided by Dr A Curry.

staff at the school who responded to a questionnaire, 71.5% recalled having had a gastrointestinal illness. Similar illnesses were seen in 31.8% of family contacts of cases and only 10.1% of family contacts of school attenders who had not been ill. In a nearby school only 6.5% reported a similar illness over the same time period. In the school attenders there was a significant association between the risk of illness and normal consumption of school water ($p < 10^{-8}$). In a study of illness among two soccer teams who had played their matches at the school there was also a highly significant association with drinking school water ($p = 10^{-6}$). Stool samples were submitted from only three cases and were found to be negative. However, serological examination of two cases showed seroconversion to Norwalk virus. The school took its water from a well. Well-water was pumped to a pressure tank. Because water was frequently spilled from this tank, the maintenance personnel had attached a hosepipe, taking this water to a floor drain. The day before the outbreak foul water had flowed into the room through the floor drain due to a blockage at the entry to the septic tank. Faecal coliforms were detected in five samples of school drinking water.

Soon after this first outbreak of Norwalk gastroenteritis, a second one occurred at a children's summer camp in Pennsylvania during July 1978 (Wilson et al. 1982). The outbreak was spread over two sessions, although some children attended both sessions. Infections occurred throughout the first session. During this first session there was 73 cases of illness, an attack rate of 28.6%. Two days after the start of the second session there was an explosive outbreak, with most cases developing over just two days. In this second session there were 100 children and 20 staff affected, giving an attack rate of 61.5%. Serological analysis showed a four-fold rise in titre to Norwalk virus in three of three sera examined. In a cohort study of campers and staff present during session 2 the only significant association was with drinking more than five glasses of water per day ($p < 0.02$) or a water containing beverage ($p < 0.05$). Fluorescein testing showed no evidence of cross-contamination in the water system. Microbiological analysis showed the presence of coliforms and faecal streptococci in the well and kitchen water. No residual chlorine was detected in tap-water.

Another school outbreak of viral gastroenteritis occurred in a school in Rio de Janeiro during May 1980 (Sutmoller et al. 1982). Of 1150 children at the school, 70.6% were absent during the outbreak. From 19 stool samples taken early in the outbreak, rotavirus was detected in 11 and *Shigella sonnei* in ten. The school took its water from one of several wells. It was found that just before the outbreak, the school had accidentally taken water from a poorly protected shallow well. Coliforms were detected in the shallow well. Residual chlorine was found to be zero in a sample from the tap.

Kaplan et al. (1982) reported an outbreak of gastroenteritis that affected about 1500 people in northern Georgia, US. The outbreak was spread over a one-week period during August 1980. In one area, known as Spring Village, the attack rate was as high as 68%. Epidemiological studies in several groups showed an association with drinking water. For example, there was an association with drinking from school water fountains in high school students who did not live in the area ($p < 0.001$) and in staff at the school ($p = 0.001$). Among residents of Spring Village there was also an association with drinking three or more glasses of tap-water ($p < 0.05$). In the area there was a textile plant which had its own water system, although two connections between the textile plant's system and the community system were known. The attack rates in the community decreased with distance from the known connections between the municipal and textile plant systems ($p < 0.001$). The water for the textile plant came from five wells and two springs. The water from one of the springs was found to be contaminated with faecal coliforms. Although the textile plant water was chlorinated, it was noted that the chlorinators were old. Normally textile plant water would not enter the municipal system because the latter was at higher pressure (110 versus 100 lb/sq in), although at times of peak demand the pressure in the municipal system fell to 80 lb/sq in.

Another town in Georgia suffered an outbreak of Norwalk gastroenteritis during January 1982 (Goodman et al. 1982). On 4 January, two days after very heavy rains, residents of about 250 homes that received water from the community system noted increased turbidity of their water. It was later that day that cases of gastroenteritis first occurred. A telephone survey indicated that people living in these homes suffered an attack rate of gastroenteritis of 63%, compared to only 9% among those having their own water supply ($p < 0.001$). The community system was supplied with water from one well and three springs. The well had been flooded during the heavy rains and one of the springs was situated within a fenced pig-pen and surrounded by several homes with septic tanks. Analysis of the water supplied by the dubiously sited spring, four days after the start of the outbreak, revealed the presence of faecal coliforms.

Two very large outbreaks of gastroenteritis, due to a novel strain of rotavirus, affected more than 12 000 adults in coal mining areas of China (Hung et al. 1984). The strain was said to be novel because it affected a particularly high proportion of adults. However, it is often the case that high attack rates in adults are a feature of many waterborne outbreaks. One epidemic affected 5942 cases (attack rate 12.8%) in an area near Laanzhou from November 1982 to February 1983. The other affected 7368 cases (attack rate 14.25%) near Jinzhou from December 1982 to January 1983. Both epidemics were explosive in onset. In the Jinzhou outbreak the attack rate was higher in just three residential districts (22.4–31.4%) compared to the others (5.4%). Furthermore, the attack rate among those who drank well-water (11.6%) was lower in high-risk areas. The main water supply to the high-risk areas was found to be heavily faecally polluted (230/ml $E.\ coli$). The outbreak quickly subsided after control of the water hygiene. No indication was given as to the reason for the failure in water hygiene.

Following several complaints about gastroenteritis to the local Department of Health on Friday, 13 March 1981, Hopkins *et al.* (1984) undertook a telephone survey of residents of two local communities in Colorado. They also examined local health centre records. In the telephone survey, 48 households were contacted, with 128 residents. Of these 128, 56 (43.8%) had been ill with diarrhoea and/or vomiting in the previous 30 days. Most people had been ill in the week starting 6 March. When analysis was restricted to those with illness starting after 6 March there was a strong correlation with drinking one or more glasses of tap-water per day against not drinking tap-water (RR 2.18, CI 1.10–4.32). Rotavirus was seen in the stool of one case and seroconversions or single high titres found in sera from several others. Environmental analysis found that a sewage works was discharging sludge solids into a creek upstream of a drinking water extract. Water treatment was also deficient in that there was no treatment prior to filtration, the filter beds were severely channelled and there had been a failure of chlorination.

The importance of ice as a vehicle for waterborne outbreaks was reinforced by two linked outbreaks in Philadelphia and Delaware during September 1987 (Cannon *et al.* 1991). Both of these outbreaks were associated with large public events. Small round structured virus was seen in one stool and serological conversions or high titre to Norwalk virus were seen in most of the 30 cases examined. In a survey of four groups who attended these events 191 people with gastroenteritis were identified, an attack rate of 31%. Illness was associated with the consumption of ice (RR 12.5, CI 8.7–18.0). The ice for both these events was provided by a single supplier. The ice manufacturing plant used water from three nearby wells and treated it with UV irradiation. On the 8 September the manufacturer's wells and septic tank had been flooded during heavy rain. Manufacture was suspended for two days while turbid water was pumped out of the wells.

Gastroenteritis affected over 900 people during a visit to a resort in Arizona between 17 April and 1 May 1989 (Lawson *et al.* 1991). Three of seven paired sera showed rising titres to Norwalk virus. In a telephone survey of 240 guests, 110 (46%) reported having symptoms. Drinking tap-water from the resort's well was significantly associated with illness (RR 16.1, CI 14.5–17.8). There was also an increasing risk with increased consumption of water ($p < 0.005$). The well-water was found to be heavily contaminated with faecal coliforms and faecal streptococci. It was discovered that, due to mechanical problems, two of the resort's five leach fields were incapable of accepting effluent at the time of the outbreak. Therefore, the remaining leach fields were subject to increased water flow. Furthermore, the wastewater chlorinator had failed because of flooding. Fluorescein dye placed in the leach fields appeared in the drinking water well. The well was drilling into flooded caverns in a limestone bedrock, which was under 60–80 m of sandstone (Figure 28.2). This sandstone had been assumed to be impervious to water.

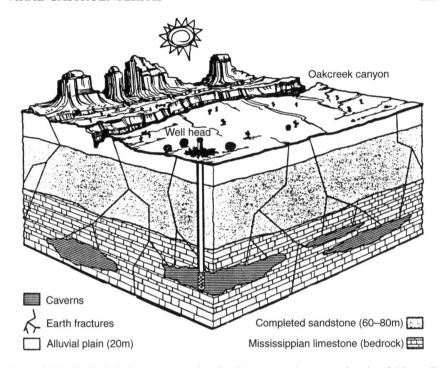

Caverns	
Earth fractures	Completed sandstone (60–80m)
Alluvial plain (20m)	Mississippian limestone (bedrock)

Figure 28.2 Geological features associated with a waterborne outbreak of Norwalk virus gastroenteritis at an Arizona resort. Reproduced from Lawson *et al.* (1991) Waterborne outbreak of Norwalk virus gastroenteritis at a southwest US resort: role of geological formations in contamination of well water. *Lancet* **337**: 1200–1204, by permission of The Lancet Ltd.

During the 1989 Christmas holiday period people staying at a caravan park at Moama, New South Wales, developed a Norwalk-like gastroenteritis (McAnulty *et al.* 1993). The authorities were alerted to this outbreak by a sudden increase in the number of people presenting to the local hospital's accident and emergency department with diarrhoea. From a review of the local hospital records it was found that 77% of patients with infective diarrhoea had stayed at a single caravan park. The authors then interviewed 351 people at the suspect park, of whom 305 (87%) reported illness. During the Christmas period up to 3000 people had been staying at the park, suggesting that about 2400 people may have been affected. There were two sources of water. Drinking water came from three above-ground rain-water tanks. Untreated river water was also pumped into two underground tanks for distribution throughout the site. Attack rates were higher in people who reported drinking the untreated water (RR 1.2, CI 1.1–1.3) and in those who reported using that water for ablutions (RR 1.3, CI 1.1–1.6). A plumber also reported that he had repaired a fracture in the sewage pipe near the underground water tanks during the time of the outbreak and that sewage had been leaking into both water tanks. High levels of faecal coliforms were detected in the untreated water, but not in the rain-water. One interesting aspect of this outbreak was that many people (26.9%) drank water from taps that were not intended for potable use.

Another ice-related outbreak affected passengers and crew aboard a cruise ship in Hawaii during February 1992 (Khan *et al.* 1994). Two separate cruises were affected. The outbreak started during the last two days of the first cruise, and within 24 hours of departure of the second cruise cases were already occurring. Approximately 30% of the 672 passengers and crew were affected. In a cohort study a significant association was found between illness and consumption of ice in passengers (RR 2.60, CI 1.03–6.55) and the crew (RR not calculable, $p = 0.05$). There was no association with water consumption. Although water was hyperchlorinated and food discarded between cruises the ice was the same. There was also a suggestion that illness during the second cruise was associated with inadequate decontamination of cabins between cruises. People who occupied a cabin on the second cruise used by an affected individual on the first were more likely to be ill even after adjusting for ice consumption (RR 1.60, CI 1.14–2.24). Design faults in the ice-making machines were identified that would potentially allow contamination either from people's hands or from sewage backup.

Recreational water associated outbreaks

Norwalk virus gastroenteritis affected students and teachers of an elementary school in Ohio during June 1977 (Kappus *et al.* 1982). All 103 primary cases took part in school trips to a picnic ground that had a swimming pool. In a cohort study of those attending the outing, all cases and 55 of 63 non-cases had been swimming in the pool ($p < 0.001$). Among swimmers there was an association between illness and swallowing pool water (OR 2.5, CI 1.1–5.6). Secondary cases were common. There was a high attack rate in family members of cases, of about 30%. The school trips were the first time that the pool had been used that season. Examination of the pool revealed that the chlorinator had been disconnected. Faecal coliforms and streptococci were isolated from pool water.

Three separate groups of people who had visited a park in Michigan during July 1979 developed a gastrointestinal illness (Baron *et al.* 1982). A telephone survey identified 314 individuals who had developed illness after visiting the park, of whom 277 (88%) had visited the park between 13 and 16 July. Among visitors to the park, there was a significant association between illness and swimming in the lake (OR 4.8, CI 1.8–12.7). Among family members of cases, there was an attack rate of 19% in those who had not visited the park. No source of pollution in the park was identified. Of 20 stool samples examined, virus-like particles similar to Norwalk virus were seen in only one

(Koopman *et al.* 1982). However, all of 11 paired sera examined showed a rising titre to Norwalk virus.

Prospective studies

Murphy, Grohmann and Sexton (1983) reported that, over several years, islanders and tourists on Norfolk Island, off the coast of Australia, suffered from a high incidence of gastroenteritis. The authors collected 28 faecal samples from individuals with gastroenteritis and found virus particles by EM in 21 (75%). Of these 21 positive identifications, 6 were rotavirus, 6 were small round virus, 5 astrovirus, 3 calicivirus and 1 adenovirus. No bacterial or viral pathogens were isolated by culture. Of 32 water samples from boreholes, 6 (29%) had faecal coliforms or greater than 10 coliforms in 100 ml. Seven vaccine strains of poliovirus and two strains of adenovirus were cultured. Rotavirus was seen once, small round viruses twice and adenovirus once by EM. The island is volcanic and made up of basaltic lava. The implication of these studies was that the high incidence of gastroenteritis was due to the leakage of sewage-polluted water through the very porous rock and into the boreholes.

Olusanya and Taiwo (1989) undertook a prospective study to determine the prevalence of rotavirus in urban children with diarrhoea at Ile-Ife, Nigeria. The study took place in the dry season, October 1985 to March 1986. All children, cases and controls, were either inpatients or attended a paediatric outpatient clinic. Of the 376 symptomatic children screened, rotavirus was detected in 57 (15.2%). Rotavirus was not detected in any of 80 asymptomatic children. The highest infection rates (40.6%) were seen in children between the ages of 7 and 12 months. Rotavirus was identified much more frequently in children from areas without a treated pipe-borne water supply (22.7% versus 7.1%, $p < 0.001$). *E. coli* were isolated from two of ten wells examined.

In a study of rotavirus-specific antibodies in Ecuadorian children, Brussow, Rahim and Freire (1992) found that antibody levels were not associated with drinking water quality or the presence of an organized sewage or sanitation system.

In their prospective epidemiological study of water-related gastrointestinal illness discussed elsewhere (Payment *et al.* 1991a, b), Payment, Franco and Fout (1994) studied the presence of Norwalk virus-specific antibodies in their two groups, one of which drank tap-water and the other tap-water after filtration through a reverse-osmosis filtration unit. Sera were taken on four separate occasions during the study period, in March, June and September 1988 and in June 1989. Norwalk infections occurred in one-third of individuals during the study, but there was no difference between the two groups in the attack rate.

29 Enterovirus Infections Including Poliomyelitis

For water virologists, enteroviruses are the viral equivalent to faecal coliforms. Like *E. coli*, the bacterial marker, enteroviruses are relatively easily culturable markers of faecal pollution. Like *E. coli*, enteroviruses can also cause disease and waterborne outbreaks in their own right.

VIROLOGY

Enteroviruses are a genus of viruses belonging to the family Picornaviridae. As the name suggests, Picornaviridae are very small RNA viruses. They are approximately 27 nm diameter, icosahedral viruses and have no envelope. Enteroviruses generally grow well in tissue culture

Traditionally, enteroviruses were classified by differences in host range, growth in cell lines and pathogenicity into one of four subgroups: polioviruses, coxsackieviruses A, coxsackieviruses B and echoviruses. These subgroups were further subdivided into a number of serotypes (Table 29.1). More recently described enteroviruses are no longer placed into one of these subgroups and are just given a serotype number. Enterovirus 72 is occasionally used for hepatitis A virus, although it is still not clear that HAV is an enterovirus.

PATHOGENESIS

The best-studied enteroviruses are the polioviruses. However, the basic pathogenic mechanism is similar for most enteroviruses. Infection usually follows the ingestion of faecally contaminated material. The infective dose is around 10^5 to 10^6 infectious particles. Initial site for replication is the submucosal tissue of the pharynx or distal small intestine. From the gut virus may then spread directly to regional cervical or mesenteric lymph nodes or via the blood to various reticuloendothelial tissues such as liver, spleen, other lymph nodes and the bone marrow. Replication may then cease. In severe illness and poliomyelitis further blood spread occurs to such target organs as the brain, skin, heart and muscles. The severity of illness is increased in the

Table 29.1 Classification and clinical effects of human enteroviruses

Subgroup	Serotypes	Human pathogenicity
Polioviruses	1–3	Aseptic meningitis; encephalitis; paralytic polio-myelitis
Coxsackieviruses A	1–24	Aseptic meningitis; encephalitis; paralytic disease; hand, foot and mouth disease; petechial rashes; herpangina; ulcerative stomatitis; lymphonodular pharyngitis; acute catarrh; pneumonitis and pleurisy; hepatitis; conjunctivitis; lymphadenitis; splenomegaly
Coxsackieviruses B	1–6	Aseptic meningitis; encephalitis; paralytic disease; maculopapular rashes; acute catarrh; pneumonitis and pleurisy; epidemic myalgia (Bornholm disease); pericarditis and myocarditis; generalized disease of the newborn; hepatitis; conjunctivitis; orchitis; lymphadenitis and splenomegaly
Echoviruses	1–34	Aseptic meningitis; encephalitis; paralytic disease; maculopapular and petechial rashes; croup; pneumonitis and pleurisy; generalized disease of the newborn; respiratory–enteric disease; gastro-enteritis; conjunctivitis
Enteroviruses	68–71	Aseptic meningitis; encephalitis; paralytic polio-myelitis; maculopapular rash; hand, foot and mouth disease; epidemic conjunctivitis

very young, pregnant, immunosuppressed and otherwise debilitated. Large amounts of virus may be excreted in the faeces and oropharyngeal secretions.

CLINICAL FEATURES

A truly bewildering array of clinical syndromes are associated with enteroviral infection (Table 29.1). In addition to those diseases where the link is proven, enteroviruses have been blamed by some authors for causing a range of other illnesses such as Guillain-Barré syndrome and 'post-viral fatigue syndrome'. Given the importance of the disease, I describe the clinical features of poliomyelitis in detail. As the features of epidemic myalgia are distinctive to coxsackievirus B, this is also discussed.

The incubation period of poliomyelitis is normally 9–12 days (range 5–35) to the onset of the prodromal illness. At least 95% of poliovirus infections are asymptomatic, and some have estimated that only 1 in 1000 infections is ever diagnosed. Abortive polio presents as an influenza-like illness, a tonsillitis or gastroenteritis, which last for just a few hours to 4–5 days at most before recovery. Those patients that go on to develop paralytic disease usually also experience a similar illness. Unfortunately, after remaining symptom-free for

2–5 days, patients develop features of meningitis: fever, headache, neck stiffness and vomiting. Muscle pain is also an early feature. After about one to two days of the meningitic illness, patients start to develop muscle weakness and eventual paralysis. The exact nature of the paralysis depends on the site affected. For spinal poliomyelitis, the degree of paralysis, which is of the flaccid type, varies from weakness of a portion of a single muscle to complete quadriplegia. For bulbar poliomyelitis the cranial nerves are affected, leading to dysphagia, dysarthria and dyspnoea. In bulbar disease circulatory and respiratory centres may be affected, leading, in severe cases, to respiratory or cardiovascular collapse. The most common complication of paralytic poliomyelitis is respiratory failure, due either to effects on the bulbar respiratory centre or to paralysis of the respiratory muscles. Pharyngeal paralysis can also lead to respiratory problems secondary to inhalation of secretions. Myocarditis has also been reported as a cause of death.

Epidemic myalgia (Bornholm disease or pleurodynia) has an incubation period of two to five days. It is characterized by the sudden onset of spasmodic pain with fever. The pain typically affects one side of the lower chest or abdomen. Illness usually lasts for four to six days, although it can last for up to three weeks. Meningitis and orchitis are occasional complications.

DIAGNOSIS

Diagnosis of enterovirus infections is often difficult and has to rest on the clinical presentation. Many, but not all, enteroviruses can be grown in tissue cell culture from throat swabs, faeces or CSF. Poliovirus is relatively easily cultured from throat and faeces, but rarely from CSF. Coxsackieviruses A do not grow readily in tissue culture and isolation of these agents used to rely on culture in sucking mice.

Serological diagnosis was primarily based on neutralization of viruses in tissue culture. As there are many different serotypes, such diagnosis is not commonly done. For poliomyelitis, the diagnosis may be confirmed by demonstrating specific antibody in CSF or a rising titre in serum. Demonstration of coxsackievirus B-specific IgM by ELISA is now frequently used, although cross-reaction between various serotypes makes this not very specific. DNA probes and PCR methods are also available but are not used routinely.

TREATMENT

No specific treatment is available for enteroviral infections. Where needed, treatment is symptomatic relief of pain. In poliomyelitis, patients should be admitted to hospital for bed rest. Where paralysis of respiratory muscles occurs, artificial ventilation will be required.

ENVIRONMENTAL DETECTION

The basic principles of virus isolation from water in environmental samples is the same as that described in Chapter 27, on viral hepatitis. PCR methods have been developed for enteroviruses although these may be no more sensitive than tissue culture (Abbaszadegan *et al.* 1993; Kopecka *et al.* 1993; Gilgen *et al.* 1995; Jothikumar *et al.* 1995; Ma, Gerba and Pepper 1995). However, Puig *et al.* (1994) found PCR to be more sensitive than cell culture at detecting enteroviruses in sewage and polluted river water. In a study of 16 sewage samples, enterovirus was detected by culture in 4 (25%) samples and by nested PCR amplification in 12 (75%). In nine river-water samples enterovirus was detected by culture in only one (11%), but in all samples by nested PCR amplification.

Moore and Margolin (1993) reported that both radioactive and non-radioactive gene probes were more sensitive than cell culture for the detection of poliovirus in water samples.

ECOLOGY

Unlike the other viruses discussed in this book, most enteroviruses are readily isolated in tissue culture cell lines. This ease of isolation is reflected in the large number of reported studies that have investigated the distribution of enteroviruses in environmental samples. This may also be why enteroviruses are used as viral markers of water quality.

Hurst (1991) reviewed the 1980–1990 English and French language literature on enterovirus isolation from waters. Enteroviruses were isolated from all 16 studies of raw surface waters reviewed. The percentage of positive samples ranged from 0.4% to 100%. Median isolation rate was 48.5% with the median of all studies average concentration being 1.4 units/l. Enteroviruses were isolated in two of three studies of groundwaters at a rate of 20.2% and 100%. Nine studies also looked at the isolation from conventionally treated water. Positive samples were found in four of these studies at rates of 7.6% and 100% in Quebec, 40.0% in Bolivia and 77.8% in Jalisco, Mexico. Hurst (1991) also reviewed five studies that looked at the removal of enteric viruses from various stages of conventional water treatment. Table 29.2 shows the median efficiency of virus removal at the different stages of water treatment.

Gilgen *et al.* (1995) used a PCR test to screen water from bathing beaches and found 7 of 40 (17.5%) samples positive. All positive samples were also positive for *Escherichia coli*. In a study of waters in Northern Ireland, Hughes, Coyle and Connolly (1992) reported enteroviruses isolated from 4 of 46 (8.7%) coastal waters in 1986 and 49 of 107 (45.8%) of similar samples in 1987. Thirty-three (62%) of the enterovirus-positive samples passed one or both of the coliform standards for bathing beaches. In 39 samples from three inland

Table 29.2 Median enteric virus removal efficiency from different stages in conventional water treatment processes. Adapted from Hurst (1991)

Stage of water treatment	Efficiency of virus removal (%)
Coagulation and sedimentation	50.4
Filtration	72.1
Coagulation, sedimentation and filtration	86.2
Post-filtration disinfection	≥ 45.0
Full treatment process	≥ 95.1

recreational waters, enteroviruses were detected in 33 (84.6%). Over a 63-month study period in Japan, Tani *et al.* (1995) found that enteroviruses were isolated throughout the year but the highest rate was during the summer, the time of peak infection in the community.

The predominant strains of enteroviruses that are isolated from the environment are those strains that happen to be circulating in the human population at the time. This is best seen in the case of polioviruses. This was seen during and after an outbreak of poliomyelitis in Finland in 1984 and 1985 (Püoyry, Stenvik and Hovi 1988). In routine sampling of sewage water during the 1970s enteroviruses, but no polioviruses, were isolated. During the peak of the epidemic, the wild-type epidemic strain was isolated from sewage from samples taken throughout the country. Soon after the start of a national immunization campaign the wild-type strain disappeared from sewage water. Continued monitoring revealed many enteroviral isolates and five vaccine-derived poliovirus isolates.

From 1980 to 1991, 268 isolations of polioviruses from sewage or river water were reported to the Japanese national surveillance scheme (Miyamura *et al.* 1992). The seasonal distribution of isolations mirrored the activity of the national vaccination campaign. Tambini *et al.* (1993) studied the distribution of poliovirus serotypes and wild and vaccine strains in children and wastewater in Cartagena, Columbia, a city with endemic poliomyelitis. The distribution of wild and vaccine strains of poliovirus and other enteroviruses was essentially the same in the faecal and wastewater surveys.

Keswick, Gerba and Goyal (1981) reported isolating enteroviruses from 10 (71%) of 14 samples of swimming pool and wading pool water in Texas. Two of the ten positive samples were taken from pools with free chlorine levels above the 0.4 ppm standard, suggesting that enteroviruses may persist for a while in adequately chlorinated swimming pools.

Survival of enteric viruses in the environment is affected by a number of factors (Fewtrell *et al.* 1994). The most important factor is probably temperature. As the ambient temperature rises from 3–5 °C to about 22–25 °C the survival of enteroviruses in marine water falls from 40–90 days to 2.5–9 days. Ultraviolet radiation also reduces survival, and survival in fresh waters is longer than in marine waters. Virus associated with solid material, such as faeces, survives longer than that which is dispersed through the water body.

EPIDEMIOLOGY

Enteroviral infections occur worldwide and can be seen as both endemic and epidemic disease. Spread may be directly from person to person via faecal-oral spread or contact with pharyngeal secretions. Spread of enteroviruses may be airborne, by contact with fomites and by waterborne spread. By contrast with the large number of studies that have looked at the isolation of enteroviruses from aquatic environments, there have been very few outbreaks of enteroviral disease linked to water.

Drinking water associated outbreaks

The only outbreak of poliomyelitis linked by an epidemiological study to water occurred in Taiwan in 1982 (Kim-Farley *et al.* 1984). Having been free of the disease for seven years, 1031 cases of paralytic poliomyelitis were reported between 29 May and 26 October. Cases occurred throughout the country and attack rates ranged from 1.3 to 15.2/100 000. The authors conducted a case-control study in two neighbouring rural areas with 32 cases and 210 controls. After univariate analysis of the study, having had no or only one dose of vaccine (OR 21.7, CI 10.5–44.9), a non-municipal water supply (OR 8.1, CI 3.0–21.7), a toilet shared with another family (OR 4.0, CI 1.9–8.3), non-municipal sewage disposal (OR 3.1, CI 1.5–6.6), a father with a non-professional occupation (OR 23.8, CI 3.4–167.3) or a father who was not a university graduate (OR 10.6, CI 1.1–103.6) were associated with increased risk of disease. After logistic regression analysis, inadequate vaccination and receipt of a non-municipal water supply remained as independent risk factors. In children who received municipal water, sharing toilet facilities with another family was still a significant risk factor.

An outbreak of pleurodynia affected 17 (20%) of the football players of a public high school in New York during the autumn of 1991 (Ikeda *et al.* 1993). Symptoms were severe and several cases attended hospital, although none was admitted. Coxsackievirus B1 was isolated from four of eight stool cultures. A cohort study was initiated among the school's football players, hockey players and cheerleaders, although as no cases of illness were reported in these two latter groups, they were excluded from further analysis. Behaviours that increased risk of illness were eating ice cubes from the team chest (RR 9.2, CI 1.3–65.5) and drinking water from the team cooler (RR 6.3, CI 1.5–25.7). These two risk factors were independently associated. The team coach remembered that an ill player had sat by the water cooler during a practice session at the start of the outbreak. The source of the infection was likely, therefore, to have been the index case, who infected the others by his use of the team ice and water cooler.

Recreational water outbreaks

Hawley *et al.* (1973) described an outbreak of coxsackievirus B5 infection at a boys' summer camp in northern Vermont in 1972. The index case was a nine-year-old boy who was admitted to hospital with conjunctivitis, sinusitis and meningitis. Including the index case, 21 of 33 campers and counsellors had evidence of viral infection. The virus was isolated from 13 of these individuals. The authors isolated virus from one of two samples of lake water, although they did not report any epidemiological study to support their hypothesis that swimming was associated with the transmission of the infection.

An outbreak of a viral illness affected children who participated in a swim class in Colorado during June 1987 (Lenaway *et al.* 1989). The case definition was fever of greater than 101 °F with at least one of the following: malaise, headache, stomach ache, nausea or diarrhoea. The authors considered this symptom complex to be enteroviral. Of 63 children who attended the class, 26 met the case definition. The attack rate for children who used the outdoor wading area was 62%, compared to 12% for those who did not (OR 12.1, CI 2.9–74.2). Inspection of the wading pool found several deficiencies, including high turbidity, too high a temperature, a low pH and an inoperative flow meter. Records of pool chlorine levels showed zero readings for five consecutive days.

Forty-six people developed vomiting, diarrhoea and headache soon after an outdoor swimming pool opened for the summer in Northern Ireland in June 1992 (Kee *et al.* 1994). A questionnaire was returned by 57 people, of whom 46 were ill. Echovirus 30 was isolated from 7 of 20 stool samples examined. Of those who were ill, 34 had swum in the pool. The 12 cases who had not been swimming were family contacts of swimmers. Among swimmers illness was higher in those who had swallowed water (86%) than in those who did not (59%), although this was not statistically significant ($p = 0.07$). Pool attendants recalled that on the opening day two children had vomited in the pool. Although attempts were made to spoon out the solids, much of the vomitus had dispersed. No other abnormality was detected and chlorine levels were satisfactory.

Prospective epidemiological studies

D'Alession *et al.* (1981) studied enteroviral excretion in children up to 15 years old attending a paediatric clinic in Madison, Wisconsin, from June to September 1977. They studied 296 children with 'enteroviral-like syndromes' and 679 well controls. Children with a febrile illness of the gastrointestinal or respiratory tract or of the central nervous system or with an undifferentiated fever were included as cases in the study. Viruses were isolated from 135 (56%) of 287 cases, of which 119 were non-polio enteroviruses. Group A coxsackieviruses were isolated from 45, group B coxsackieviruses from 29, echoviruses from 39 and untypable enteroviruses from 6. A history of swimming was obtained from all cases and controls. Children from whom an enterovirus was isolated were more likely to have swum exclusively on a beach than controls (OR 2.359, CI 1.462–3.807). Those who only swam in a swimming pool were not at increased risk (OR 1.053, CI 0.681–1.629). Case children from whom no virus was isolated did not differ from well controls.

Shortly after an epidemic of echovirus type 4 in Israel, Fattal *et al.* (1987) studied enteroviral antibody levels in agricultural workers. Residents of kibbutzim that used partially treated wastewater for irrigation purposes had higher levels of antibody to echovirus type 4 but not to other enteroviruses, most notably in the 0–5 year age group ($p < 10^{-5}$).

In a study of 109 individuals who took military diving courses in 1991 and 1992 in France, serological and cultural examination for enteroviruses was done at the start and again every 15 days thereafter (Garin *et al.* 1994). In addition, 49 non-diving controls were investigated, and environmental samples were taken from the area. Enteroviruses were detected by molecular hybridization in 9 (31%) of 29 water samples. At the start of the course, it was found that divers were significantly more likely to be positive to coxsackieviruses B4 and B5 than controls ($p < 0.05$), suggesting that diving may be a risk factor for these infections. During the course 15% of divers and 10% of controls seroconverted to at least one positive, but this was not statistically significant.

COMMENTS

Despite the observation that enteroviruses are widespread in the water environment, there have been relatively few documented reports of outbreaks of enterovirus disease linked to water consumption or contact. This discrepancy is probably because waterborne outbreaks are grossly under-reported as the majority of infections are asymptomatic. Even when symptoms develop, the clinical features of enteroviral disease are very varied, making diagnosis difficult. Furthermore, most waterborne outbreaks will be lost in the general level of endemic disease.

30   Adenoviral Infections

Although adenoviruses mostly cause acute respiratory infections and/or conjunctivitis in humans, there is currently considerable interest in this group of viruses because they have been shown to cause tumours in animals. The only waterborne outbreaks reported in the literature have been associated with inadequately chlorinated swimming pools.

VIROLOGY

Of all the viruses that have been associated with waterborne spread, adenoviruses are the only DNA viruses. The virus particle has no envelope, only an icosahedral protein coat or capsid. The intact virus has a diameter of 70–80 nm.

Human adenoviruses have been classified into six subgenera (A to F) based on SDS-polyacrylamide gel-electrophoresis patterns, now confirmed by DNA homology studies. The human adenoviruses have also been classified into 47 serotypes. Table 30.1 shows the relationship between subgenera and serotypes. Most serotypes grow well in standard cell culture line. The exception is the fastidious adenoviruses serotypes 40 and 41, which cause gastroenteritis. These viruses only grow in cell culture of transformed cells.

PATHOGENESIS

Adenoviruses can affect cells in one of three ways. In a lytic infection the virus infects the cell, replicates to produce up to a million new viruses and then kills the cell by lysis to release new infective particles. This type of infection occurs in epithelial cells and is probably the basis of most clinical human infection. Alternatively, the virus can infect the cell and become latent. Latency results in relatively slow replication and release of virus from the cell. The mechanism of latency is unclear but it tends to occur in lymphoid cells. In the third type of infection viral replication does not proceed at all, but the viral DNA becomes integrated into the host-cell DNA. The host cell can then be transformed into a cancer-like cell. This is the basis for tumour formation as described in animals.

Table 30.1 Classification of human adenoviruses. Adapted from Baum (1995)

Subgenus	Serotype	Human illness
A	12	Meningoencephalitis
	18,31	
B	3	Acute febrile pharyngitis; adenopharyngo-conjunctival fever; pneumonia; follicular conjunctivitis; fatal infection in neonates.
	7	Acute febrile pharyngitis; adenopharyngo-conjunctival fever; acute respiratory disease with pneumonia; fatal infection in neonates; meningoencephalitis
	11	Follicular conjunctivitis; haemorrhagic cystitis in children
	21	Haemorrhagic cystitis in children; fatal infection in neonates
	14	Acute respiratory disease with pneumonia
	16	
	34,35	Acute and chronic infection in patients with immunosuppression and AIDS
C	1,2	Acute febrile pharyngitis; pneumonia in children; intussusception
	5	Acute febrile pharyngitis; pertussis-like syndrome; intussusception; acute and chronic infection in patients with immunosuppression and AIDS
	6	
D	8,19,37	Epidemic keratoconjunctivitis
	9,10,13,15,17,42	
	19,20,22–29	
	30	Fatal infection in neonates
	32,33,36,38,	
	39,42–47	Acute and chronic infection in patients with immunosuppression and AIDS
E	4	Respiratory infection
F	40,41	Diarrhoea

CLINICAL FEATURES

Adenoviruses can cause a variety of clinical syndromes (Table 30.1). Adenoviral gastroenteritis was discussed in Chapter 28, on viral gastroenteritis. So far the outbreaks of adenovirus disease associated with water have been of pharyngitis and/or conjunctivitis. I will restrict myself to describing only these illnesses.

For adenoviral disease the incubation period is very varied, between 4 and 24 days. This is seen in the prolonged outbreak curves of the outbreaks described below.

In adenoviral keratoconjunctivitis, the onset may be sudden or insidious. The conjunctivitis is usually bilateral and the patient complains of pain, photophobia, blurred vision and headache. There is occasionally fever. The illness may persist for one to four weeks.

Pharyngoconjunctival fever is characterized by an acute onset of conjunctivitis, pharyngitis, rhinitis, cervical lymphadenitis and fever of up to 38 °C.

DIAGNOSIS

Diagnosis is made on the basis of clinical features, and the isolation of adenovirus from throat or conjunctival swabs. The diagnosis may be confirmed later by the demonstration of rising anti-adenovirus antibody levels by complement fixation tests.

TREATMENT

There is no specific treatment available, but virtually all cases recover. Supportive measures to reduce fever and manage pain may be needed.

ENVIRONMENTAL DETECTION

The basic methodologies for the isolation of viruses from environmental samples were described in Chapter 27 and will not be repeated here. Puig *et al.* (1994) described a nested PCR amplification method which was able to detect adenovirus in all of 9 river water and 16 sewage samples tested.

ECOLOGY

As with all other viruses, adenoviruses can be found in the environment where contamination by human faeces or sewage has occurred. However, most studies have either not detected adenoviruses or only in a relatively small percentage of samples (Hurst 1991; Tani *et al.* 1995). As already mentioned, using PCR Puig *et al.* (1994) detected adenovirus in all of 9 river water and 16 sewage samples. Adenoviruses were isolated from one swimming pool during the investigation of an outbreak of disease.

EPIDEMIOLOGY

The non-enteric adenoviral infections are usually spread directly or indirectly through infected secretions. Airborne spread through coughing and sneezing is probably common. The only waterborne outbreaks of adenoviral illness have been associated with swimming pools. Indeed, outbreaks of adenoviral disease have been linked to swimming pools since the 1950s.

In 1973 members of a swimming club were unable to compete because of a large number of cases of conjunctivitis (Caldwell et al. 1974). A case-finding questionnaire survey identified 44 cases with onset dates ranging from 4 to 23 January. The highest attack rates (33%) were in individuals who had been swimming in a local Kansas pool. Viral culture of conjunctival and throat swabs of eight cases were positive for adenovirus type 7 in at least one site in six. All affected cases had been swimming late in the day or in the evening. Inspection of the pool records showed that the filter sump pump had failed in December. Without this pump, the normal practice of automatic chlorination every hour failed. While the pump was out of action the pool attendant tested chlorine levels each morning and then added sufficient hypochlorite power as needed. No more chlorine was added during the day. It would appear that this led to inadequate chlorine levels towards the end of the day and so permitted transmission of infection.

An outbreak of pharyngoconjunctival fever affected 72 individuals who had attended a private recreational facility in Georgia during the summer of 1977 (D'Angelo et al. 1979). Case onset was distributed throughout August. All cases were members of a private club. Among members of the club the attack rate was significantly higher in those who had used the pool ($p < 0.001$). Furthermore, there was a linear relationship between the attack rate and number of visits per week to the pool ($p < 0.005$) and also the time spent in the pool ($p < 0.01$). Adenovirus type 4 was isolated from conjunctival or throat swabs in 20 of 26 cases sampled. The same virus was also isolated from two of four samples of pool water. Chlorine was added manually to the pool once or twice a day. The investigators noted that no records were kept of chlorine levels and that no regular schedule of water testing was followed. It would appear that inadequate chlorination was a factor in the cause of the outbreak.

Another outbreak of adenoviral disease linked to a private recreation centre swimming pool occurred in Georgia in 1977 (Martone et al. 1980). In a survey of swimming team members and their families, 54 cases were identified with onset dates throughout June and July. The illness was characterized by sore throat, fever, anorexia and headache. Conjunctivitis was present in only 35%. A subsequent survey of 99 randomly selected families living in the community identified 69 individuals (attack rate 18%), of whom 18 had been previously identified. Adenovirus type 3 was isolated from 19 of 24 people sampled. Illness was significantly associated with frequency of attending the local swimming pool ($p < 0.001$). Again, the investigators found that the pool was chlorinated by daily manual addition of hypochlorite and that a temporary failure in the filtration system had led to an increase in turbidity secondary to probable algal overgrowth.

An outbreak of pharyngitis with conjunctivitis affected at least 77 people in Oklahoma State in July 1982 (Turner et al. 1987). These cases were identified in two telephone surveys, the first of 5% of telephone listings and the second of 50% of people who had season tickets to the local swimming pool. In the first survey the attack rate was higher in swimmers than in non-swimmers (RR 10.8, $p < 0.001$). This finding was confirmed in the second survey. There was also a correlation between attack rate and the number of hours spent each week at the pool ($p < 0.01$). Furthermore, people who remembered swallowing pool water were more likely to be ill (RR 2.1, $p < 0.01$). Five of seven viral cultures from ill cases were positive for adenovirus type 7a. During early July the normally automatic chlorination system had failed and chlorination was being done by hand. No permanent records of chlorine levels or dosing were kept.

31 Chemical Poisoning and Drinking Water

Drinking water and recreational waters, whether taken from mains or private supplies or from natural sources, are always dilute solutions of a mix of chemicals. Some of these chemicals will have been deliberately introduced to improve water quality and safety, others will have been present in the source water and yet others will have been accidentally introduced to the supply or source. The problem is in identifying which chemicals pose a threat to human health.

Part of the problem in writing this chapter was knowing what to include. There has been a considerable amount of information about the potential and actual affects on human health of chemicals in drinking water. Much information will have been obtained as a result of toxicological studies in animals. Other information will have been derived from the known effects of human exposure associated with non-water routes, such as may occur in certain occupational exposures. Other information will have come from the study of individuals who have been exposed to chemicals in drinking or recreational water. This latter source of information provided the basis for this chapter.

As with previous chapters, I tend to restrict my review to those papers that have reported on epidemiological studies of human exposure. The papers reviewed in this chapter have been grouped by the main chemical under investigation. Where applicable, those studies investigating the results of chronic exposure are discussed separately from those investigating acute poisoning. Any discussion of the possible carcinogenic role of chemicals in drinking water is left until the next chapter. Similarly, the discussion of any effect of drinking water on the outcome of pregnancy is left until the chapter specifically concerned with this issue.

More detailed reviews of toxicology of potential waterborne chemical contaminants are given elsewhere (Fawell 1993; World Health Organization 1984).

ALUMINIUM

Aluminium is the most common metal element in the earth's crust, where it exists mainly as aluminium silicate. It is present in all soils, water and plant and animal tissues. Aluminium is one of the agents used in water treatment, where it acts as a chemical coagulant to assist in the removal of particulate materials. The current EC recommended maximum limit is 0.2 mg/l, although this level was set for aesthetic rather than toxicological reasons. Above this level complaints of discoloration increase. Levels of aluminium in finished water above 0.3 mg/l usually indicate faults in the treatment process. Even at the EC limit aluminium consumption from drinking water would probably only represent about 2% of total daily intake.

Aluminium is said to be poorly absorbed from the gut and rapidly excreted by the kidneys so that acute toxicological effects from oral ingestion are thought not to occur, but see below for a discussion of the Camelford incident. Rats administered high doses of aluminium (2.5 mg/kg/day) for six months showed only minimal signs of toxicity (Krasovskii, Vasukovich and Chariev 1979). There is no animal evidence of mutagenicity. However, aluminium toxicity has been described in patients undergoing renal dialysis, usually when levels are high in the dialysis water. This takes the form of osteomalacia (Ward et al. 1978; Parkinson et al. 1979; O'Brien, Moore and Keogh 1990) or dementia (Alfrey, Legendre and Kaehny 1976; Rozas, Port and Easterling 1978; Parkinson et al. 1979) if the aluminium concentration in the dialysate exceeded 0.1 mg/l.

Acute exposure: The Camelford incident

Undoubtedly the most notorious water exposure incident of recent years in the UK was that due to the accidental contamination of the water supply to the Cornish town of Camelford on 6 July 1988 (Rowland et al. 1990). The accident happened when a relief driver poured 20 tons of aluminium sulphate into the contact chlorine reservoir. The incident was not discovered for a few days so an estimated 20 000 individuals were exposed to high levels of aluminium and other chemicals, most notably lead and sulphate. From estimates of exposure made from the known peak concentrations of aluminium, the authors of the original report estimated that individuals would have had to drink several litres of water per day to positively absorb the metal. Nevertheless, 500 questionnaires were sent to households within the exposed area and 500 to controls in a non-exposed area. Even with the intense amount of public interest in the contamination incident, the response rate was only 44.6%. Half of the respondents in the exposed area stated that they experienced unusual symptoms after the episode compared to 10% of people in the control sample (RR 4.2, CI 3.3–5.4). Virtually all of the acute symptoms asked about in the questionnaire were reported significantly more commonly from respondents in the exposed area (headache, nausea, vomiting, diarrhoea, fever, cold, excessive tiredness, blurred vision, painful mouth/tongue, bad breath, earache, difficulty passing urine, chest pain, stomach ache, painful joints, pain in muscles and skin rashes). The only symptom to be reported more commonly from the exposed area, in relation to other reported symptoms, was joint pain. It was notable that significantly more individuals reported illness in the exposed area before the contamination incident ($p <$ 0.001). The authors concluded that the results of their study were consistent with a causal relationship between symptom reporting and the water contamination incident. Rather diplomatically, they stated that they could not identify whether the causal mechanism was pharmacological, toxicological or psychological. They did note that such incidents inevitably cause considerable anxiety and stress.

The comments about the improbability of absorption of aluminium reported by Rowland et al. (1990) were cast into some doubt by a report of the investigation of two patients who had been exposed to the contaminated water (Eastwood et al. 1990). Both patients had been well prior to the incident, reported acute symptoms at the time of the incident and were still unwell six months later. Aluminium concentrations in blood and urine samples were normal. The only abnormalities found were infrequent lines of positive staining with solochrome azurine of bone biopsy samples. This histological appearance was compatible with an acute period of increased aluminium absorption.

A few years later Owen and Miles (1995) reported a longer term follow-up of hospital discharge rates after the incident (in the UK discharges from, rather than admissions to, hospital are recorded). The authors compared standardized hospital discharge rates in the Camelford population with that of the whole of the Cornish population. The discharge rate from Camelford rose from being below average in the year 1987–1988 to being above average in the year 1989–1990 and remained high up to at least the year 1992–1993. No single specific diagnosis was responsible for this increase.

Powell et al. (1995) reported a study of toxic metal concentrations, other than aluminium, in individuals who had been present during the toxic incident. The authors were testing the hypothesis that the low pH generated during the incident would have dissolved other potentially toxic metals into the supply. The first study identified 14 individuals who complained of a variety of symptoms, including loss of concentration, poor short-term memory and musculo-skeletal pains. This study was conducted some 31 months after the incident and all had normal blood or serum concentrations of magnesium, iron, copper, zinc and lead. One individual whose hair was sufficiently long to have been present during the time of the incident had hair tested. The concentration of lead in the hair was higher at the distal end, hair that would have been formed at the time of the incident. Another female also had a higher concentration of mercury in the hair estimated to have grown at the same time.

The health implications of this incident have been open to significant debate and some dispute between health professionals and the local population. The publication of the second of two official reports published into this incident

(Lowermoor Incident Health Advisory Group 1989, 1991) stimulated an editorial in the *British Medical Journal* (Coggon 1991). In that editorial the question of the difficulty of conducting an unbiased epidemiological study after such incidents was raised. The author suggested that the situation was similar to that of a doctor trying to reassure an anxious patient. This led to a brisk complaint that the health services had not adequately investigated the incident (Lawson 1991).

Tohani *et al.* (1991) also reported the accidental addition of aluminium sulphate to a mains water supply in 1988. However, peak concentrations were much lower (1.8 mg/l) and the duration of contamination was much shorter. Nevertheless, one individual reported a skin rash after bathing in the affected water. Skin testing with aluminium sulphate was unable to replicate the rash. The patient reported that she was allergic to cheap jewellery, and skin testing with nickel and cobalt showed strong allergy to both metals. The authors suggested that the aluminium sulphate reduced pH so that these metals were dissolved from the distribution system, so causing her rash.

The Camelford incident will become a classic example for public health doctors in the problems raised. As has been seen throughout this book, standard epidemiological methods suffer from serious problems of bias when individuals are aware of an environmental exposure and already consider this exposure harmful. Even when expert medical opinion is that no health risk exists, the local population may not be reassured. To support their doubts they need only refer to one of the many recorded situations where expert medical opinion has been proven to be wrong. In such situations standard epidemiological studies will almost inevitably be seriously flawed. Even when no direct toxicological effect exists, statistically significant associations between reported illness and the popular suspect exposures are likely to be found. Even when no such association is found, the local press and population are likely to denounce the study or the investigators. If an association is found, the mechanism for this will then be open to debate. Possible explanations include a real effect due to a direct toxicity, a real effect due to psychological factors, or an artefactual finding due to deliberate or unconscious over-reporting of illness or exposure.

Aluminium and dementia

One of the more worrying correlations between long-term water quality and human ill health is the suggestion that dementia may be higher in people who have higher aluminium contents in their drinking water. This suggestion first came from findings of aluminium encephalopathy in patients on haemodialysis. There have been several epidemiological studies that have set out to investigate this relationship.

In a study of 386 patients admitted to hospital from 1982 to 1985 with fracture of the hip from health authorities in Tyneside, northeast England,

Table 31.1 Relative risks of effect of aluminium concentration on incidence of Alzheimer's disease

Reference	Aluminium (mg/l)	Risk estimates (OR or RR)
Martyn et al. (1989)	0–0.01	1 (RR)
	0.02–0.04	1.5 (1.0–2.2)
	0.05–0.07	1.4 (1.0–1.9)
	0.08–0.11	1.3 (0.9–2.0)
	>0.11	1.5 (1.1–2.2)
Flaten (1990), males	<0.05	1
	0.05–0.2	1.15
	>0.2	1.32
Flaten (1990), females	<0.05	1
	0.05–0.2	1.19
	>0.2	1.42
Neri and Hewitt (1991)	<0.01	1
	0.01–0.099	1.13
	0.10–0.199	1.26
	≥0.200	1.46
	(χ^2 for trend = 12.24, p = 4.7×10^{-4})	
Forbes, Hayward and Agwani (1991)	<50th centile	1
	>50th centile	1.07
Jacqmin et al. (1994)	0–0.003	1
	0.003–0.006	1.02
	0.006–0.018	0.62
	0.018–0.940	0.84
	(χ^2 for trend = 12.31, p = 4.5×10^{-4})	
Forster et al. (1995)	<0.05	1.2 (0.67–2.37)
	0.05–0.09	0.8 (0.42–1.50)
	0.10–0.15	0.8 (0.42–1.71)
	≥0.15	1.0 (0.41–2.43)

there was no difference in mental test score between residents of North and South Tyneside (Wood et al. 1988). North Tyneside had aluminium concentrations in the water ranging from 0.18 to 0.25 mg/l compared to <0.05 mg/l in South Tyneside. However, the use of aluminium in the north had only started in 1982.

In the UK, Martyn et al. (1989) conducted an ecological survey of rates of Alzheimer's disease in the 40–69 year age group of 88 county districts of England and Wales. Rates were calculated from records of computerized tomographic (CT) scanning units. Aluminium concentrations, which were all within accepted limits, were obtained from water company records. After accounting for distance of residence from a CT unit, the relative risk of Alzheimer's disease was greater in those counties with aluminium levels greater than 0.01 mg/l (Table 31.1). There was no gradient with increasing concentration above 0.02 mg/l.

In an ecological study from Norway, Flaten (1990) compared death certificate reports of dementia and aluminium in water supply in 454 municipalities. Municipalities were classified as to whether their water supplies contained <0.05, 0.05–0.2 or >0.2 mg/l of aluminium. Highly significant associations were found between rates of dementia, but not Parkinson's disease and amyotrophic lateral sclerosis, and aluminium concentrations over four separate time periods between 1969 and 1983. Relative risks for 1974 to 1983 are shown in Table 31.1.

Neri and Hewitt (1991) reported a case-control study of 2344 patients with Alzheimer's disease or pre-senile dementia aged over 55 years and discharged from Ontario hospitals. These were compared with 2232 patients with non-psychiatric illness. They compared cases and controls for drinking water aluminium concentration at home. There was an increase in the estimated relative risk for concentrations above 0.01 mg/l ($p < 0.05$) although no confidence intervals were given.

Further support for the association between aluminium and dementia was given by Forbes, Hayward and Agwani (1991), who also reported from Ontario cases of any mental impairment in a group of elderly males. They found that mental impairment was commoner in those individuals whose water contained aluminium in excess of the 50th centile (OR 1.07) (Table 31.1). This association held up in a multivariable logistic regression model which included aluminium, fluoride (OR 0.58, $p < 0.05$), pH, water source, educational achievement and number of moves (Forbes and McAiney 1992). Impaired mental functioning was more common in those taking high aluminium water (OR 1.86, $p < 0.01$) and in those moving home more than twice in 30 years (OR 1.47, $p < 0.05$), and less common in those taking high fluoride water (OR 0.58, $p < 0.05$), surface water sources (OR 0.36, $p < 0.05$), those with alkaline pH (7.85–8.05) water (OR 0.43, $p < 0.05$) and those with post-secondary education (OR 0.41, $p < 0.01$). The suggestion that fluorine in water supplies may be protective against mental impairment will be mentioned further below.

In an earlier study of Alzheimer's disease, eight of nine patients who were born in Bonavista Bay, Newfoundland, came from the same area. Frecker (1991) set out to investigate whether this cluster could be confirmed by looking at death certifications for the years 1985 and 1986. He found that the community with the highest rate of dementia deaths was the one with the highest aluminium concentration in drinking water (0.165 mg/l). However, dementia death rates in the other communities did not correlate with aluminium concentrations.

Wettstein et al. (1991) investigated the issue more directly by examining 805 individuals aged 81–85 years. Of these people, 400 had lived for at least 15 years in a low-aluminium water area (0.004 mg/l) and 405 in a high-exposure (0.098 mg/l) area. There was no significant difference between the two populations as defined by tests of mnestic and naming skills. The authors suggested that their results did not support a role for aluminium in causing dementia.

Jacqmin *et al.* (1994) conducted a survey of 3777 French men and women aged 65 years and over. They investigated the impact of water aluminium, calcium, fluoride and pH. In the univariate analysis the prevalence of cognitive impairment actually declined with increasing Al concentration, although most waters had low levels (<0.018 mg/l) (Table 31.1). When the impact of pH was taken into account, there was a negative association between aluminium and cognitive impairment in alkaline waters (pH 8.5), but a positive association in neutral waters (pH 7.0). In the multiple logistic model with occupational data, age, sex, educational level, calcium, aluminium and pH there was a relationship with log aluminium concentration (OR 5.2, CI 1.1–25.1). In a model without the educational and occupational data there was an increased risk but the confidence intervals included unity (OR 5.4, CI 0.8–38.4).

Finally, Forster *et al.* (1995) reported a case-control study of 109 cases of pre-senile Alzheimer's disease and 109 age- and sex-matched controls. Only univariate analyses were reported. Alzheimer's sufferers were significantly more likely to have a first-degree relative with the disease (OR 2.5, CI 1.05–6.56), any relative with dementia (OR 2.1, CI 1.01–4.55) and any relative aged less than 65 years with dementia (OR 8.0, CI 1.07–348). They found no significant association between aluminium concentration and mental impairment (Table 31.1).

The issue of whether aluminium in drinking water predisposes to dementia remains open. The findings of dementia in patients on haemodialysis provide strong supportive evidence but not proof of a link. Most of the epidemiological studies that have supported an association have been of the ecological type. Few have demonstrated a clear dose–response curve and more analytic studies have given mixed results, with the strength of evidence being against an association. Nevertheless, an association cannot yet be dismissed.

ARSENIC

Arsenic is an extremely toxic metal that occurs in many environments, although usually in very small concentrations. It has several uses as, for example, ant poisons, insecticides, weed killers and medically. It has a long tradition of use for homicide. The current EC limit for arsenic in drinking water is 0.05 mg/l.

The pathogenicity of arsenic is thought to be due to the binding of sulphydril enzymes, which then interrupts cellular metabolism.

After oral intake, the symptoms of acute poisoning are initially gastrointestinal. Two to three hours after an oral dose there is sudden vomiting, and copious watery diarrhoea, which may be bloody. Dehydration may develop quickly, leading to death from circulatory collapse. If death does not occur, jaundice and renal failure may develop after a couple of days. The fatal dose may be as low as 100 mg.

Chronic poisoning is manifest by anorexia, diarrhoea and weight loss. If poisoning continues, other features include typical skin changes such as bronzing and hyperkeratosis of the palms and soles, peripheral neuritis, and cardiac, renal and liver changes. There is still some debate over the effect of chronic arsenic exposure on peripheral vascular disease. This is reviewed by Engel et al. (1994).

The diagnosis is made from history of exposure, clinical features and quantification of arsenic levels in blood or urine. In acute exposure, X-rays may show the compounds, as they are radio-opaque.

Treatment is by removal from source, gastric lavage in acute cases, and specific antidotes (dimercaprol and penicillamine). If the patient survives a week, the prognosis is good.

Acute exposure

An outbreak of acute poisoning affected nine members of a family who lived on a farm in Virginia in 1979 (Armstrong et al. 1984). There were two deaths. The only person not affected was an 18-month-old child who only drank shop-bought drinks. All drinking water came from an outdoor well, which was found to contain 108 mg/l of arsenic. There was a significant correlation between urine arsenic levels and daily consumption of well-water ($r = 0.85$). Neighbours' wells had very little arsenic present. No source of contamination could be found.

Another family outbreak affected a husband and wife who had recently moved into a rural home in upstate New York in 1987 (Franzblau and Lilis 1989). The house had not been lived in for some years. Water from the family's well was found to have a high arsenic concentration, 9–10.9 mg/l. Most neighbours' wells had low concentrations of arsenic. The well was situated downhill of an abandoned mine. Samples of ore taken from near to the mine entrance contained concentrations of arsenic of up to 32.1 mg/l.

Chronic exposure

Perhaps the best-known area to suffer from increased arsenic in drinking water is the southwest coast of Taiwan. Chronic arsenism, due to consumption of artesian drinking water, is endemic, and several studies from this area have investigated the correlation between arsenic in drinking water and various diseases. This group of papers is discussed first.

Blackfoot disease is the name give to a peripheral vascular disease endemic to the southwest coast of Taiwan. The disease usually begins with numbness or coldness in the feet, but the hands can also be affected. Eventually pain develops at rest and gangrene sets in. Over a thirty-year survey the case fatality rate was found to be 66.5% of which two-thirds were due to cardio-vascular causes (Tseng 1989). There is a dose–response relationship with disease risk and duration of using affected water. However, following a review of the literature, Ko (1986) did not accept that arsenic is the cause of blackfoot disease; he suggested that the incidence of disease actually increased after the installation of a new water supply. It is not known whether his opinion has changed in the light of more recent evidence.

Chen et al. (1988) reported a case-control study of 305 patients with blackfoot disease. In the multivariate model, they found that duration of consumption of artesian well-water (0 years, OR 1.00, 1–29 years OR 3.04, $\geq$30 years OR 3.47, $p < 0.001$), evidence of arsenic poisoning (OR 2.77, $p < 0.01$), a positive family history of blackfoot disease (OR 3.29, $p < 0.01$) and not eating vegetables each day of the week (OR 1.43, $p < 0.05$) were all independently associated with the risk of blackfoot disease.

To investigate further the association between blackfoot disease and arsenic in water Tseng et al. (1995) studied the microvascular circulation of apparently normal individuals living in villages with and without the affected artesian water. Using laser Doppler flowmetry, they showed that men in the affected villages had poorer circulation in the foot even in the absence of obvious disease.

Lai et al. (1994) reported a study of the prevalence of diabetes in 891 adults in Taiwan. They found a significant association between diabetes prevalence and both the duration of exposure to the contaminated artesian water and the calculated lifetime exposure. In a multivariate model including age, sex, body mass index and physical activity at work they found a significant association with cumulative arsenic exposure; 0 mg/l-years (OR 1.0), 0.1–15 mg/l-years (OR 6.61, CI 0.86–51.0) and $\geq$15 mg/l-years (OR 10.05, CI 1.30–77.9). In a similar study by the same authors (Chen et al. 1995) an association was found between cumulative exposure to arsenic and hypertension. In a multivariate model including age, sex, diabetes, proteinuria, body mass index and fasting triglyceride levels there was a significant correlation with increasing dose.

There have also been reports of chronic arsenism from many other parts of the world. The city of Antofagasta, Chile, received water containing high concentrations of arsenic (0.8 mg/l) over the years 1958–1970 (Borgoño et al. 1977). In the early 1960s the first cases of dermatological arsenism were noted in children. These children also suffered from increased incidence of bronchopulmonary disease, hyperkeratosis, chronic cough, lip herpes, Raynaud's syndrome, acrocyanosis, angina, hypertension, chronic diarrhoea and abdominal pain. High levels of arsenic were found in hair samples whether or not the children had dermatological evidence of arsenism. Six years after a new treatment plant had been built, arsenic levels in hair were much lower.

After discovering arsenic levels of up to 10 mg/l in the well-water supply to a residential area near Fairbanks, Alaska, Harrington et al. (1978a) undertook a survey of 211 residents of the area (a 91% response rate). Water samples collected from people's homes ranged from 0.001 to 2.45 mg/l (mean

0.224 mg/l). In those who drank well-water there was a strong correlation between urine and water arsenic levels, and between hair and water levels. The authors did not identify any clinical or haematological abnormality that could be attributed to chronic arsenic exposure.

Cebrián et al. (1983) compared the prevalence of signs of chronic arsenism in two populations, one with a low (0.007 mg/l) and the other a high (0.41 mg/l) concentration of arsenic in drinking water. The exposed population was more likely to suffer cutaneous signs of arsenism: hypopigmentation (RR 8.0), hyperpigmentation (RR 6.4), palmoplantar keratosis (RR 36.0), papular keratosis (RR 13.3) and ulcerative zones (RR 3.6). The exposed population was more likely to suffer from nausea (20.9% versus 6.0%), epigastric pain (27.4% versus 8.2%), colic (17.9% versus 7.2%), diarrhoea (16.9% versus 9.1%), headache (27.7% versus 14.2%) and oedema (6.1% versus 1.3%). Furthermore, within the exposed population those with cutaneous signs were also more likely to suffer from these same symptoms.

A study of volunteers from Nevada compared chromosomal abnormality rates in individuals whose drinking water contained between 0.05 and 2.275 mg/l of arsenic with those whose water contained less than 0.05 mg/l (Vig et al. 1984). The authors found no difference in chromosomal aberrations between the two groups. Those who were in the high-exposure group reported symptoms compatible with arsenism in 31% compared to 19% of the low-exposure group although this did not quite reach statistical significance ($p = 0.064$).

Arsenical dermatitis is seen in villages in west Bengal, where it is associated with water from tube wells (Chakraborty and Saha 1987). This problem was first identified in 1983 but since then more cases have come to light. The authors surveyed 6 villages of 14 known to be affected. Arsenical dermatitis was identified in 197 (25.1%) individuals in the survey. Also, the authors were told of three deaths due to ascites, which they suspected was due to arsenism. Arsenic was detected at levels of greater than 0.05 mg/l in 55 (77.5%) of water samples from tube wells. Arsenic concentrations in tube well water associated with affected families ranged from 0.20 to 2.00 mg/l (mean 0.64 mg/l). In the water samples from non-affected families the mean arsenic concentration was 0.21 mg/l. The investigators were unable to ascertain the source of the contamination.

Foy et al. (1992–93) surveyed residents of a tin and wolfram mining area in southern Thailand. They found dermatological evidence of chronic arsenism in 9% of adults. Concentrations of arsenic from shallow well-water ranged from 0.02 to 2.7 mg/l. The source of the contamination was probably slag heaps from the mines.

In an ecological study covering 30 US counties over the years 1968–1984, Engel and Smith (1994) compared mean arsenic concentrations in drinking water with mortality from diseases of the arteries, arterioles and capillaries. The standardized mortality ratios for those counties exceeding 0.02 mg/l arsenic were 1.9 (90%CI 1.7–2.1) for females and 1.6 (90%CI 1.5–1.8) for males.

Undoubtedly arsenic in drinking water other than at very low concentrations has a significant adverse health impact. This concern is further strengthened by studies of arsenic and cancer reviewed in the next chapter.

BARIUM

Barium is an alkaline earth metal that rarely exists in the metallic form because it is so reactive with water. The insoluble salt, barium sulphate, is used as a contrast medium for X-ray examination of the gastrointestinal tract. Other salts of barium are soluble. They are sometimes used as pesticides. The EC limit for barium in water is 1.0 mg/l.

The soluble salts of barium are acutely toxic. Features of acute poisoning include gastroenteritis, weakness, paralysis, convulsions and myocarditis. The fatal dose for an adult is between 500 and 1000 mg. It is thought that the barium ion affects muscle cell membranes so that the muscle fibre is stimulated indiscriminately. Treatment involves supportive care and the use of the anti-dote, sodium sulphate.

Concerns about the safety of barium in drinking water come from the observation that it increases systolic blood pressure in rats (Perry *et al.* 1983). This was supported by an ecological study that showed significantly high death rates in communities whose water contained 2–10 mg/l of barium compared to those containing <0.2 mg/l (Brenniman *et al.* 1979). However, a second ecological study of two communities in Illinois, one of which had a mean barium level of 7.3 mg/l and the other 0.1 mg/l, found no difference in the rates of hypertension between the two communities (Brenniman *et al.* 1981). Wones, Stadler and Frohman (1990) studied the impact of changing oral intake of barium on 11 healthy males over a 10-week period. There was no impact on known risk factors for cardiovascular effects, including blood pressure, plasma cholesterol or lipoprotein levels, or arrhythmias. The authors concluded that drinking-water barium had no apparent effect on cardiovascular risk factors at levels of 5 and 10 mg/l.

COPPER

Copper is one of the most widely used metals, especially in plumbing, where it is used for domestic pipes. It is ubiquitous in the environment and water and is present in many foods. Copper is an essential trace element for many physiological processes. The European limit for copper in drinking water is 3.0 mg/l.

Several papers prior to 1970 have described outbreaks of illness linked to excess copper in water or drink. Spitalny *et al.* (1984) reported recurrent episodes of vomiting and abdominal pain in a father and two daughters in a family of four in northwestern Vermont. These bouts of illness usually followed 10 to 20 minutes after drinking water that was noted as having a blue tint. The water came from a spring and was distributed in a copper main. The concentration of copper in the water supply was 7.8 mg/l. Copper levels in the hair of the affected children were elevated, as were those in hair samples from a neighbouring family, but not in a family supplied from a cast iron main. The water was acidic (pH 5.8) and corrosive (Langelier index – 3.59). The bouts of vomiting stopped as soon as the family stopped using tap-water for drinking.

Schramel *et al.* (1988) reported the development of severe liver disease in three children in two unrelated families. All three developed disease in the first year of life and two died. Histological examination revealed micronodular liver cirrhosis similar to that seen in Indian childhood cirrhosis. There was a high copper concentration in the liver. Drinking water was obtained from wells, and transported to the house in copper pipes. Copper levels in the well-water was low, but at the tap it was 3.4 mg/l. Von Mählendahl and Lange (1994) presented two further cases, one of whom died, in similar situations.

An unusual cause of vomiting, abdominal pain and eventual renal failure was presented in a Nigerian man living in California (Sontz and Schwieger 1995). This man developed illness after consuming green water, a traditional Nigerian drink used in religious ceremonies, to induce vomiting. Among other things, it contained alcohol and 13 390 mg/l of copper.

Although copper is generally considered to be non-toxic, these reports confirm that high copper concentrations in drinking can have both acute and chronic effects. Soft, acidic waters can dissolve significant amounts of copper from pipes. The potential risk of liver disease in young children led Sidhu, Nash and McBride (1995) to propose a reduction in the US standard for copper in drinking water from 1.3 mg/l to 0.3 mg/l, only 10% of the current European standard.

FLUORIDE

In its elemental form, fluorine is greenish-yellow gas which is slightly heavier than air. It is one of the halogens. In its gaseous form and as many of its compounds it is extremely corrosive and poisonous. Fluorine compounds have many industrial uses. The European limit for fluoride in water varies according to ambient temperature, but in the UK it is set at 1.5 mg/l.

Acute ingestion of excess fluorides results in salivation, nausea, vomiting, abdominal pain and diarrhoea followed by weakness, muscle spasm and convulsions. Death is by respiratory paralysis. Diagnosis of acute poisoning is on the clinical and epidemiological features; urinary fluoride estimations may also help.

Chronic poisoning, with the ingestion of more than about 6 mg of fluorine per day, results in a condition known as fluorosis. Fluorosis results in weight loss, anaemia, brittle bones, joint stiffness and mottling of the teeth. Diagnosis of fluorosis is by examination of the teeth and by radiological examination showing osteosclerosis and calcification of ligaments.

Treatment of acute fluoride poisoning is by giving intravenous calcium gluconate with oral milk of magnesia. If this form of calcium is not available then any soluble oral form of calcium, such as milk or calcium gluconate or lactate solution plus magnesium sulphate, is suitable. Supportive measures include treatment of shock and giving milk or cream every few hours to reduce oesophageal pain. Treatment of fluorosis is the removal of the patient from continuing exposure.

Fluorine is the only chemical that is deliberately added to drinking water for therapeutic gain. Once fluoride is incorporated into tooth enamel it reduces the solubility of the enamel and protects the tooth from decay. Recent reviews of the benefits of fluoridation include those of Ripa (1993), Murray (1993) and Lewis and Banting (1994). Fluoride is, however, the focus of one battle between some sections of the population, who see this as mass medication and an infringement of their civil liberty. There has been considerable and often ill-informed debate about the real and potential hazardous effects of fluorine in drinking water. This review is limited to a discussion of those properly conducted epidemiological studies.

Acute poisoning

Hoffman *et al.* (1980) reported an outbreak of abdominal pain, nausea and vomiting at a New Mexico elementary school during November 1978. In a survey of students and staff at the school, 34 (16.4%) cases were identified out of 207. There was a significant association between illness and drinking school water ($p < 0.001$). The school supply came from a private well. Concentrated sodium fluoride was added to this water with the aim of increasing fluoride levels to the range 1–5 mg/l. Analysis of two water samples after the incident showed fluoride levels of 375 and 93.5 mg/l. Examination of the fluoridation system revealed faults that allowed excess fluoride to be pumped directly into the supply.

In November 1979, an employee at a waterworks in Maryland failed to close a control valve of the machine that metered the addition of hydrofluosilicic acid to the water supply (Waldbott 1981). This led to the distribution of water at approximately 30 mg/l for up to about 18 hours. Because the water company did not inform the health authorities about this accident, the first that was known was when eight patients on dialysis developed headache, nausea and vomiting. On the basis of a telephone survey, the author estimated that some 5000 people would have been ill out of a population of 35 000.

During August 1980, the head teacher of a school in Vermont reported that people who attended a market at the school had developed nausea and vomiting (Vogt et al. 1982b). A telephone survey of 40 vendors who had attended the market identified 22 cases out of 82 individuals. Cases were significantly more likely to have drunk beverages made from the school's water supply ($p < 0.0001$). On inspection, the fluoride concentration in the water supply was 1041 mg/l. The school had a small on-site fluoridator, which had been accidentally left on.

During March 1986, excess hydrofluosilicic acid was pumped into a small community water supply for 12 hours (Petersen et al. 1988). The cause of the error was an inadvertently opened valve. Measured fluoride was 42–51 mg/l. Copper was also increased at 25–41 mg/l, presumably due to increased mobilization of copper from pipe work due to the low pH. Soon after excess fluoride started to be added, customers started to complain about abnormal taste, and dermatological and gastrointestinal symptoms. A house to house survey found an attack rate of 18%. There was a strong association between gastrointestinal illness and water consumption (RR 23, CI 5.7–92.4). There were also correlations between itching and having a bath (RR 4.2, CI 1.7–10.7) or having a shower (RR 2.4, CI 1.1–5.0).

In another incident, this time in Alaska during May 1992, there was a death (Gessner et al. 1994). A total of 91 affected people were identified. In addition to the death of a 41-year-old male, a 37-year-old female had to be evacuated by air to a regional hospital. The median time between water consumption and onset of illness was seven minutes. In a case-control study, cases were more likely to live in the area supplied by the affected system (OR 7.1, CI 1.7–33.4), to drink water from the affected system (OR 18.5, CI 3.7–125.4) and to have drunk water from the affected system on three specific days (OR 75.9, CI 16.1–419.1). The attack rates for individuals satisfying these three risk criteria were 63%, 71% and 91%, respectively. The estimated fluoride level during the period of most illness was 150 mg/l. The man who died was estimated to have taken a dose of 17.9 mg/kg. Environmental inspection of the suspect water supply revealed several failings. The supplier was not complying with regulations requiring the submission of monthly fluoride levels to the state. The operator could not correctly perform fluoride assays. The operator had not responded to requests from the local health officers to unplug the fluoride pump. There were also several mechanical and electrical defects identified in the fluoridation system.

Fluorosis

Fluorosis develops from continued high oral or respiratory intake of fluorides. Fluorosis has been classified as being associated with drinking water, food and the burning of certain types of coal. However, in many situations children are often exposed to fluoride from more than one source. There have been many studies of the incidence of fluorosis in relation to fluoride concentrations in water and other sources. In the space available for this topic, I do not want to review all of the many papers that have been written an the issue. Recent reviews include those of Li (1993) and Lewis and Banting (1994). I will, however, mention a few that have attracted my particular attention.

Chandra *et al.* (1980) reported a significant correlation between dental fluorosis and water fluoride in India and suggested optimal concentrations between 0.34 and 1.05 mg/l, levels significantly below that which would cause fluorosis in more temperate countries.

Haimanot *et al.* (1987) studied the prevalence of endemic fluorosis in farms and villages in the Ethiopian rift valley. Water in that area came from wells, the fluoride concentration of which ranged from 1.2 to 36.0 mg/l. Severe dental mottling was seen in 32% of children, and 80% showed some degree of dental fluorosis. Severe crippling skeletal fluorosis was identified in some areas, the prevalence of which was shown to be linearly related to water fluoride and duration of exposure. An exposure to water with at least 8 mg/l of fluoride for at least ten years was necessary before severe skeletal fluorosis developed.

The suggestion that recommended levels of fluoride in water based on western experience would not be appropriate to hot countries was further strengthened by a Kenyan study (Manji, Baelum and Fejerskov 1986). The authors found a 100% prevalence of dental fluorosis in children exposed to water with only 2 mg/l fluoride. Furthermore, half of the children had severe damage in at least half of their teeth.

In Senegal when the concentration of fluoride in water was 1.1 mg/l the prevalence of mild dental fluorosis in children aged 7–16 years was 68.5% (Brouwer *et al.* 1988). When the concentration reached 4 mg/l the prevalence reached 100%. In a community whose drinking water contained 7.4 mg/l kyphosis was common and radiographic examination of three adults confirmed skeletal fluorosis.

The residents of the Ikeno district of Japan were accidentally exposed to water containing 7.8 mg/l of fluoride for a period of 12 years. After discovery of the excess level, concentrations were reduced to just 0.2 mg/l. Surveys of children in the area showed that increased prevalence of dental fluorosis was present only in those children aged 7 years or less at the start of the high dose period or aged 11 months or more at the end. Furthermore, the severity of fluorosis depended on the duration of exposure to the excessive level.

In a study of 14-year-old children living in four areas of Sri Lanka, Warnakulasuriya *et al.* (1992) found that the prevalence of dental caries was reduced by 43% in those whose water had fluoride concentrations between 0.6

and 0.79 mg/l compared to those whose water had less than 0.4 mg/l. However, of those children drinking water with less than 1.0 mg/l, 41% still had dental fluorosis, of whom 9% had severe lesions. The authors recommended a maximum limit for hot countries of 0.8 mg/l.

Chen *et al.* (1993) studied rates of dental and skeletal fluorosis in two Chinese villages before and after the water source was changed from a high fluoride content artesian well supply to river water. In the first village tap-water fluoride in 1984 was 5.5 mg/l; the overall prevalence was 96% for dental fluorosis and 82.1% for skeletal fluorosis. Seven years after changing supply the tap-water fluoride was then only 0.4 mg/l and the prevalence of dental and skeletal fluorosis had fallen to 57.8 and 46.0%. In the second village changing supply did not seem to affect the concentration of fluoride at the tap, which was 3.1% before and afterward. Pre and post rates of dental fluorosis were 100% and 83.7%. The prevalence of skeletal fluorosis increased from 71.1% to 86.0%. The reason for the continuing high fluoride levels in the second village was found to be damaged pipes allowing entry of hot spring water with a very high fluoride content into the supply.

In a study in San Luis Potosi, Mexico, Grimaldo *et al.* (1995) sought risk factors for endemic fluorosis. Of 401 samples of tap-water, 61% had fluoride levels above 1.2 mg/l and 4% above 4 mg/l. The prevalence of moderate and severe dental fluorosis increased in relation to tap-water fluoride levels. In children whose tap-water was <0.7 mg/l this was 25%, while in children whose water was >2.0 mg/l it was 82.76%. Prevalence of any degree of dental fluorosis in these two groups was 69% and 98%. Additional sources of fluoride were found to include certain soft drinks and bottled waters. It was noted also that boiling increased water fluoride concentrations.

Despite the problems with fluorosis described above and elsewhere, fluoride does offer considerable protection against dental caries. The protective effect of fluoride in drinking water seems to be greater in poorer communities, as for example in the study by du Plessis *et al.* (1995). This showed that black children experienced a reduction of 50–80% in the prevalence of dental caries when fluoride in water was 0.2–0.9 mg/l. The prevalence of fluorosis in black children in the peak fluoride area was 16%.

I have already referred to work by Forbes, Hayward and Agwani (1991) and Forbes and McAiney (1992) under the discussion of aluminium and dementia, which suggested that fluoride in drinking water may be protective against dementia. Perhaps the first study to identify a negative correlation between water fluoride and dementia was reported by Still and Kelley (1980). In a case-control study, cases were patients admitted to South Carolina Department of Mental Health Hospitals from July 1971 to June 1979 from one of three counties. There was a significant *negative* association with living in the county with highest water fluoride (4.18 mg/l) compared to the two counties with lower levels (0.61 and 0.49 mg/l) ($p < 0.0001$). This topic is further discussed and reviewed by Kraus and Forbes (1992).

HARDNESS

The hardness of a water is caused by the presence of divalent cations, the major contributions being from calcium (Ca^{2+}) and magnesium (Mg^{2+}). The total hardness of a water is usually expressed in milligrams per litre of $CaCO_3$. Although exact definitions vary, hard waters usually have a concentration of >200 mg/l while soft waters are usually <75 mg/l. Soft waters are usually more corrosive in dissolving metals, such as copper and lead, from the distribution system. Hard waters cause scaling and reduce the lathering of soap. Current EC regulations give a minimum hardness value of 60 mg Ca/l.

Calcium and magnesium, the chief chemical components of hardness, are not in themselves acutely toxic at anywhere near the doses that could be dissolved in water. However, the health effects of hardness have received more interest than most other topics in water chemistry. In particular, many studies have identified a negative association between water hardness and deaths from cardiovascular disease. During the past twenty years there have been numerous studies reported in the literature that have confirmed this association. It would be inappropriate to discuss more than just a few of these. Significant reviews were published by Comstock (1979), Masironi and Shaper (1981) and Shaper (1994).

One of the more influential studies of water hardness and cardiovascular mortality was the British Regional Heart Study (Pocock *et al.* 1980). This was an ecological study of 253 towns in Great Britain investigating the impact of water hardness, rainfall, temperature and socioeconomic factors on death rates from stoke and ischaemic heart disease. There was a two-fold difference between the lowest and highest death rates. After adjustment for other variables, cardiovascular mortality in very soft water areas (25 mg/l) was found to be about 10–15% higher than in areas with medium hard water (170 mg/l). Increased hardness above this latter level had no further protective effect. This was compatible with the conclusions of previous studies.

This general conclusion has stood the test of time in several different countries, including the USA (Comstock, Cauthen and Helsing 1980; Greathouse and Osborne 1980), South Africa (Derry, Bourne and Sayed 1990), Sweden (Rylander, Bonevik and Rubenowitz 1991; Nerbrand *et al.* 1992; Oreberg *et al.* 1992) and Italy (Leoni, Fabiani and Ticchiarelli 1985; Bernardi *et al.* 1995). However, while confirming the same association in Sweden as other authors, Gyllerup *et al.* (1991) found that cold was more significant and that water hardness did not greatly improve predictive power when added to any model already containing cold. The association in Scotland also seems to be much weaker (Smith and Crombie 1987; Crombie *et al.* 1989).

The exact mechanism for this small but consistent protective effect of water hardness on cardiovascular death rates is not fully proven. What is clear is that hardness *per se* is unlikely to be protective. One possible explanation is that soft waters are more likely to be corrosive and dissolve trace metals such as copper and lead from water distribution systems.

Over the period reviewed there have been several studies investigating a possible relationship between water hardness and urolithiasis (renal stones). A negative association between reported incidence rates of urinary stones and water hardness was reported from the US by Sierakowski, Finlayson and Landes (1979) and from Finland by Juuti and Heinonen (1980). In the UK no such association was demonstrated in an ecological study comparing rates in 18 towns (Power, Barker and Blacklock 1987). In a case-control study Shuster *et al.* (1982) compared home tap-water hardness in 2295 patients with urinary stones with that of controls. Cases were drawn both from a hard-water and a soft-water area. They found no difference in water hardness between the cases and the controls. In a door to door survey of 38 805 people in rural and urban India, the prevalence of urolithiasis was higher in soft water areas but this was not statistically significant (Singh and Kiran 1993).

LEAD

When one thinks about problems with chemicals in drinking water, probably the first to come to mind is lead. Lead is a dense, blue-grey metal that is widely distributed throughout the environment. It has been used by man in large quantities for centuries for a variety of purposes. It was used extensively for water distribution pipes and is still, inappropriately, used as a component of solder to join pipes. The EC standard for lead in drinking water is currently 50 mg/l, although this is likely to be reduced in the near future. In industrialized countries, lead in tap-water usually comes from lead pipes or solder, frequently from inside the dwelling itself. Lead levels are often higher in softer, more acidic, and so more aggressive waters. Where the main source of lead is domestic plumbing, the concentration at the tap does not remain constant through the day. The first draw water in the morning usually has the highest lead concentration. Hence it is good practice to flush cold water to waste at the start of the day in houses with older plumbing.

Acute lead poisoning is very uncommon and usually only follows the ingestion of certain salts and is due to irritation of the gastrointestinal tract. Features include experience of a metallic taste, vomiting, abdominal pain and diarrhoea. The main problem with lead is chronic exposure. This presents much more insidiously. Features of chronic poisoning include a metallic taste in the mouth, constipation, abdominal pain and peripheral nerve palsies. Severe cases, especially in children, may present with encephalopathy, leading to coma and convulsions. Typical blue lead lines may be seen on the gums.

Diagnosis of lead poisoning is made on clinical features and the demonstration of elevated blood lead levels. In chronic poisoning, radiological examination may show transverse bands at the growing margin of long bones.

Chronic lead poisoning may require chelation therapy with calcium disodium edetate. Dimercaprol may also be added in severe cases and in cases of encephalopathy.

The main area for debate is whether relatively low levels of lead, below that needed to cause obvious illness, have any adverse effect on children. It is suggested that low levels of lead exposure impairs neuropsychological performance (Needleman et al. 1979; Needleman and Gatsonis 1990; Pocock, Smith and Baghurst 1994). The weight of evidence from these and other epidemiological studies would support this suggestion.

One of the problems with writing about lead in water and disease in the context of this chapter is that lead in drinking water is rarely the sole contributor to total lead intake. Lead intake can come from paint, dust, soil, petrol and foods (Mushak and Crocetti 1989). Nevertheless, several studies have reported a strong association between blood lead and lead in drinking water (Marcus 1986; Davies et al. 1990; Jin et al. 1995), although water lead is not always the most significant source (Cambria and Alonso 1995).

Symptomatic lead poisoning associated with high lead levels in drinking water still occurs. Shannon and Graef (1989) reported a case of plumbism in a 13-month-old infant whose powered baby milk was made with tap-water containing 130 mg/l. These same two authors subsequently reported a four-year survey of lead intoxication within Massachusetts during the first year of life (Shannon and Graef 1992). Of 50 children with plumbism, they found that nine (18%) had acquired the metal from infant formula prepared from tap-water. Household renovation was associated with 40%, and 20% had eaten paint chips. In children aged between 18 and 30 months no cases were associated with drinking water. Most (87%) were associated with eating paint chips.

NITRATE

Nitrates are widely distributed in soil, water and plants and are found in most foods and drinking waters. The excess nitrate in water may come from agricultural sources, because nitrates form the basis of many fertilizers. They can also come from domestic and industrial effluents, and decaying animal and vegetable matter. Conventional water treatment processes have very little impact on the concentration of nitrate in water. Excess nitrate in water seems to be an increasing problem for users of groundwater supplies in some rural areas, particularly for shallow groundwaters. For example, 18% of private wells in Iowa (Kross et al. 1993) and 39% of dug or bored wells in Minnesota exceed the limit of 10 mg/l (Johnson and Kross 1990). This latter study found that 22% of drilled wells and 16% of driven wells exceeded the limit.

Nitrites are also widely distributed, but in much lower concentrations than nitrate. Conversion from one to the other occurs readily in the environment.

This conversion can also occur in the body, and nitrite is probably responsible for acute symptoms. Current European standards for nitrate and nitrite are 50 mg NO_3/l and 0.1 mg NO_2/l.

Symptoms of acute poisoning include headache, vomiting, flushing of the skin, hypotension, collapse, convulsions and coma. In infants methaemoglobinaemia can develop after exposure to high levels of nitrate. Methaemoglobinaemia occurs when the ferrous ion of haemoglobin is oxidized to the ferric form. This form of haemoglobin is less effective at carrying oxygen. The earliest clinical feature is cyanosis, but after 30–40% of haemoglobin has been converted to methaemoglobin there is weakness and exertional dyspnoea. After about 60% has been converted, respiratory depression and stupor develop. Death may follow soon after. Diagnosis of acute nitrate poisoning is aided by the demonstration of methaemoglobin in blood samples. Treatment is by giving oxygen and possibly the antidote, which is methylene blue or ascorbic acid.

In the period of interest for this book, there have been several reports of individual cases of methaemoglobinaemia. For example, Grant (1981) surveyed Nebraska for the years 1973–1978. Over a third of Nebraska's 93 counties had water sources with nitrate concentrations over 10 mg/l. During the period of the study only one case of nitrate-induced methaemoglobinaemia was reported and that child resided in Iowa, a neighbouring state. Three months after the survey a second case was reported. This child had drunk water from the well on the family's farm. In a survey of 2175 physicians in those counties with reported high water nitrate, 910 (41%) responded to the questionnaire. Of these 910, 33 said that they had seen nitrate-induced methaemoglobinaemia, although most cases were mild and responded to changes in water use. Johnson et al. (1987) reported a fatal case of methaemoglobinaemia in an infant associated with a private well containing 150 mg/l of nitrate. Knobeloch et al. (1993) reported a non-fatal case in a child associated with a well-water concentration of 58 mg/l.

Craun, Greathouse and Gunderson (1981) reported a study of 102 children aged one to eight years in Washington County, Illinois, an area where over 70% of wells had nitrate concentrations above the EPA limit of 22 mg/l as NO_3-N. Although children from high nitrate areas did have slightly higher methaemoglobin levels this was not statistically significant and all were within the normal range.

Nitrate is the chemical that appears in drinking water closest to its hazardous concentration, even if only in infants. Nitrate is a particular risk for families taking shallow well-water in agricultural areas. The best advice to any mother is to breast-feed. If a household takes water from a private well it is good advice to check nitrate levels before a baby is born to ensure that it complies with existing standards. I would not advocate bottle-feeding infants unless the water used to make up the feed was well within the current standard.

Two studies have looked at whether nitrate in drinking water may be linked to diabetes mellitus. The first was an ecological study of 63 counties in Colorado (Kostraba *et al.* 1992). In this study, between 1978 and 1988, incidence rates for children under 18 years old were determined for each county and compared with a weighted average nitrate level for the county. They found that counties whose water nitrate was 0.77–8.2 mg/l were significantly more likely to have higher diabetes incidence rates than those whose water nitrate was 0–0.084 mg/l. This suggestion was not supported in a case-control study from Finland (Virtanen *et al.* 1994). These workers reported a study of 684 diabetic children and their parents along with 595 control children. No difference was reported in nitrate intake from water, although cases did have a small but significant increase in total daily nitrate intake from other sources (0.9 mg versus 0.8 mg, $p < 0.001$).

SODIUM

Sodium salts are also widely distributed in the environment, being present naturally and as a result of human activity. The concentration of salt in oceans is about 30 g/l. Salt is a major component of all living things, and is added to food to increase palatability. Thus, salt intake from water forms only a proportion of the daily intake. The current European limit is 150 mg/l.

The relative importance of drinking-water sodium depends on the sodium concentration in water and the total sodium intake from all sources. Perhaps the most useful discussion on the relative importance of water sodium is contained in the *Guidelines for Drinking-Water Quality* by the World Health Organization (1984). In a typical diet, an adult may consume 5000 mg of sodium per day; at such a consumption level, the relative importance of sodium in drinking water is minimal. However, in those on restricted sodium diets, because of renal or heart disease, and in the very young the contribution of sodium in drinking water increases (Table 31.2).

In adults acute poisoning from sodium chloride is virtually unheard of due to the efficient way that the kidneys handle sodium. Furthermore, salt has been used therapeutically as an emetic, and large oral intakes will usually induce vomiting, with the ejection of much of the salt. However, hypernatraemia may develop in the very young and in those with impaired renal function. Clinical features of hypernatraemia may include cerebral and pulmonary oedema with convulsions, muscle twitching and breathlessness. Diagnosis is by the analysis of serum electrolytes. Treatment is by judicious water replacement and possibly dialysis.

The possibility that high water sodium levels are a factor in sudden infant death (cot death) was suggested in a study by Robertson and Parker (1978). Over a 30-year period changes in water treatment practices led to an initial increase from 11 to 129 mg/l for chalk sources and from 47 to 157 mg/l for

Table 31.2 The relative contributions of water salt to the daily diet. Adapted from World Health Organization (1984)

Sodium concentration in water (mg/l)	Relative proportion of salt from drinking water/Intake from food (%)			
	Special restricted diet (500 mg Na/d)	Low sodium diet (2000 mg Na/d)	Typical diet (5000 mg Na/d)	Infant aged 0–2 months (250 mg Na/d)
20	7	2	1	7
50	17	5	2	17
100	28	9	4	29
200	44	17	7	44

Based on the assumption of 2 l water per day for adults and 1 l per day for infants.

limestone sources. After 10 years further changes resulted in a drop to 79 and 128 mg/l for chalk and limestone sources, respectively. In the 10 years before the increase the cot death rate was 18.0 per 10 000 live births. During the period of highest water sodium it was 32.5 per 10 000 live births and during the 10 years after the slight fall it was 21.7 per 10 000 live births. There was no similar change in mortality rates in nearby towns with no change in water sodium levels.

Most concern about drinking-water sodium has been related to the chronic effects of continuous exposure to high sodium concentrations over time. Comprehensive recent reviews include those of Hoffman (1988) and Muntzel and Drueke (1992).

Tuthill and Calabrese (1979) reported a survey of the blood pressure of high school children in two Massachusetts communities. One community was served by a high sodium (107 mg/l) water supply and the other by a low sodium (8 mg/l) supply. After adjustment for other risk factors the authors reported a significant excess of both systolic and diastolic blood pressures in males (systolic, 4.78 mmHg, $p < 0.001$; diastolic 1.77 mmHg, $p = 0.078$) and females (systolic, 4.82 mmHg, $p < 0.01$; diastolic 4.31 mmHg, $p = 0.001$). Hallenbeck, Brenniman and Anderson (1981) reported an identical survey in two Chicago communities (405 versus 4 mg Na/l). They found no difference in the systolic blood pressures between the two groups, although diastolic blood pressure was slightly lower in females (2.02 mmHg, $p = 0.013$) and males (1.60 mmHg, $p = 0.061$) in the low-salt community.

Calabrese and Tuthill (1981) followed up their initial report by an experimental study where they randomly allocated children from their high sodium community to one of three groups. Each group received bottled water for three months. The first group received their own community water, the second group received water from the low sodium community but with added salt and the third group received water from the low sodium community but without added salt. In girls there was a consistent decline in both systolic and diastolic blood pressure in the low sodium bottled water group. This effect was not seen in boys.

Further support for the relationship between water sodium and increased blood pressure came from the Netherlands (Hofman, Valkenburg and Vaandrager 1980). In a study of 348 schoolchildren aged 7.7–11.7 years, mean systolic and diastolic blood pressures were higher in the children from high water sodium communities, although differences were low, 1–4 mmHg.

However, the positive results of these studies have not been found in several other studies (Bierenbau et al. 1975; Punsar et al. 1975; Armstrong et al. 1982; Faust 1982; Pomrehn et al. 1983; Lackland et al. 1985; Welty et al. 1986). For example, Bierenbau et al. (1975) found blood pressure in adults in Kansas City, KS, was higher than in Kansas City, MO, despite the fact that sodium levels were higher in the latter city (46 versus 25 mg/l). Welty et al. (1986) surveyed 342 Gila Bend Papago Indians and 375 non-Indians in Arizona during the summer of 1983. They were all aged 25 years or greater and lived in an area with 440 mg/l of sodium in the water supply. Blood pressures in the white population were generally lower than in the corresponding age groups for the US white population. There was also no correlation between water intake and blood pressure.

To a large extent, any minor effect that drinking-water sodium has on blood pressure is not important unless it translates into increased cardiovascular morbidity. Greathouse and Osborne (1980) reported a study of 4200 adults from across the US. They interviewed and examined the individuals and took water samples from their homes. Interestingly, they found a negative association between drinking-water sodium and cardiovascular mortality rates.

The evidence that higher concentrations of sodium in drinking water, at levels that would still be palatable, causes disease in humans has not been proven. Indeed, the balance of evidence is against sodium in drinking water being a risk factor for hypertension or cardiovascular disease. This is probably because, for most healthy adults, drinking-water sodium contributes only marginally to daily sodium intake. Nevertheless, for the very young and those on severely reduced sodium intakes for medical reasons, water sodium levels can cause problems when moderately elevated. This latter group should consider alternatives to straight tap-water if sodium levels are much above 50 mg/l.

ORGANIC CHEMICALS

Organic chemicals are those chemicals based on the carbon atom. Within this class of chemicals are a huge range of different compounds including proteins, vitamins, drugs, several disinfectants, petroleum products, herbicides and pesticides. Many organic chemicals have significant physiological effect, often at very low doses.

The health implications of organic micropollutants of drinking water sources generate considerable anxiety. This concern is exacerbated by the observation that water pollution by organic chemicals from industrial and agricultural sources is probably much more frequent now than it was 20 years ago, although it must be said that part of this apparent increase in water pollution is because analytical chemists are now much better at detecting various organics at low levels. However, despite being the focus of much of the public and professional concern about water safety, very little is known about the real health risks of pollution of drinking water from this group of compounds. In comparison to the many publications that have reported on inorganic pollution, there have been lamentably few good epidemiological studies of the effects of organic pollutants.

Chlordane

Chlordane is a chlorinated hydrocarbon pesticide. The safe limit for acute exposure is 0.5 mg/m^3. I can find reports of two instances where public water supplies were contaminated. The first occurred during March, 1976 and affected the supply to 42 homes in Chattanooga, Tennessee (Harrington et al. 1978b). The incident was first noted when residents in the affected area reported that the water had turned milky and smelt of insecticide. Chlordane was found in water samples at concentrations of up to 1 200 000 µg/l. The source of contamination was one of the homes, where chlordane had been used to treat termites in the foundations. It was noted that water pressure in the mains was lowest at this point and this would have been lower after using a large volume of tap-water to dilute the chlordane. Of 105 people interviewed, 71 (68%) gave a history of illness over the four days after the contamination. However, only 13 of these individuals described symptoms compatible with known features of chlordane poisoning. Symptoms included nausea, vomiting, abdominal pain, dizziness, blurred vision, irritability, paraesthesia and muscle dysfunction. All individuals recovered within 48 hours.

The second incident of chlordane contamination occurred on 7 December 1980 in Pittsburgh, Pennsylvania (Silverman et al. 1981). The source of contamination was thought to be deliberate injection of the pesticide through a stopcock normally used for the insertion of testing devices. In all, the number of individuals living in the affected areas was thought to be about 10 500. However, for most individuals, concentrations were much lower than in the previous incident. The highest concentration, 6600 µm/l, was recovered from a dead-end water line near the source of contamination. Other samples gave concentrations ranging from 0 to 905 µm/l, with 44 of 70 positive samples showing less than 1 µg/l. An epidemiological survey of the most affected census tract and a matched but non-affected area found 4–13% of exposed residents complaining of one or more of the following symptoms: nausea, diarrhoea, abdominal pain, skin and eye irritation, headache, dizziness and sore throat. In the non-exposed population only 1–4% of individuals reported these same symptoms ($p < 0.05$). Other symptoms of chlordane poisoning such as vomiting, sweating, seizures, tingling or muscle aches were not increased in the exposed individuals. There was no increase in attendance at hospital. Chlordane was not detected in serum samples.

Phenol

Phenol is a weakly acidic aromatic compound, C_6H_5OH. It has a long therapeutic use, being one of the first antiseptics used in modern medicine. Its common name was carbolic acid. The exposure limit is 5 mg/l and the fatal dose is 2 g. The current European limit for phenols is 0.5 $\mu g/l$.

In July 1974 there was an accidental spillage of 37 900 l of phenol after a derailment in southern Wisconsin (Baker et al. 1978). This caused contamination of nearby wells, and concentration of phenol in well-water reached a peak of 1130 mg/l in one such well. Most individuals continued to consume well-water until poor taste developed, when they switched to other water sources. People in the area affected by the spill were significantly more likely to complain of diarrhoea, mouth sores and a burning mouth than controls ($p < 0.01$). There was a strong correlation between noticing a bad taste and the presence of these symptoms in the study group. Six months later no differences were noted between people in the affected area and controls after a physical examination, nor were there any differences in the urinary excretion of phenols. The authors concluded that although short-term toxicity did occur, no longer-term sequelae were present.

A kitchen facility of a Georgia hospital was affected by poor tasting water, which was traced to phenol leaching from an inadequately cured phenolic resin liner that had been installed recently (Trincher and Rissing 1983). Many employees and patients developed nausea, vomiting and/or diarrhoea. However, phenolic compounds were not detected in urine samples and it is unclear whether there was a link between the illness and the phenol.

Jarvis et al. (1985) reported an incident in January 1984 in North Wales. The River Dee was polluted with an unknown quantity of chemical, mainly phenol and a much smaller amount of 2-ethyl-hexanol from an industrial site. During chlorination much of this phenol was converted to mono-, di- and trichlorophenols, giving the water a strong medicinal taste. Estimated concentrations of chlorophenol in two service reservoirs were 84.7 and 39.4 $\mu g/l$ and those of phenol were 10.3 and 4.7 $\mu g/l$ on the day after the pollution incident. Concentrations fell to zero over the next few days. The investigators conducted a postal questionnaire survey of an exposed and an unexposed community. At the time of the survey it was not general public knowledge which areas had been affected. The exposed community had highly significant excess in reporting of diarrhoea, nausea, vomiting, abdominal pain, headache, rash, malaise and other symptoms (most $p < 10^{-5}$). These symptoms were still significantly more common in the exposed group even after standardizing for the effect of noticing a bad taste in the water. All illness was self-limiting with recovery within, at most, 48 hours. Only 0.8% of those who reported symptoms sought medical attention.

Trichloroethylene

Trichloroethylene (TCE) (C_2HCl_3) is a clear, colourless liquid which is widely used as an industrial solvent, degreasing agent and dry-cleaning fluid. It was previously used as an anaesthetic agent but is now considered too dangerous for this use. The exposure limit is 50 mg/l and the fatal dose is estimated to be 5 ml. The current EC limit for TCE in drinking water is 30 μg/l. Reflecting its widespread use, TCE is one of the more commonly identified organic pollutants of groundwaters. The main effect of TCE exposure is depression of the central nervous system.

Following the finding of a dump of toxic chemicals in a wooded area near Londonderry Township, Pennsylvania, TCE was detected in water samples from nearby homes at concentrations ranging from 2.6 to 140 μg/l (Logue et al. 1985). It was thought that these chemicals had been dumped 23 years or more before their discovery. Following a public meeting, the Department of Health conducted a health survey of 14 affected households (61 individuals) and 23 non-affected households (66 individuals). Exposed individuals were significantly more likely to report eye irritation ($p < 0.005$), diarrhoea ($p < 0.05$) and sleepiness ($p < 0.025$). Within the exposed group only, there was a slight trend for symptomatic individuals to have been exposed to higher concentrations of TCE in their water but this was not statistically significant.

Also in Pennsylvania, 1900 gallons of TCE were accidentally released onto the ground when a pipe ruptured in July 1979 (Landrigan et al. 1987). Subsequent well-water samples taken from within 1 km of the site were as high as 183 000 μg/l, mean 130 000 μg/l during August. In May the following year mean levels were still 6350 μg/l. In November 1979, 13 local residents whose well-waters contained the highest levels were examined. Two were found to have TCE in urine samples, although one of these two worked as a degreaser operator in a factory. The other only drank bottled water, so the source of TCE was not obvious.

Kilburn and Warshaw (1992) reported a study of 362 individuals who drank well-water from a contaminated aquifer over a prolonged period in Tucson, Arizona. The principle contaminant was TCE, which was probably related to cleaning metal parts during aircraft refitting operations near a local airport. In addition to TCE, other pollutants included trichloroethane and chromium. The authors took blood samples and administered a health questionnaire, designed to identify symptoms of systemic lupus erythematosus (SLE), to the exposed population and 158 non-exposed controls. The exposed population was significantly more likely to report arthritis of over three months' duration

(26.5 versus 22.8%, p = 0.009), Raynard's phenomenon (39.8 versus 27.9%, p = 0.009), a malar rash on exposure to sunlight (5.0 versus 1.3%, p = 0.04), skin lesions (17.7 versus 6.3%, p = 0.008) and seizure (9.1 versus 2.5%, p = 0.007). Blood samples from the exposed population were also more likely to be positive for antinuclear antibodies, a diagnostic test for SLE. These same authors subsequently reported a laboratory study of the neurophysiological responses of 170 people from this exposed population and 68 controls (Kilburn and Warshaw 1993). The exposed individuals gave significantly impaired neurophysiological tests such as sway speed with eyes open and closed, blink reflex latency, eye closure speed and two-choice visual reaction time. They were also significantly impaired for neuropsychological reactions such as intelligence scores, recall of stories and visual recall, among others.

Mixed pesticides

Current European standards for total pesticides and related products in drinking water are 0.5 μg/l, but no single compound should exceed 0.1 μg/l.

Clark *et al.* (1982) studied a population in Tennessee whose water had become contaminated by leachate from a 300 000 barrel pesticide dump. Various pesticides were involved. Chemicals identified in water samples included hexachlorocyclopentadiene, heptachlorobicycloheptene, carbon tetrachloride and tetrachloroethylene. There were significant differences in biochemical tests of liver function between the exposed population and controls, although few cases had liver function tests outside of the normal range. Nevertheless, these results suggested some sub-clinical toxic effect on the liver.

Pesticides in water and Parkinson's disease

One of the more interesting lines of epidemiological investigation within this area in recent years has been those studies that have investigated a possible link between drinking water and Parkinson's disease. Parkinson's disease is a chronic, slowly progressive neurological disease that usually presents in later life. The average age of onset is about 55 years and it is rare in patients under 40 years old. Clinical features include tremor at rest, rigidity of muscles, akinesia (a general poverty and slowness of movement) and postural instability, leading to falls. Mental disturbances are common and dementia develops in some.

The first report of an association between Parkinson's disease and drinking water was made by Rajput *et al.* (1984) in Saskatchewan, Canada. This included a description of all 15 of their patients with early onset Parkinson's disease (EPD) who had been born and raised locally. All 15 had been born and raised in communities with populations of fewer than 140 and all had used well-water exclusively. Two years later they published data on all 21 cases of EPD born and raised in Saskatchewan (Rajput *et al.* 1986). Of these

21 cases, 19 had spent their first 15 years exclusively in rural communities ($p =$ 0.0154). The use of well-water during childhood was also significantly associated with EPD ($p = 0.003$). Subsequent analyses were unable to detect any differences in inorganic or organic chemicals in water samples from the wells used by patients in their youth and other drinking water supplies (Rajput *et al.* 1987).

The results of this early work has been confirmed by some but not all subsequent studies. Barbeau *et al.* (1987) also reported an ecological study from Canada. This time they estimated the prevalence of Parkinson's disease in Quebec from assurance data, from sales of the drug levodopa and from death certification. In nine rural hydrographic basins there was a correlation ($r = 0.967$) between the prevalence of the disease and the use of pesticides in the area.

Stern *et al.* (1991) conducted a case-control study of 80 patients with old onset (>60 years) and 69 young onset patients (<40 years) and the equivalent number of age- and sex-matched controls. They found no association between Parkinson's disease and well-water use. Furthermore, when adjusted for past history of head trauma, an apparent slight positive association with rural living became negative (OR 0.5).

Jiménez-Jiménez, Mateo and Giménez-Roldán (1992) reported a case-control study of 128 cases of Parkinson's disease and 256 age- and sex-matched controls from the Madrid area of Spain. Although there was no significant difference in the proportion of cases and controls who reported exposure to well-water, cases were more likely to have been exposed for 30 or more years (32.0 versus 21.1%, $p < 0.02$). Although cases were more likely to report exposure to pesticides for periods of at least a year, this was not statistically significant (33.6 versus 27.3%, $p = 0.2$). Cases were also more likely to have lived in rural areas up to the age of 30 (52 versus 38%, $p < 0.05$). Only univariate analyses were reported.

In a further case-control study from Spain, Morano *et al.* (1994) investigated 74 patients with Parkinson's disease and 148 age- and sex-matched controls. The conclusions were in line with the earlier study by Jiménez-Jiménez, Mateo and Giménez-Roldán (1992). There was little difference in the proportion of cases and controls who reported exposure to well-water for a year or more, although more cases reported exposure for over 40 years (73.0 versus 49.3%, $p < 0.001$). Rural living for at least 50 years was also significantly associated with disease (56.8 versus 34.5%, $p < 0.002$). Exposure to pesticides for at least a year was also more common in cases, although this did not quite achieve statistical significance (54.0 versus 40.5%, $p = 0.056$).

In the context of studies of Parkinson's disease and environmental factors, Semchuk and Love (1995) studied the effect of misclassification errors. They interviewed 40 cases, 77 controls and one proxy respondent (spouse or offspring) for each case and control. They demonstrated that using data from mixed cases and proxies could cause significant misclassification of exposure variables, perhaps explaining the differing results of the above studies, although not suggesting whether pesticides in well-water is a risk factor or not.

One must be very cautious about giving too much significance to these studies. Few of the studies, whether ecological or case-control, have attempted to account for potentially confounding factors. The two Spanish studies relied only on univariate analyses. Also, other studies have found no association between Parkinson's disease and well-water consumption (Aquilonius and Hartvig 1986; Wechsler et al. 1991). The evidence is not strong.

COMMENTS

Undoubtedly, chemical contamination of drinking water supplies is of great concern to consumers in the west. Yet even despite all the work reported in this chapter, the overall impact of chemical contaminants in drinking water on human health remains unclear, even in the west, where most of the work has been done. For example, the direct toxicological effects of the aluminium incident at Camelford are still open to debate. If the picture is unclear in the west, it is more so in those tropical countries where health systems are inadequate and environmental controls are weak. There is a very real need for detailed research into the health problems of water and environmental contamination in many countries.

32 Cancer and Water

The issue of the relationship between drinking water and cancer has generated more studies than almost any other issue in epidemiology. Compared to epidemiological studies investigating the relationship between microbial disease and water, those that have set out to study cancer are much more technically complex. Furthermore, their interpretation has often been subject to much debate in the scientific literature. Many of the published studies could be classified as to the main agent being hypothesized as causing malignant disease. Thus, this chapter is broken down into these broad areas.

Before going any further, it is important to stress that reviews of studies on cancer may be subject to significant selection bias. In this chapter, I am relying on published work. It has often been suggested that epidemiological studies that find a significant association between a putative carcinogen and disease are more likely to be published than ones that come up with a negative result. Therefore, simply relying on published work may over-emphasize the significance of any factor.

RADIOACTIVITY

Epidemiological studies of the effect of radioactivity in drinking water on health have concentrated on the presence of radium, especially radium-226. Radium is derived from the radioactive decay of uranium and itself decays into radon and eventually into stable lead:

$$^{234}U \rightarrow\ ^{230}Th \rightarrow\ ^{226}Ra \rightarrow\ ^{222}Rn \rightarrow\ \ldots \rightarrow\ ^{206}Pb$$
$$\text{Uranium Thorium Radium \quad Radon} \qquad\qquad \text{Lead}$$

Radium is a silvery white metal that oxidizes immediately on exposure to air. Salts of radium are soluble in water.

Bean *et al.* (1982a) used cancer register data for the whole of Iowa to calculate age-standardized cancer rates for each municipality or group of municipalities. This was part of a larger ecological study, which used reports of cancer data from the years 1969–1971 and 1973–1978 (Bean *et al.* 1982b). For this part of the study only 28 municipalities of between 1000 and 10 000 population, whose water came from wells greater than 500 ft deep and whose water had not been softened were analysed. The 28 towns were ranked according to their mean level of radium-226 in samples taken between 1958 and 1979. On the first analysis incidences of lung and bladder cancer in males and breast and lung cancer among females were higher in those towns with a radium-226 level exceeding 5.0 pCi/l. After adjusting for other potentially confounding variables, such as medium income, percentage of manufacturing workers, percentage of agricultural workers and fluoride levels, a significant relationship remained between lung cancer in males and radium-226 (p = 0.028).

Florida has one of the world's largest deposits of natural phosphate, which contains substantial quantities of uranium-238, radium-226 and radon-222. In an ecological study, Lyman, Lyman and Jackson (1985) estimated the level of radio contamination of groundwater by sampling water from 50 private wells in 27 Florida counties. Among the 27 counties 12.4% of water samples exceeded the maximum recommended concentration for total radium (5.0 pCi/l). Ten counties were classified as high-exposure counties, because more than 10% of water samples exceeded 5.0 pCi/l. The incidence of leukaemia was based on 1980 census data and reports to the Florida Cancer Data Service and standardized for age, sex and race. A significant excess of total leukaemia (p < 0.001) and acute myeloid leukaemia death rates was seen in the high-exposure counties (p < 0.001). There was a similar trend for deaths due to leukaemia. This study prompted a flurry of letters to the journal in which it was published. Wishart (1986) pointed out that the risk of leukaemia was still very low in Florida and that suggestions for public health changes based on the tentative findings of a single study were premature. Stebbings, Lucas and Toohey (1986) wrote to point out the weaknesses in ecological correlation studies, most notably that geographical associations do not prove causation and instead may cause confusion.

O'Brien, Decouflé and Rhodes (1987) analysed mortality data from the same counties as Lyman and colleagues over a longer, five-year, period from 1978 to 1982. Although they also found a significant excess of deaths from acute myeloid leukaemia, this was not as statistically significant (RR 1.4, CI 1.16–1.68). These authors doubted that the relatively low lifetime exposures of residents of these high-risk counties could cause significant excess leukaemia deaths and suggested that the explanation should rest with other potential causes.

Using data from the study of radium in water and cancer reported earlier by Bean *et al.* (1982a), Fuortes, McNutt and Lynch (1990) investigated the relationship between radium-226 and leukaemia. This study used actual levels of radium in the towns' supply as the indicator of exposure. They found a slight positive trend for both total leukaemia and acute myeloid leukaemia. However, confidence limits were wide and statistical significance was not achieved. The results were consistent with either no effect or only a small effect.

Collman, Loomis and Sandler (1991) looked at the effect of groundwater radon on cancer death rates in North Carolina. In this study, however, they looked at childhood cancers over the years 1950–1979. Rates were standardized for age and sex. Data on radon in groundwater supplies came from publicly available information. Counties were ranked according to geometric mean radon concentrations into low (0–228 pCi/l), medium (229–1375 pCi/l) and high (1376–10 692 pCi/l) exposure. There was an increase in all cancer deaths in both medium (RR 1.16, CI 1.05–1.28) and high (RR 1.23, CI 1.11–1.37) regions. There was also a significant increase in leukaemia deaths in medium (RR 1.26, CI 1.08–1.47) and high (RR 1.33, CI 1.13–1.57) exposure counties. It is interesting to note that these relative risks for fatalities are similar to those reported by previous authors.

Approaching the problem from a different direction, Hoffmann, Kranefield and Schmitz-Feuerhake (1993) started to investigate a cluster of cases of leukaemia in children living within 20 km of a uranium processing plant. Within the 20-year period, 1970–1989, 31 cases were diagnosed compared to an expected 27. The ratio of observed to expected cases was highest in those children living within 5 km of the plant. The investigators identified that a stream that contributed to the drinking water in the area had high levels of α-emitting nucleotides. The authors constructed a theoretical model suggesting that some of these excess leukaemia cases may be related to such contamination of drinking water. However, sampling of the water supply itself suggested lower levels than had been assumed in the model. The difference between observed and expected cases in the report was not great, thus the suggestion that this was an abnormal cluster is open to doubt.

Finkelstein (1994) has conducted one of the few case-control studies of radium in drinking water. A total of 335 people who had died from bone cancer while under the age of 25 years were identified as cases. Controls were randomly matched to case based on sex, age and year of death. After exclusions 283 cases and 285 controls were included in the study. Radium was present at a level of 7.0 mBq/l or greater in the birthplace of 15.2% of cases and 10.2% of controls (OR 1.58, CI 1.01–2.5). This study was well designed and found an association that was significant at the $p = 0.05$ level. However, statistical significance was only just achieved and, as Finkelstein pointed out, difficulties in assessing exposure risk may have biased the results one way or another.

Comments

Most of the studies reported here are ecological and I would certainly echo the warning of Stebbings, Lucas and Toohey (1996) about interpreting associations in such studies as indicating causation. However, the three studies by Bean *et al.* (1982a), Fuortes, McNutt and Lynch (1990) and Collman, Loomis and Sandler (1991) all found similar levels of association between groundwater radium and leukaemia. Although not conclusive, this would suggest that the association is real.

NITRATE

Nitrates are salts of nitric acid and they are usually soluble in water. High nitrate levels in many drinking waters are thought to be derived largely from agricultural activity. Concern about the carcinogenic potential of nitrates in drinking water comes from the suggestion that they may be converted into nitrosamines in the stomach. Nitrosamines have been shown to have significant oncogenic potential in animal studies.

An early case-control study of patients discharged from hospital in the Department of Nariño, Columbia was reported by Cuello et al. (1976). The authors identified 276 patients with stomach cancer, who had been discharged from hospital or died in the years 1968–1972. The same number of age- and sex-matched controls were chosen from patients discharged from hospital with a diagnosis other than disease of the gastrointestinal tract. Histories of water use were identified from interviews with patients or their relatives. Samples of urine and well-water were obtained for analysis. Increased cancer risk was associated with two areas compared to cities and a third rural area. Those areas with the highest rate of stomach cancer had high nitrate levels in groundwater and urine, although this was not tested for statistical significance. Mean well-water nitrate levels in the high-level areas were 12.5 and 39.0 g/l.

A descriptive epidemiological (ecological) study of gastric carcinomas was reported from the Piemonte region of Italy by Gilli, Corrao and Favilli (1984). They identified cases of gastric cancer from hospital discharge data for the years 1976–1979 and used this to identify which of 1199 had incidences of gastric carcinoma that were significantly above the regional mean. They also found the mean nitrate content in drinking waters for all communities. They were able to show that 40% of those communities with >20 mg/l nitrate in drinking water had standardized hospital discharge rates of >200 compared to only 16.8% of those communities with nitrate concentrations of <20 mg/l. Using a chi squared test for trend, this was highly significant ($p < 0.001$).

Beresford (1985) used census data, mortality reports and available water quality data in an ecological study of 253 urban areas in the UK. Despite the fact that many of the towns included in the study had water supplies that exceeded EC guide levels for nitrate in drinking water (26 mg/l as N), there was no association between standardized mortality ratios for stomach cancer and nitrate levels in water.

An ecological study of cancer deaths in the Hungarian county of Borsod was reported by Takács (1987). This study included areas where the nitrate levels were very high, over 100 mg/l. Although no significance tests were used, there did appear to be a correlation between the incidence of malignant tumours of the gastrointestinal tract and nitrate levels in water, although the mortality data was not standardized for age.

A case-control study was undertaken in Wisconsin by Rademacher, Young and Kanarek (1992). They looked at all gastric cancer deaths from 1982 to 1985. Controls were matched for age, sex and year of death. The nitrate levels analysed were values for the address at which the patient was living at the time of death. Nitrate levels for public water sources were taken from publicly available information. Nitrate levels in private wells were analysed by the investigators. The authors found no relationship between gastric cancer and water nitrate levels, despite the finding that many supplies had nitrate levels above guide limits.

Weisenburger (1993) studied the incidence of non-Hodgkin's lymphoma (NHL) in eastern Nebraska during 1984. He identified 159 cases. Two populations were examined: 25 counties with less than 10% of wells exceeding the guide limit of 10 mg/l nitrate and 25 counties with 20% or more well-waters exceeding the guide limit. The incidence rate of NHL was higher in those counties with higher failure rates (21.0 versus 11.6/100 000).

The concentration of nitrate in drinking water in the province of Valencia, Spain, is said to be the highest in Europe (Morales-Suarez-Varela, Llopis-Gonzalez and Tejerizo-Perez 1995). The authors conducted an ecological study of 258 municipalities within the province grouped according to whether their drinking water contained 0–25, 25–50 or greater than 50 mg/l of nitrate. The authors then calculated age-standardized mortality for each municipality during the period 1975–1980 for stomach, bladder, prostate and colon cancer for each sex (where appropriate) over three age bands (<55, 55–75 and >75 years). Comparing groups with the <25 mg/l municipalities, they found no increased risk in the 25–50 mg/l municipalities. In the >50 mg/l nitrate municipalities they found increased relative risk of stomach cancer in the 55–75 year age group for males (RR 1.91, CI 1.36–2.67) and females (RR 1.81, CI 1.15–2.87) and for prostate cancer in the 55–75 year age group (RR 1.86, CI 1.2–2.88) and the over 75 age group (RR 1.80, CI 1.15–2.82). No other results were significant.

Comments

In researching this section, only one properly conducted and analysed case-control study was found (Rademacher, Young and Kanarek 1992). This found no association between nitrate and stomach cancer. The evidence from the other, predominantly ecological, studies is at best conflicting. The paper by Morales-Suarez-Varela, Llopis-Gonzalez and Tejerizo-Perez (1995) is interesting in that it illustrates a danger in multiple analyses. Significant tests were performed on 33 age, sex and cancer type groups. The probability that at least one would be significant at the 0.05 level is high (0.816). With the evidence presented here one must conclude that nitrate in drinking water that complies with current EC standards (50 mg/l) does not cause stomach cancer. The evidence that nitrate levels in excess of this limit cause cancer is at best weak.

ARSENIC

Arsenic is an extremely toxic semi-metal with an atomic weight of 74.9. Poisoning from arsenic in drinking water is well described. That arsenic may be carcinogenic for humans has come from studies that have looked at ingestion from medicines, 'wine substitutes', drinking water and by inhalation (Bates, Smith and Hopenhayn-Rich 1992).

Water supplies in Lane County, Oregon, are know to have relatively high arsenic levels (mean 8.6 μg/l, range 0–2150 μg/l (Morton et al. 1976). In an ecological study the authors reviewed records of histology material from skin cancers for the years 1958–1971 and used this data to calculate cancer incidence rates in various areas of Lane County. They found no obvious relationship between the incidence of skin cancer and mean water arsenic levels. Nevertheless, one patient was reported who had previously had documented arsenic poisoning from the consumption of well-water (Wagner et al. 1979). After a latent period of 14 years she developed multiple basal cell carcinomas.

An area of southwest Taiwan suffers from having high levels of arsenic in its artesian well-water. The residents of this area are prone to blackfoot disease, a vascular disorder thought to be caused by arsenic. Chen et al. (1988) reported that patients with blackfoot disease are more likely to suffer a higher prevalence of cancers of the bladder, skin, lung and liver then would be expected from the local population. Wu et al. (1989) reported an ecological study of 42 villages in the area where arsenic levels in well-water for the years 1964–1966 were known. Population and mortality data covered the years 1973–1986. There was a highly significant ($p < 0.001$) association between arsenic levels in water and bladder, skin and lung cancers for both males and females and for kidney cancer in females. There were also statistically significant ($p < 0.05$) associations for kidney, liver and prostate cancers in men. Significant effects were seen for arsenic levels over 0.30 mg/l.

One of the most convincing studies of the relationship between arsenic in drinking water and cancer deaths was a historical cohort study of 454 individuals who were identified as using well-water containing arsenic in 1959 (Tsuda et al. 1995). The study covered the 33 years up to 1992. The study covered a small town called Namiki-cho in Japan, where a small factory had been producing king's yellow (arsenic trisulphide) for over 40 years. Wastewater from the factory had contaminated wells in the area. The problem came to light in 1959 when a young boy was diagnosed as suffering from chronic arsenism. In a survey of 383 residents at the time, 97 had at least one clinical feature of arsenism. Sampling 34 wells found that 11 wells had concentrations in the range 1.0–3.0 mg/l, 17 in the range >0 and <1.0 mg/l and in 6 arsenic was not detected. Tsuda *et al.* (1995) identified 443 individuals whose exposure to arsenic in drinking water was known from the 1959 government investigation. These individuals were classified according to whether exposure was <0.05 mg/l, 0.05–0.99 mg/l or ≥1 mg/l. Age- and sex-standardized mortality rates were calculated for each group for all deaths, all cancer deaths and various cancers. In the ≥1 mg/l group, excesses were seen in all deaths (SMR 1.58, CI 1.12–2.22), all cancer deaths (SMR 3.63, CI 2.25–5.71) and in cancer of the lung (SMR 15.69, CI 7.38–31.02), urinary tract (SMR 31.18, CI 8.62–91.75), liver (SMR 7.17, CI 1.28–26.05) and uterus (SMR 13.47, 2.37–48.63), but not colon (SMR 0, CI 0–17.11). SMRs were not raised in the group exposed to 0.05–0.99 mg/l. Cancer deaths in two nearby control areas were not raised. Interestingly, the authors also found synergistic effects with smoking.

Bates, Smith and Cantor (1995) reported a case-control study investigating the association between bladder cancer and arsenic ingestion in Utah. This time the authors tried to get a measure of total arsenic exposure and bladder exposure to arsenic. Arsenic levels in the 88 study towns were undetectable in 18, 1–<2 µg in 43, 2–<10 µg in 20, 10–<50µg in 6 and ≥50µg in 1. A total of 117 cases and 266 age-, sex- and geographically-matched controls were included in the study. No relation was found between arsenic exposure and bladder cancer. However, it must be noted that the concentration of arsenic in drinking water was much lower than found in other studies mentioned.

Comments

The evidence in favour of arsenic in drinking water, at concentrations over 0.3 mg/l, being a potent carcinogen appears to be very strong. Despite reservations about ecological studies, the strength of association between cancer death and arsenic in the study of Wu *et al.* (1989) is very high ($p < 0.001$). Furthermore, the cohort study reported by Tsuda *et al.* (1995) is very convincing in a way that ecological studies can never achieve. The negative results from the American studies must be interpreted in the knowledge of the relatively low concentrations of arsenic. The evidence would suggest that arsenic in drinking water at concentrations of less than 0.1 mg/l probably does not increase cancer risk substantially.

FLUORIDE

Hrudey *et al.* (1990) investigated the incidence of osteosarcoma in two Canadian cities, one of which fluoridated the water in 1967 and the other did not until 1989. The authors found no difference between the two.

ASBESTOS

Asbestos is a fibrous silicate compound that was formerly widely used in building and engineering for its insulation and heat retarding properties. There are two principal classes of asbestos, the amphiboles and the serpentines. About 95% of the world supply of asbestos is chrysotile, a member of the serpentine class. The role of asbestos in causing asbestosis, a severe lung disease, and lung cancer after inhalation is well known.

In 1980, Kanarek *et al.* published an ecological study of age-adjusted cancer incidence ratios for 1969–1971 in the San Francisco area. The cancer incidence ratios for 722 census tracts, over the three-year period 1969–1971, were compared with measured chrysotile asbestos counts in drinking water. Asbestos is a naturally occurring contaminant of water in the area. For analysis the census tracts were grouped according to these asbestos counts. Data from 35 diagnostic groups were analysed for whites, non-whites, combined races, and male and female (210 statistical tests in all). There were 36 significant associations, mainly in whites. Some of these associations were impressive. For example the association for trachea, bronchus and lung was $p = 10^{-6}$. When log-linear multiple regression analyses were performed with possible confounding factors such as socioeconomic variables significant associations were found for all sites ($p = 0.043$), stomach ($p = 0.044$), peritoneum ($p = 0.002$), all respiratory ($p = 0.001$) and trachea, bronchus and lung ($p < 0.001$) in males. In females significant associations included oesophagus ($p = 0.020$), stomach ($p = 0.024$), digestive related organs ($p = 0.004$), gall bladder ($p = 0.001$), pancreas ($p = 0.005$), peritoneum ($p = 0.009$), pleura ($p = 0.010$), corpus uteri ($p = 0.025$) and kidney ($p = 0.021$). This study generated significant criticism in the letters pages of the relevant journal. Most of the criticism seemed to be around the handing of potentially confounding factors such as the choice of socioeconomic indicators and the suggested lack of allowance for possible population densities and occupational factors (Browne 1982; Higgins 1981). Tarter, Cooper and Freeman (1983) used complex modelling techniques to investigate the impact of population density. The conclusions were that the trend remained, although the morbidity density was bimodal for high-exposure census tracts, while it was unimodal for low exposure. The epidemiological relevance of this observation is unclear.

The authors of the above study repeated the work with data from an additional three years, making six in all (Conforti *et al.* 1981). Broadly similar findings were made, although certain cancers that were not found to be associated in the earlier study were now found to be significant, and others found to be significant in the earlier study were no longer. Conforti (1983) reanalysed this data a year later to take account of population density. Including population density in the regression analyses did not affect their conclusions.

Polissar *et al.* (1982) conducted a similar ecological study to those of Kanarek and colleagues, but this time in the Puget Sound region of western Washington. Asbestos contamination of drinking water in this region was associated with one river due to natural sources. This study was based on incidence data from 1974 to 1977 and mortality data from 1955 to 1975. The authors calculated 332 odds ratios for neoplasm risk and concluded that although several cancers had elevated OR values, no more were significant at the 0.05 level than would have been expected by chance. They concluded that the study did not support an effect of asbestos on cancer incidence.

Polissar, Severson and Boatman (1983, 1984) then went on to report a case-control study conducted in the same area. They interviewed 382 individuals or their relatives taken from the local tumour registry and unmatched population controls from the same area. Exposure to asbestos was calculated from water company data, based on residence and occupational histories. Only two cancers were found to give statistically significant results, pharyngeal cancers in males (RR 2.99, lower CI 1.43) and stomach cancer in males (RR 1.71, lower CI 1.06). The relative risks for females for these cancers were 0.26 and 0.65, respectively. The authors concluded that given the number of statistical analyses undertaken, these results were compatible with no oncogenic risk from asbestos in the area.

In another ecological study, Millette *et al.* (1983) looked at the impact of asbestos derived from man-made sources in the form of asbestos-cement pipe for water distribution mains. It was noted that in some areas the pipe was deteriorating, and asbestos material had been recovered from a customer's tap. The authors assessed the exposure risk of 40 census tracts as none, low or high depending on which type of mains pipe was in use. There were no significant associations between asbestos risk and cancer mortality.

Staying with the potential risk of asbestos-cement piping, Sadler *et al.* (1984) looked at the incidence of 11 cancers in Utah communities. Of these communities, 14 had used asbestos cement pipe for 20 years or more and 27 had never used such pipes. Standardized incidence rates (SIRs) were calculated from Utah cancer registry data. There were increased SIRs for only two cancers, kidney cancer in men and leukaemia in women. SIRs were significantly low for cancer of the colon in both sexes. Overall there were significantly fewer cancers in the potentially exposed group.

An ecological study of cancer mortality rates in 66 Canadian cities, discussed in more detail below, found no association between any of 13 cancers and asbestos contamination of drinking water (Wigle *et al.* 1986).

In November 1985, the New York State Department of Health was alerted to high levels of asbestos leachate in the public drinking water of Woodstock Town (Howe *et al.* 1989). This was due to deterioration of an asbestos-cement pipe. Standardized cancer rates were calculated for the area from state cancer registry data. The authors identified a total of 127 cancers, a low SIR of 0.9 (CI 0.8–1.1). Only 1 of 42 comparisons showed a significant excess, buccal cancer (SIR 3.0, CI 1.2–6.1). The authors concluded that there was no evidence that this incident was associated with an increased cancer risk.

Finally, Andersen, Glattre and Johansen (1993) reported a study of Norwegian lighthouse keepers whose water had come from rain-water collected from asbestos tiled roofs. The fibre content of these water supplies ranged from 1760 to 71 350 million fibres per litre. It was not clear when the tiles had begun to deteriorate. The authors identified a cohort of 690 workers employed in the period 1920–1966. In the cohort there were no more cases then would have been expected from the incidence of those cancers in the general population. However, in the group that had been exposed more than 20 years ago, there was a significant increase in the SIR for cancers of the stomach (SIR 241, CI 120–431) (11 cases observed versus 4.57 expected).

Comments

The studies reported in this section have certainly been conflicting. The strongest evidence comes from the San Francisco Bay studies (Kanarek *et al.* 1980; Conforti *et al.* 1981). However, I find this study design and the analysis very difficult to follow. The other studies have generally been negative, except where one would expect chance to throw up some significant results from the sheer number of analyses performed. It would appear that the weight of evidence is against asbestos in drinking water being carcinogenic.

ORGANIC CONTAMINANTS

Organic chemicals are those chemicals with a basic carbon structure. In drinking water organic chemicals can include oils, petroleum products, solvents and pesticides. They would also include so called chlorination by-products formed by the action of chlorine on organic compounds. This latter group of organic chemicals are discussed in their own section. In 1979, Wilkins, Reiches and Krusé (1979) produced a useful review of studies on organic chemical pollution and health. Anyone interested in studies up to that time should consult that paper.

The Iowa drinking water study already discussed also looked at the relationship between cancer incidence of indices of contamination (Isacson *et al.* 1985). Towns were grouped according to the concentration of volatile organic compounds in finished groundwater supplies. There was a significant association between 1,2-dichloroethane and the incidence rates of male colon cancer ($p = 0.009$) and male rectal cancer ($p = 0.02$). However, given the number of different associations examined, the latter is of doubtful significance.

In 1979, contamination of well-water from industrial solvents was discovered in Woburn, Massachusetts (Byers *et al.* 1988). The main pollutant found was trichloroethylene (267 μg/l). The contamination had probably existed for several years before discovery. Between 1969 and 1979 there were 12 cases of leukaemia in Woburn, compared to the expected 5.3. There was also a significant association between access to the contaminated water and the incidence of childhood leukaemia.

Griffith *et al.* (1989) did a study of the health effects of hazardous waste sites and cancer mortality in the USA. The authors identified 593 waste sites in 339 US counties with analytical evidence of contaminated groundwater as the sole source of drinking water. Cancer incidence rates for the years 1970–1979 in these counties were compared with 2726 control counties. Unlike many ecological studies, these authors used a Bonferroni procedure to account for the large number of statistical tests performed. They found significant excess ($p < 0.002$) deaths in hazardous waste site counties for cancers of the lung, bladder, oesophagus, stomach, large intestine and rectum in males and for lung, breast, bladder, stomach, large intestine and rectum in females.

Following a health department report that suggested a link between water contamination with dibromochloropropane (DBCP) and leukaemia and gastric cancer in Fresno County, California, Wong *et al.* (1989) conducted further ecological and case-control studies. Mean DBCP levels in the census tracts ranged from 0.0041 to 5.7543 μg/l. In the ecological study census tracts were grouped in seven groups depending on mean DBCP levels. Leukaemia and gastric cancer death incidences were based on data covering 1960–1983. No association was found in the ecological study. In the case-control study, cases were deaths from these two diseases from 1975 to mid-1984. Controls were other fatalities stratified for age, race and year of death. A living relative or other contact was interviewed for each case and control. For the gastric cancer study, 263 cases and 1044 controls were included. For the leukaemia study there were 259 cases and 1161 controls. There was no relationship between gastric cancer or leukaemia and DBCP levels.

Cancer maps of Illinois have consistently shown areas of high mortality from bladder cancer in the northwest of the state. A case search of hospital records was used to calculate standardized cancer incidence ratios for eight northwestern counties (Mallin 1990). While none of the counties showed an excess SIR, it was noted that a single zip code area of 43 000 people had an increased SIR for bladder cancer in males (SIR 1.4, CI 1.1–1.9) and females (SIR 1.8, CI 1.2–2.7). Within this area this excess was restricted to a single community of 13 000 people (males SIR 1.7, CI 1.1–2.6; females SIR 2.6, CI 1.2–4.7). Investigation of possible environmental factors for this cluster found that two of four drinking water wells were located within half a mile of a waste dump. Industrial solvents, especially trichloroethylene, had been detected in both wells.

Fagliano *et al.* (1990) reported an ecological study in New Jersey of the incidence of leukaemia in populations exposed to volatile organic chemicals (VOC) in drinking water. Twenty-seven towns where more than 90% of the population were served by the public water supply were rated as having low, medium and high exposure to non-trihalomethane volatile organics. A significant association was found between drinking water VOC and leukaemia in females (SIR 1.53, CI 1.02–2.21) but not in males.

From 1980 to 1982 it was noted that a single region of north central Saudi Arabia contributed far more referrals for oesophageal cancer then other regions (Amer et al. 1990). This observation stimulated a prospective case-control study for the years 1983–1987. Comparing 531 case-matched pairs showed that there was a significant excess of cases of oesophageal cancer throughout the time period ($p < 0.001$). When cases of oesophageal cancer from Gassim were compared with cases from elsewhere, the only significant positive correlation was in drinking from well-water ($p < 0.05$). Analyses of well-water from the Gassim region found traces of petroleum oil in five of six samples.

During November 1987, high concentrations of chlorophenols (70–140 $\mu g/l$) were found in tap-water in a village in southern Finland (Lampi et al. 1992). The source of the contamination was thought to be a local sawmill. A nearby lake was also found to be contaminated. A case-control study was done in the wider Tiirismaa health care district, which included the affected village. Cases were residents who presented with one of several cancers between 1967 and 1986. Controls were matched for sex, age and residence within the Tiirismaa health district at the times of diagnosis of the case's cancer. There was a significant excess of cases of both soft tissue sarcoma and non-Hodgkin's lymphoma in the affected village. However, the numbers of cases were very small, only six sarcomas. In the case-control study, the only significant association reported was the association of fish from the polluted lake and non-Hodgkin's lymphoma. However, the number was again small (three cases versus one control).

Aschengrau et al. (1993) reported a population-based case-control study in a population exposed to tetrachloroethylene that was leaching into the water from the inner vinyl lining of certain asbestos-cement mains pipes. Concentrations in some low-use pipes were as high as 7750 $\mu g/l$, although in medium- and high-use sites concentrations only reached 80 $\mu g/l$. A case-control study recruited 79 cases of bladder cancer, 42 of kidney cancer and 44 of leukaemia diagnosed between 1983 and 1986. Random controls were selected from the same population. Delivered doses were estimated from residential history, and knowledge of the flow, age, state of repair and size of the mains pipes. The authors claimed that they had found an elevated risk of both leukaemia and bladder cancer. However, the 95% confidence intervals of both of these were wide and included unity. For example, they suggested an association between bladder cancer and exposure based on an odds ratio of 4.03, but with 95% confidence intervals of 0.65 to 25.10. There was, however, an association between leukaemia and above 90 percentile of exposure (OR 8.33, CI 1.53–45.29), although this was based on only three cases. Therefore, any conclusions of a significant association based on this study must be open to serious doubt. Ramlow (1995) subsequently criticized the study methodology on several grounds.

During 1985 a small cluster of cases of leukaemia was identified in a small area of the Netherlands (Mulder, Drijver and Kreis 1994). The area of concern is one of the world's main centres for flower cultivation and pesticides are used intensively. Fourteen patients under the age of 40 were identified between 1975 and 1989; six had acute lymphoid leukaemia, one acute myeloid leukaemia, six non-Hodgkin's lymphoma and one Hodgkin's lymphoma. Four age- and sex-matched controls were identified for each case. Significant associations were found between disease and involvement in do-it-yourself activities (OR 5.5, CI 1.1–26.6), exposure to petroleum products for three hours per week or more (OR 8.0, CI 2.2–129.9) or having a father who had occupational exposure to petroleum products for three hours per week or more (OR 9.0, CI 1.0–66.1). Furthermore, swimming in a local pond was also significantly associated (OR 5.3, CI 1.3–17.4) with illness. This pond had been contaminated with pesticides and petroleum products in the 1970s.

Comments

One of the problems in summarizing this section is the differing nature of the pollutants and diseases investigated. This is reflected in the very different conclusions that can be drawn from the individual studies. For an ecological study, the paper by Griffith et al. (1989) on hazardous waste sites is convincing. However, although organic pollutants are likely, the exact chemical nature of the pollutants remains unclear. Of the other studies the paper by Amer et al. (1990) on oesophageal cancer in Saudi Arabia is also convincing. There is certainly a case to answer for organic pollution in drinking water, although the exact risk can not yet be estimated.

WATER SOURCE

As discussed in the earlier chapter on water supply, most water for consumption comes from either groundwater sources (wells and springs) or surface water sources (streams, rivers and lakes). Waters from these two main sources differ considerably in their chemical nature and in the risks of contamination. This section discusses those few papers that have looked at the effects differing sources of supply may have on health. One of the problems in assessing these different health effects is knowing how they may be mediated. For example, surface waters are often more polluted and have higher organic load, so require more chlorination. On the other hand, groundwaters are increasingly found to be polluted by various organic and inorganic chemicals. Because groundwaters are generally assumed to be safe, they may be subject to minimal treatment, which may not reduce the concentration of any polluting chemical. At this point we shall also consider those studies that have considered a possible relationship between wastewater reuse and malignant disease.

A case-control study in Louisiana looked at the relationship between cancer of the colon and rectum and the consumption of water sourced from the Mississippi River (Gottlieb, Carr and Morris 1981). A total of 3718 deaths from either cancer were identified between the years 1960 and 1975. A similar number of matched controls were also identified. Water consumption was estimated from water billing data for each family and categorized as mostly surface, some surface, possible surface and least surface water sources. Using least water consumption as the base, surface water consumption was associated with cancers of the rectum (OR 2.0, CI 1.49–2.88) but not colon cancers (OR 0.96, CI 0.75–1.24). Rectal cancers were also more common below Orleans than above (OR 1.82, CI 1.01–3.26). When chlorination was included in the analysis, it was found to give some borderline additional effect to source ($p = 0.05$) for rectal cancer.

In the Louisiana study reported above, the effect of water below Orleans may have been due to the reuse of wastewater. Frerichs, Sloss and Satin (1982) specifically studied the impact of wastewater reuse on health in four areas of Los Angeles county. This was an ecological study of two areas that had received recycled water since 1962 and two that had not. Standardized mortality ratios were calculated for each of the four areas. Of four specific malignancies investigated, those of stomach, colon, rectum and bladder, only cancer of the rectum was raised in both communities that used recycled water. This was not, however, quite significant ($p = 0.08$).

In the Iowa study referred to already in this chapter, Bean et al. (1982b) compared the incidence of cancers in different municipalities and attempted to link this to information about the water supplies to those municipalities. Significant differences in cancer incidence rates were seen between municipalities using groundwater and surface water for cancer of the lung (males $p = 0.0088$; females $p = 0.0128$) and rectum (males $p = 0.0005$; females $p = 0.0001$).

Beresford (1983) reported an ecological study of the potential impact of wastewater reuse on cancer incidence in 14 London boroughs. Cancer incidence data were collected from the appropriate cancer registers covering the years 1968–1974. The source of water for each borough was determined as well-water (mean reuse 1%), Thames/well mixture (9%) and Thames water (14%). In addition, social factors such as social class distribution, housing condition, employment type and local immigration were also taken into account. Significant associations were found between reuse and stomach cancer ($p < 0.01$) although this was reduced after the effect of social factors was taken into account ($p = 0.08$). All urinary cancers in males ($p < 0.05$) and females ($p < 0.01$) and bladder cancers in males ($p < 0.05$) were also associated with reuse when social factors were not included, but disappeared when they were. A major problem with the study design was that it was impossible to distinguish between the effect of water reuse and surface water.

Morin *et al.* (1985) estimated the proportion of surface to groundwater supplies to each of 473 of the largest US cities. They then determined the mortality rates for cancer and other causes over a 20-year period. The authors found a significant association between cancer mortality and surface water use ($p < 0.001$). This association remained significant when the effects of other variables were taken into account (log of population density, population change, percentage of non-whites, median school years achieved by the population over 25 and percentage of males) ($p < 0.05$). From this study the authors estimated a small but significant excess of cancer deaths of 2% in communities receiving 100% surface water compared to those receiving 100% groundwater, after the effects of social variables had been taken into account.

In a similar ecological study, this time in the UK, Carpenter and Beresford (1986) identified the water source to 238 urban areas in England, Wales and Scotland. Sex-specific standardized mortality ratios for oesophagus, stomach, intestine, bladder and all urinary cancers were calculated for the years 1969–1973. The proportions of water supplied to each area from groundwater, natural springs, upland water and lowland spring water was determined. Data on 14 possible confounding factors were obtained from the 1971 census. After including appropriate socioeconomic factors in the model, associations were found between the proportion of upland waters examined and cancers of the stomach ($p < 0.001$) and intestine ($p < 0.01$), although no such association was found in males.

In a case-control study of bladder cancer in ten areas of the US, Cantor *et al.* (1987) looked at the impact of beverage consumption and drinking water source. Included in the study were 2116 white male cases, 689 white female cases and 3892 controls. Cases were aged 21–84 years and had newly diagnosed and histologically confirmed cancer of the bladder in the 12 months beginning December 1977. The study authors also investigated water sources and treatment for 1102 water utilities. There was a significant association between daily tap-water consumption and bladder cancer in males ($p < 0.0001$). This association did not quite achieve significance in the female group ($p = 0.08$). The odds ratio in males for consumption of ≥ 1.96 l/day compared to ≤ 0.80 l/day was 1.4 (CI 1.2–1.8) and in females it was 1.29 (CI 0.9–1.8). In multiple regression analysis there was also a significant association with years of residence with a chlorinated surface water source, as the ORs for tap-water consumption were highest in the groups taking this water for 40 years of more.

In one of the few cohort studies in the area of drinking water and cancer, Yu *et al.* (1993) reported a study of oesophageal cancer in Linxian, China. The cohort was a group of 13 808 individuals (7025 males and 6783 females) who had participated in a screening exercise for oesophageal cancer in 1974. During the 1974 screening a questionnaire about various social and dietary variables was administered. In 1989, 13 610 of these people or, if they had died, their nearest relative were interviewed about subsequent illness. Significant age- and sex-adjusted relative risk factors with a negative association with oesophageal cancer included: education (OR 0.82, CI 0.71–0.94), use of water from wells (OR 0.82, CI 0.69–0.99) and consumption of fresh vegetables (OR 0.66, CI 0.44–0.99). Significant positive factors were a positive family history (OR 1.92, CI 1.70–2.18) and consumption of pork (OR 1.37, CI 1.11–1.68). Given that 24 possible risk factors were included in the analysis a p value of only 0.038 is not conclusive for a water association.

Comments

Despite the fact that several of the studies reported in this section are ecological, there does appear to be a small but frequently significant association between the consumption of surface water and cancers of the bladder and possibly of the rectum. In particular, the study by Cantor *et al.* (1987) stands out as one of the few really sound investigations of the relationship between cancer and drinking water ever done. The authors were able to demonstrate a significant dose–response effect on bladder cancer for tap-water consumption and for chlorinated surface water. I find this study convincing.

The problem with the studies that looked at wastewater reuse was that it was not possible to distinguish between any effect of surface water against well-water and reused water against well-water. Although not intended to look at water reuse, the finding by Gottlieb, Carrand and Morris (1981) of excess mortality below New Orleans compared to above may suggest an effect.

While the overall results of these studies would suggest an excess of cancers from surface water consumption, it is not clear what mechanism may be involved. It may be that surface waters are more at risk of chemical or other pollutants, which are in themselves carcinogenic. However, a plausible explanation may be that surface water frequently contains more organic material and therefore requires higher chlorine doses. The potential impact of chlorination on cancer incidence is discussed below.

CHLORINE AND CHLORINATION BY-PRODUCTS

To a certain extent, there is a large overlap between the papers considered in this section and those considered in the previous one. As already discussed, one of the explanations for differences in health effects between surface waters and groundwaters may be due to greater concentrations of chlorination by-products in the former. In this section I consider those studies that have specifically set out to investigate the effects of chlorine or chlorination by-products. Many different chlorination by-products have been described in drinking water. However, the commonest are the trihalomethanes (THM).

THMs are single carbon compounds with the general formula CHX_3 where X represents any halogen. The four common THMs found in water are chloroform ($CHCl_3$), bromodichloromethane ($CHBrCl_2$), dibromochloromethane ($CHBr_2Cl$) and bromoform ($CHBr_3$). The formation of THMs during chlorination depends on the presence of organic compounds such as humus in the finished water, temperature and pH. There have been a large number of studies reported in the literature that have investigated the association between chlorination of water supplies, trihalomethanes and various cancers. Cantor (1982) reviewed the available epidemiological evidence for carcinogenicity of chlorinated organics in drinking water up to about 1980. This review only considers publications since then.

Wilkins and Comstock (1981) reported an ecological study of the association between water source and cancer in Maryland. The study was restricted to white males and females over 25 years who had a diagnosis of cancer during the 12 years starting on 16 July 1963. Altogether 14 553 males and 16 227 females were included in the analyses. Water sources were classified into high, intermediate and low exposure to trihalomethanes based on how much surface and groundwater was included in the study. The authors found no statistical association between the incidence of any specific cancer and any of the three drinking water cohorts.

Young, Kanarek and Tsisatis (1981) did a death certificate-based case-control study of female cancer mortality in Wisconsin. They identified 8029 cancer deaths and the same number of non-cancer death controls matched for age, year of death and county of residence for the years 1972–1977. Details of water treatment were obtained by questionnaire from the appropriate water superintendents, and water was then classified as having no, low, medium and high chlorine dose. The authors analysed for 11 specific cancers and found an association only between water chlorination and cancer of the colon (OR 1.51, CI 1.06–2.14) for high-dose exposure and (OR 1.53, CI 1.11–2.11) for low-dose exposure. Given the number of statistical tests reported, the lack of any dose response and the only marginal statistical significance, this should probably be taken as a negative response. The following year Kanarek and Young (1982) reported a reanalysis of the mortality data while attempting to get a better indicator of trihalomethane exposure. They compared colon cancer mortality in areas with unchlorinated water with that in areas with chlorinated water without organic contamination (OR 1.41, p = 0.03) and chlorinated with organic contamination (OR 1.41, p = 0.03). Colon cancer was also significantly higher in areas with chlorinated surface water (OR 2.81, p = 0.01). Unfortunately, confidence intervals were not given.

Some years later this same group reported a prospective case-control study of colon cancer in Wisconsin (Young, Wolf and Kanarek 1987). Cases and controls were taken from reports to the cancer registry. Included in the study were 366 cases of colon cancer, 785 controls with other cancers and 654 general population controls. This study attempted to gain an estimate about lifetime THM exposure, and as well as obtaining residential information, it identified drinking water habits for cases and controls. The study found no support for the hypothesis that THM consumption was associated with colon cancer.

A very similar case-control study in Louisiana investigated the effect of water chlorination on 17 cancer death causes in 11 349 cases (Gottlieb and Carr 1982; Gottlieb, Carr and Clarkson 1982). Deaths were between 1960 and 1975. The authors found an association between chlorination and breast cancer (high versus no chlorination OR 1.58, CI 1.09–2.29; low versus no chlorination OR 1.61, CI 1.13–2.30). However, they noted a possible confounding factor in that family size varied with chlorination due to the effect of rural families. They also noted an association between chlorination and rectal cancer (high versus no chlorination OR 1.68, CI 1.17–2.42) but not with colon cancer.

An ecological study of age-standardized cancer mortality rates in 66 Canadian cities was reported by Wigle et al. (1986). Mortality data were extracted from the national mortality database for the years 1973–1979 and water quality data from three national surveys of urban drinking water quality. Thus, some 13 cancers were each compared with 9 indices of water quality. Not surprisingly, given the vast number of statistical comparisons done, there were several apparently significant correlations. The authors claimed a positive correlation between trihalomethane levels and cancer of the stomach ($p < 0.01$) and prostate ($p < 0.05$) and a negative correlation with ovarian cancer ($p < 0.05$). This study highlights some of the dangers of epidemiological fishing exercises: where vast numbers of comparisons are made, many apparently significant associations are likely to arise purely by chance. This merely adds to the dangers of using ecological studies to infer causation of malignant disease.

Cech et al. (1987) reported an ecological study of chlorination by-products in drinking water and cancer mortality rates in Houston. In this situation the city traditionally took its water from lightly chlorinated groundwater sources until 1954, when a more heavily chlorinated surface water source was developed, which has gradually replaced the original well-water. The degree of exposure to chlorinated surface water was estimated for each census tract as: (i) on groundwater throughout, (ii) switched to surface water in 1954, (iii) switched to surface water between 1954 and 1969 and (iv) switched to surface water around 1971. Trihalomethane concentrations were also determined for these areas. The authors were not able to demonstrate any effect of the switch from groundwater to chlorinated surface water on the incidence of bladder cancers in the four areas.

A case-control study in Massachusetts investigated the effect of two different chlorination procedures, chlorination and chloramination, on bladder cancer (Zierler et al. 1988a). The authors interviewed 614 informants of individuals who had died of primary bladder cancer and of 1074 individuals who had died of other causes. Cases were more likely than controls to have lived all (OR 1.3, CI 1.1–1.7) or most (OR 1.2, CI 1.0–1.5) of their lives in communities supplied by chlorinated water.

Ijsselmuiden *et al.* (1992) performed a case-control study of pancreatic cancer in Maryland. They used the geographical estimates of trihalomethane exposure presented in the earlier Maryland study (Wilkins and Comstock 1981). The investigators identified 101 cases and 206 controls. Cases were older than controls and were more likely to smoke and to drink chlorinated municipal water. The odds ratio for chlorinated water consumption, adjusted for age and smoking, was 2.18 (CI 1.20–3.95).

An ecological study of gastrointestinal and urinary tract cancers was based on 56 Finish municipalities (Koivusalo *et al.* 1994). By a complex formula taking into account water quality parameters and water treatment and disinfectant practices, the authors were able to estimate the mutagenicity of the water. With adjustment for potentially confounding factors, bladder cancer was significantly associated with water mutagenicity (RR 1.17, CI 1.03–1.31). Cancers of the kidney, stomach, colon and rectum were not associated. The following year the same authors reported analyses for several more cancers using the same water mutagenicity estimates (Koivusalo *et al.* 1995). After accounting for potentially confounding variables they reported an association with Hodgkin's lymphoma (RR 1.21, CI 1.02–1.40) but not with liver, pancreatic and soft tissue cancers, nor with leukaemia or non-Hodgkin's lymphoma.

Morales-Suarez-Varela *et al.* (1994) reported an ecological study covering all 261 municipalities in the province of Valencia, Spain. They compared mortality rates for stomach and bladder cancer in those municipalities receiving lightly chlorinated groundwater and those receiving heavily chlorinated surface water. No significant difference was found between the two.

Comments

Taking those studies that investigated chlorination directly with those in the previous section that looked at surface water versus well-water, one must again conclude that the evidence for any specific carcinogenic affect is either not significant or at best minimal. In a meta-analysis of publications up to 1988, Morris *et al.* (1992) calculated that the pooled relative risk estimate for exposure to chlorination by-products for bladder cancer was 1.21 (CI 1.09–1.34) and that for rectal cancer was 1.38 (CI 1.01–1.87). I would certainly agree that the evidence in favour of a link to bladder cancer appears stronger. It is, furthermore, supported by Cantor *et al.* (1987) and Zierler *et al.* (1988a). However, the negative results in the Houston study (Cech *et al.* 1987) may suggest a factor associated with certain surface waters rather than chlorination by-products. The case-control study suggesting an association between chlorination and pancreatic cancer needs to be investigated further (Ijsselmuiden *et al.* 1992).

33 Adverse Pregnancy Outcomes and Water

An adverse pregnancy outcome occurs when any pregnancy does not result in a live, healthy baby. Those studies that have investigated the association of water consumption or contact with abortion (miscarriage) or foetal abnormality are discussed in this chapter. I divide the discussion into papers investigating the impact of inorganic chemicals, chlorination by-products and other organic chemicals in drinking water. I also briefly discuss those looking at the suggestion that living near the sea causes foetal abnormality. The reader is also referred to the chapter on cyanobacterial disease.

INORGANIC CHEMICALS IN DRINKING WATER

Several studies in the UK have investigated the relationship between water hardness and congenital malformations of the central nervous system. One of the earliest was an ecological study by Lowe, Roberts and Lloyd (1971). The authors collected data on all live births in 48 local authority areas of South Wales during the years 1964–1966. They found a negative correlation between the rate of CNS abnormalities with mean total hardness ($p < 0.01$). They also analysed data from 1963–1967 death certificates in 58 boroughs in England and Wales. There was a negative correlation between the death rate from anencephalus and mean total hardness, but this was not statistically significant. A statistically significant correlation was seen between the anencephalus death rate and calcium concentration in the wider study ($p < 0.05$). However, possible confounding factors included the finding that in South Wales the softer water tended to be supplied to the poorer mining-based communities.

In a similar study in three areas around Liverpool, UK, Fielding and Smithells (1971) found no correlation between water hardness and anencephalus, either between areas of different water hardness or in the same area during changes in water hardness.

Bound et al. (1981) noted that during the period 1957–1961 the incidence of anencephalus on the Fylde peninsular, northwest England, was almost twice the national average. Furthermore, there were rather more cases of anencephalic babies in North Fylde, than in nearby South Fylde. Blackpool, which is between North and South Fylde, had intermediate incidence. Up to 1962 the water had been soft throughout the year, but after that time there was an increase in hardness. There was a notable decline in the incidence of anencephalus to coincide with this increase in hardness, which was greater than that seen in the rest of the northwest.

One of the areas of contention in the late 1970s and early 1980s was a possible relationship between anencephalus and magnesium in drinking water. The first suggestion came from an ecological study of rates of anencephalus in 36 Canadian cities by Elwood (1977), who noted a small association between rates and magnesium concentrations in drinking water. He suggested that this association was unlikely to be causal. Two years later Archer (1979) wrote a paper reanalysing Elwood's data in which he was strongly critical of Elwood's conclusions. Archer concluded that while the strongest associations were with city growth rates and horizontal electromagnetic flux, there was some association with drinking water magnesium. Elwood (1979) responded to Archer's criticisms and made some of his own regarding Archer's analyses. The reader will by now be aware of the difficulties in the interpretation of the results of ecological studies. As has been pointed out on more than one occasion, no ecological study can be taken as proof for or against a hypothesis for various reasons. The debate reported here seems less relevant in the context of the basic weaknesses of ecological studies. Elwood and Coldman (1981) eventually settled the dispute in a case-control study of 468 deaths from anencephalus and 4129 live birth controls. Although there was a significant association with longitude ($p < 0.001$), latitude ($p < 0.01$) and family income ($p < 0.05$), there was no association with water manganese levels or, indeed, any of nine trace metals in drinking water.

A case-control study was conducted in southern Australia into foetal abnormality and maternal drinking water source (Dorsch et al. 1984). The authors reviewed the birth records of three hospitals over the period 1951–1979 and identified 22 989 registered births. From these, 258 malformed babies were matched by maternal age and month of birth to a normal baby. The home of each case and control was then visited to identify the source of drinking water. Sufficient information was available on 218 matched pairs. Drinking water came from rain-water, a lake or boreholes. In the multivariate analysis, risk of malformation was higher in male babies (RR 1.6, CI 1.1–2.4) and was also significantly associated with source of drinking water ($p = 1.1 \times 10^{-4}$). Compared to those using rain-water, the relative risk in those drinking lake water was 4.9 (CI 2.1–11.7) and in those drinking borehole water was 4.3 (1.4–13.8). In a univariate analysis the authors also found a significant association between malformations and nitrate levels in drinking water. Compared to those drinking water with less than 5 mg/l, the relative risk in those drinking 5–15 mg/l was 2.6 (CI 1.6–4.1) and in those drinking >15 mg/l it was 4.1 (CI 1.3–13.1). There was also a seasonal variation in the relative risk of malformation in those drinking borehole water, with the greatest risk compared to rain-water for conception during the spring (RR 7.0, CI 1.6–63.5) and summer (RR 6.3, CI 2.2–24.7) compared to winter (RR 0.9, CI 0.4–2.3) and autumn (RR 3.0, CI 0.9–12.8). The authors claimed that this was consistent with a water hypothesis, as women would have drunk more water during the hotter summer months. Arbuckle, Hewitt and Sherman (1986) raised some concerns about the paper, mostly in relation to the calculation of nitrate exposure data.

A further case-control study, this time in New Brunswick, Canada, set out to specifically investigate the relationship between nitrate levels in water and defects of the central nervous system in babies (Arbuckle *et al.* 1988). The investigators identified 130 babies born with a CNS malformation between 1973 and 1983 and 264 controls matched for date of birth and county of residence. Where possible, water samples were obtained from each home and a questionnaire administered. A full logistic regression model for CNS malformation tested the confounding effects of mother's age, birth order, water source and mother's birthplace on any relationship between nitrate levels and CNS birth defects. There were more CNS birth defects in women drinking higher nitrate level water from wells (0.1 mg/l versus 26 mg/l) but this did not achieve statistical significance (OR 2.30, CI 0.73–7.29). In public water and spring water sources there was no excess, but nitrate levels were generally lower.

Zierler *et al.* (1988b) studied the relationship between various chemicals in maternal drinking water and congenital heart disease in Massachusetts. They identified 440 cases of congenital heart disease in babies born between 1 April 1990 and 31 March 1983. The authors used routinely collected information on the concentrations of arsenic, barium, cadmium, chromium, lead, mercury, selenium, silver, fluoride, nitrate and sodium in water supplies. There was a significantly small prevalence of heart disease in those mothers with higher intake of selenium (OR 0.62, CI 0.40–0.97). No other associations were obvious. However, the actual concentrations of pollutants were not particularly high.

As discussed in a previous chapter, a large amount of aluminium sulphate was accidentally added to the public water supply in north Cornwall in July 1988. To determine whether this incident had a deleterious affect on pregnancy outcomes, Golding *et al.* (1991) compared the outcomes of 92 pregnancies in women in the affected area with those of women in the same area completed before the incident (*n* = 68) and with those of women in an unaffected area (*n* = 193). There was no excess of perinatal death, low birth weight, pre-term delivery or severe congenital malformation in exposed pregnancies. There was, however, an increased risk of talipes (*p* = 0.01). The authors concluded that there was no evidence of significant risk to foetal health from this incident.

A large study of late adverse pregnancy outcomes among women delivered in Massachusetts between August 1977 and March 1980 identified 1039 cases of congenital abnormality, 77 stillbirths and 55 neonatal deaths as well as

1177 healthy controls (Aschengrau, Zierler and Cohen 1993). This study was based on a prior one that looked at a variety of maternal behavioural factors but with the addition of data on water quality from routine sources. The authors tested the three adverse outcomes against 13 chemicals, pH, Langelier index, water source and water treatment. After adjustment for confounding variables, none of the indicators was statistically significant, although still-births were higher in women exposed to chlorinated surface water (OR 2.6, CI 0.9–7.5) and detectable lead levels (OR 2.1, CI 0.6–7.2). The incidence of neonatal deaths was lower in women exposed to fluoride (OR 0.4, CI 0.2–1.0).

Gupta et al. (1995) studied two groups of 50 children in India. The first group lived in two areas with fluoride levels of 4.5 mg/l and 8.5 mg/l, compared to the WHO recommended maximum level of 1.5 mg/l. The second group lived in Jaipur City, with levels below the WHO limit. Children in the first group all demonstrated clinical and dental fluorosis and some showed skeletal fluorosis, while no children in the second group had fluorosis. After radiological examination 44% of the high-exposure group showed spina bifida occulta compared to only 12% of the low exposure group ($p < 0.001$).

Comments

Of the five studies reported in this section, the first study by Dorsch et al. (1984) is certainly suggestive of a link between nitrate and adverse outcome. That their conclusion was not supported in subsequent studies does not exclude the hypothesis, as nitrate levels were generally low. However, high nitrate levels in both surface water and groundwater sources usually indicate agricultural activity. High nitrate levels may be a proxy for other organic pollutants. The findings in the elegant study by Gupta et al. (1995) certainly need further investigation involving clinically apparent spina bifida.

CHLORINATION BY-PRODUCTS IN DRINKING WATER

The reader will be aware of the considerable interest of researchers in possible relationships between chlorination by-products, especially the trihalomethanes, in drinking water and various cancers discussed in the previous chapter. Several authors have also looked to see whether a relationship exists between adverse pregnancy outcomes and chlorination by-products.

Tuthill et al. (1982) reported a study of the incidence of foetal abnormality, neonatal jaundice, and foetal and neonatal mortality in two communities. The study looked at data from the 1940s in two Massachusetts communities, one of which used high-dose chlorine dioxide disinfection and the other chlorination. There was no significant difference in adverse outcomes between the two communities.

Kramer *et al.* (1992) reported a population-based case-control study of the association of trihalomethanes in drinking water and low birth weight, prematurity and intrauterine growth retardation in Iowa for 18 months from 1 January 1989. The authors compared levels of four trihalomethanes against each of the three adverse outcomes. The only significant association was found between chloroform and intrauterine growth retardation. Compared to babies of mothers with no detectable chloroform in their water, there was an increased risk in mothers drinking 1–9 μg/l (OR 1.3, CI 0.9–1.8) and those drinking $\geq$10 μg/l (OR 1.8, CI 1.1–2.9). An association with $\geq$10 μg/l of dichlorobromomethane did not achieve statistical significance (OR 1.7, CI 0.9–2.9). However, given the number of statistical tests performed, the statistical validity of these results is unclear.

Another population-based case-control study, this time in northern Carolina, investigated the relationship between adverse pregnancy outcome with water source and trihalomethane levels (Savitz, Andrews and Pastore 1995). Cases included medically treated miscarriage, and pre-term and low birth weight babies. The controls were the next live birth. Telephone interviews were conducted to identify a range of possible risk factors, including amount and source of drinking water. The authors tested each of the three adverse outcomes against water source, amount consumed each day, trihalomethane concentrations in water and daily dose of trihalomethane. No single variable reached statistical significance, although there was a consistent trend towards poorer outcomes in women who drank no water each day. Miscarriage rates were slightly increased among women who reported drinking bottled water (OR 1.6, CI 0.6–4.3), although this was not statistically significant.

A survey of all 80 938 singleton live births and 594 singleton foetal deaths in 75 New Jersey towns identified cases of low birth weight, very low birth weight and pre-term births (Bove *et al.* 1995). Cases of congenital abnormality were also identified. Data on trihalomethane levels were taken from routine water company records; information on other risk factors was taken from birth or death certificates. The authors conducted comparisons between 9 contaminants and 13 outcomes, making 117 comparisons. No significance tests were performed. Instead, odds ratios were calculated with 50%, 90% and 99% confidence intervals. Any OR greater than 1 was deemed to be relevant. The authors argued that because they were not presenting significance tests but OR ratios, any conclusions drawn would not be invalidated by the issue of the large number of comparisons. I am afraid that, although I am aware of the debate about the relevance of significance tests and confidence intervals, I am very firmly in the camp that demands one or the other. As such, I do not accept the authors' assertions that the number of comparison issues does not affect the validity of their study. I cannot, therefore, interpret this study, but I doubt that it shows any *significant* correlation.

Comments

My interpretation of the sum of these studies is that any association between trihalomethane levels and adverse pregnancy outcome is at best not proven. Indeed, I suggest that the balance of evidence is that trihalomethane levels at concentrations found in these studies do not adversely affect pregnancy.

ORGANIC CHEMICALS IN DRINKING WATER

There have been several studies that have reported on the effects of organic pollution incidents of water sources on pregnancies. Most of these reports seem to come from California, but this probably reflects enhanced surveillance and monitoring in that state rather than any real excess.

In November 1981, a leak of solvents from an electronics plant contaminated groundwaters with trichloroethane (Deane *et al.* 1989; Swan *et al.* 1989). Concentrations in the water reached 8800 μg/l. The possibility that there may be problems for pregnancies in the area emerged when a local resident wrote to the water company reporting nine cases of adverse outcome. An initial review of birth records found no excess, although as congenital abnormalities are greatly under-reported, this may not have been too surprising. Two epidemiological studies were conducted. The first looked at pregnancy loss in 191 pregnancies in the exposed areas compared with 210 in a similar but non-exposed area (Deane *et al.* 1989). Significant risk factors for spontaneous abortion were: living in the exposed area (OR 2.3, CI 1.3–4.2), drinking cold tap-water (OR 2.1, 1.3–3.5) and drinking alcohol (OR 1.5, 1.2–1.9). These associations remained significant when analysing only doctor-confirmed spontaneous abortions. There was also an increasing trend for abortion with increasing daily water consumption in both communities. No abortions occurred in women of either community who did not drink cold tap-water. In the second study the investigators looked at the incidence of major cardiac abnormalities at the time of exposure and afterwards (Swan *et al.* 1989). At the time of exposure the incidence of cardiac abnormality was 2.7 per 1000 live births in Santa Clara County and 5.6 per 1000 live births in the exposed community (RR 2.2, CI 1.2–4.0). During the post-exposure period there was no excess risk in the affected community compared to the rest of the county (RR 0.5, CI 0.2–1.7).

The findings from these first two studies were thrown into doubt shortly afterwards when the investigators expanded the area of study to include a second exposed and non-exposed community (Wrensch *et al.* 1990a). Spontaneous abortions were actually lower in the new exposed community relative to the new unexposed community at the time of the exposure (OR 0.3, CI 0.1–1.1). However, women who reported drinking home cold tap-water, whether in an exposed or non-exposed community, were at a significant increased risk of spontaneous abortion (OR 4.6, CI 1.9–10.8). The conclusion drawn was that whatever caused the excess abortions in the first study community was unlikely to be due to exposure to the solvent. This conclusion was further strengthened by reports of hydrogeological studies that confirmed the new community as one which would have had an identical exposure to the first (Wrensch et al. 1990b).

Data from the original study by Deane et al. (1989) were reanalysed a few years later to identify risk of abortion with water consumption (Deane et al. 1992). In the 346 pregnancies from both exposed and non-exposed communities there was an increasing risk of spontaneous abortion with increasing daily tap-water consumption ($p = 0.04$). There was also an increased risk of birth defect but this proved not to be statistically significant. This trend was confirmed by analysis of the expanded study by Wrensch et al. (1990) on two more communities (Wrensch et al. 1992). Again, there was a strong association between reported use of cold tap-water and spontaneous abortion (OR 4.0, CI 1.8–9.1). There was no such trend in women who reported using water filters. Despite these strong associations, the authors expressed doubt that the association between tap-water consumption and spontaneous abortion was causal. The study was conducted at a time of great publicity about the water quality issues after a known contamination incident, so many women may have believed tap-water to be harmful, wherever they lived. This may have had a significant bias effect on the assessment of water consumption.

Data from another Californian study, which was originally designed to investigate the impact of aerial spraying of crops with pesticide, was used to investigate the impact of tap-water consumption on spontaneous abortion (Hertz-Picciotto et al. 1989). Questionnaires were sent to 470 women who had experienced spontaneous abortion and 1239 who had had live births. The authors used a Cox proportional hazards regression model and determined that consumption of tap-water had a hazard ratio of 1.5 (CI 1.1–2.0). Other risk factors were maternal age over 30, a history of prior foetal loss, use of video display terminals and not responding to the original mail questionnaire. The results suggested that the protective effect of drinking bottled water was higher in women drinking groundwater.

Yet another study in California was conducted into the association between dibromopropane contamination of drinking water and birth outcome between 1978 and 1982 (Whorton et al. 1989). This was an ecological study where rates of low birth weight and congenital abnormalities were determined for various census tracts, and this correlated with DBCP exposure category. There was no significant correlation between exposure and either of the adverse outcomes investigated.

Goldberg et al. (1990) reported a study undertaken not in California but in Arizona, the state next door. In 1973 it was noted that one-third of children with congenital heart disease in Tucson Valley came from a small area with less than 10% of the population. In 1981 it was noted that most of this area corresponded with an area of polluted groundwater due to industrial chemicals, especially trichloroethylene. The authors identified 707 parents of children who had been living in Tucson Valley at the time of conception. A random telephone survey found that only 10.5% of the Tucson population had lived or worked in the contaminated area compared to 35% of case parents ($p < 0.005$). During the period of contamination, parents living in the contaminated area were three times more likely to have an affected child, but this returned to unity after the affected well was closed.

Comments

The California studies exemplify many of the problems facing public health epidemiologists investigating population exposures. Often it is a cluster of health events that draws attention to the problem. Clusters may be expected to occur randomly with considerable frequency within the world or even within a large country such as America. When a cluster is identified, people look for exposures to blame, and once a suspect exposure has been identified unbiased studies become virtually impossible if the local media has decided the cause in advance. Only when careful analysis, and reanalysis, of the data – as in the Santa Clara study – is done can it be shown that the presumed factor is in fact not responsible.

LIMB REDUCTION DEFECTS AND COASTAL AREAS

As an example of the difficulties that popular epidemiology can create, a UK national newspaper reported on 9 January 1994 a cluster of babies with limb reduction defects (James 1994). The affected babies were all born on the Isle of Wight in 1989 and 1990. It was suggested in the initial report that the only common risk factor was swimming in the sea during pregnancy. Over the next three weeks the same newspaper reported five other clusters of babies, generating considerable national and international interest and anxiety. This interest led to the publication of three short reports in the *Lancet*, which compared the risk of limb reduction defects between coastal and inland populations in the UK, Latin America and Italy (Botting 1994; Castilla and da Graça Dutra 1994; Mastroiacova *et al.* 1994). All three studies analysed routinely recorded data and all three found no difference between coastal and inland populations.

References

Abbaszadegan M, Gerba CP and Rose JB (1991) Detection of Giardia cysts with a cDNA probe and applications to water samples. *Appl Environ Microbiol* **57**:927–931.

Abbaszadegan M, Huber MS, Gerba CP and Pepper IL (1993) Detection of enteroviruses in groundwater with the polymerase chain reaction. *Appl Environ Microbiol* **59**:1318–1324.

Abdel-Hameed AA, Ahmed A-G, Elturabi MK, Mohamedani AA and Magzoub MEMA (1993) An outbreak of dracunculiasis in central Sudan. *Ann Trop Med Parasitol* **87**:571–577.

Abdel-Wahab MF, Strickland GT, El-Sahly A, El-Kady N, Zakaria S and Ahmed L (1979) Changing pattern of schistosomiasis in Egypt 1935–1979. *Lancet* **i**:242–244.

Adak GK, Cowden JM, Nicholas S and Evans HS (1995) The Public Health Laboratory Service national case-control study of primary indigenous sporadic cases of campylobacter infection. *Epidemiol Infect* **115**:15–22.

Aggarwal R and Naik SR (1994) Hepatitis E: intrafamilial transmission *versus* waterborne spread. *J Hepatol* **21**:718–723.

Agulla A, Merino FJ, Villasante PAM, Saz JV, Diaz A and Velasco AC (1987) Evaluation of four enrichment media for isolation of *Campylobacter jejuni*. *J Clin Microbiol* **25**:174–175.

Aho M, Kurki M, Rautelin H and Kosunen TU (1989) Waterborne outbreak of campylobacter enteritis after outdoors infantry drill in Utti, Finland. *Epidemiol Infect* **103**:133–141.

Akogun OB (1990) Water demand and schistosomiasis among the Gumau people of Bauchi State, Nigeria. *Trans R Soc Trop Med Hyg* **84**:548–550.

Alary M and Joly JR (1991) Risk factors for contamination of domestic hot water systems by legionellae. *Appl Environ Microbiol* **57**:2360–2367.

Alary M and Joly JR (1992) Comparison of culture methods and an immuno-fluorescence assay for the detection of *Legionella pneumophila* in domestic hot water devices. *Curr Microbiol* **25**:19–23.

Alary M and Nadeau D (1990) An outbreak of campylobacter enteritis associated with a community water supply. *Can J Public Health* **81**:268–271.

Aldom JE and Chagla AH (1995) Recovery of cryptosporidium oocysts from water by a membrane filter dissolution method. *Lett Appl Microbiol* **20**:186–187.

Aleksic S and Bockemuhl J (1988) Serological and biochemical characteristics of 416 *Yersinia* strains from well water and drinking water plants in the Federal Republic of Germany: lack of evidence that these strains are of public health importance. *Zentralb Bakteriol Mikrobiol Hyg (B)* **185**:527–533.

Alexander LM, Heaven A, Tennant A and Morris R (1992) Symptomatology of children in contact with sea water contaminated with sewage. *J Epidemiol Community Health* **46**:340–344.

Alfrey AC, Legendre GR and Kaehny WD (1976) The dialysis encephalopathy syndrome. Possible aluminium intoxication. *N Engl J Med* **294**:184–188.

Al-Majed S, Bakir TMF, Al-Aska A and Ayoola B (1990) An outbreak of acute hepatitis A infection in rural Saudi Arabia. *Trop Gastroenterol* **11**:202–205.

Al-Qarawi SM, Bushra HE, Fontaine RE, Bubshait SA and El Tantawy NA (1995) Typhoid fever from water desalinized using reverse osmosis. *Epidemiol Infect* **114**:41–50.

al-Riyami A, Haynes LG and Campbell AM (1991) The construction of a monoclonal diagnostic system for the detection of *Vibrio cholerae*. *FEMS Microbiol Immunol* **3**:25–31.

Alugupalli S, Larsson L, Slosarek M and Jaresova M (1992) Application of gas chromatography–mass spectrometry for rapid detection of *Mycobacterium xenopi* in drinking water. *Appl Environ Microbiol* **58**:3538–3541.

Amaro C, Biosca EG, Fouz B and Garay E (1992) Electrophoretic analysis of heterogeneous lipopolysaccharides from various strains of *Vibrio vulnificus* biotypes 1 and 2 by silver staining and immunoblotting. *Curr Microbiol* **25**:99–104.

Amer MH, El-Yazigi A, Hannan MA and Mohamed ME (1990) Water contamination and esophageal cancer at Gassim Region, Saudi Arabia. *Gastroenterology* **98**:1141–1147.

Andersen A, Glattre E and Johansen BV (1993) Incidence of cancer among lighthouse keepers exposed to asbestos in drinking water. *Am J Epidemiol* **138**:682–687.

Anderson DC, Folland DS, Fox MD, Patton CM and Kaufmann AF (1978) Leptospirosis: a common-source outbreak due to leptospires of the grippo-typhosa serogroup. *Am J Epidemiol* **107**:538–544.

Andre-Fontaine G, Peslerbe X and Ganiere JP (1992) Occupational hazard of unnoticed leptospirosis in water ways maintenance staff. *Eur J Epidemiol* **8**:228–232.

Anon (1995) Dracunculiasis. *Weekly Epidemiol Rec* **70**:125–132.

Anon (1996) Strength of association between human illness and water: revised definitions for use in outbreak investigations. *Commun Dis Rep Weekly* **6**:65,68.

Aquilonius SM and Hartvig P (1986) A Swedish county with unexpectedly high utilization of anti-parkinsonian drugs. *Acta Neurol Scand* **74**:379–382.

Araujo RM, Arribas RM, Lucena F and Pares R (1989) Relation between *Aeromonas* and faecal coliforms in freshwaters. *J Appl Bacteriol* **69**:439–444.

Arbuckle TE, Hewitt D and Sherman GJ (1986) Congenital malformations and maternal drinking water supply in rural South Australia: a case control study. *Am J Epidemiol* **124**:344.

Arbuckle TE, Walters D, Sherman GJ, Lo B and Corey PN (1988) Water nitrates and CNS birth defects: a population-based case-control study. *Arch Environ Health* **43**:162–167.

Archer VE (1979) Anencephalus, drinking water, geomagnetism and cosmic radiation. *Am J Epidemiol* **109**:88–97.

Arcos ML, de Vicente A, Morinigo MA, Romero P and Borrego JJ (1988) Evaluation of several selective media for recovery of *Aeromonas hydrophila* from polluted waters. *Appl Environ Microbiol* **54**:2786–2792.

Arias CR, Garay E and Aznar R (1995) Nested PCR method for rapid and sensitive detection of *Vibrio vulnificus* in fish, sediments and water. *Appl Environ Microbiol* **61**:3476–3478.

Arif M, Qattan I, Al-Faleh F and Ramia S (1994) Epidemiology of hepatitis E virus (HEV) infection in Saudi Arabia. *Ann Trop Med Parasitol* **88**:163–168.

Armstrong BK, Margetts BM, McCall MG, Binns CW, Campbell VA and Masarii JR (1982) Water sodium and blood pressure in rural school children. *Arch Environ Health* **37**:236–245.

Armstrong CW, Lake JL and Miller GB Jr (1983) Extraintestinal infections due to halophilic vibrios. *South Med J* **76**:571–574.

Armstrong CW, Siudyla EA, Stroube RB, Miller GB Jr and Rubio T (1984) Outbreak of fatal arsenic poisoning caused by contaminated drinking water. *Arch Environ Health* **39**:276–279.

Aschengrau A, Zierler S and Cohen A (1993a) Quality of community drinking water and the occurrence of late adverse pregnancy outcomes. *Arch Environ Health* **48**:105–113.

Aschengrau A, Ozonoff D, Paulu C, Coogan P, Vezina R, Heeren T and Zhang Y (1993) Cancer risk and tetrachloroethylene-contaminated drinking water in Massachusetts. *Arch Environ Health* **48**:284–292.

Ashdown LR (1979) An improved screening technique for isolation of *Pseudomonas pseudomallei* from clinical specimens. *Pathology* **11**:293–297.

Atherton F, Newman CPS and Casemore DP (1995) An outbreak of water-borne cryptosporidiosis associated with a public water supply in the UK. *Epidemiol Infect* **115**:123–131.

Baer GM, Walker JA and Yager PA (1977) Studies of an outbreak of acute hepatitis A: 1. complement level fluctuation. *J Med Virol* **1**:1–7.

Baffone W, Bruscolini F, Pianetti A, Biffi MR, Brandi G, Salvaggio L and Albano V (1995) Diffusion of thermophilic campylobacter in the Pesaro–Urbino area (Italy) from 1985 to 1992. *Eur J Epidemiol* **11**:83–86.

Bahl MR (1976) Impact of piped water supply on the incidence of typhoid fever and diarrhoeal diseases in Lusaka. *Med J Zambia* **10**(4):98–99.

Baine WB, Herron CA, Bridson K, Barker WH Jr, Lindell S, Mallison GF, Wells JG, Martin WT, Kosuri MR, Carr F and Voelker E Sr (1975) Waterborne outbreak at a public school. *Am J Epidemiol* **101**:323–332.

Baker EL, Landrigan PJ, Field PH, Basteyns BJ, Bertozzi PE and Skinner HG (1978) Phenol poisoning due to contaminated drinking water. *Arch Environ Health* **33**:89–94.

Balarajan R, Raleigh VS, Yuen P, Wheeler D, Machin D and Cartwright R (1991) Health risks associated with bathing in seas water. *Brit Med J* **303**:1444–1445.

Bandyopadhyay S, Khera AK, Banerjee K, Kar NJ and Sharma RS (1993) An investigation of an outbreak of viral hepatitis in a residential area of Dehli. *J Commun Dis* **25**:65–70.

Bannister BA, Begg NT and Gillespie SH (1996) *Infectious Disease.* Blackwell Science, Oxford.

Barbeau A, Roy M, Bernier G, Campanella G and Paris S (1987) Ecogenetics of Parkinson's disease: prevalence and environmental aspects in rural areas. *Can J Neurol Sci* **14**:36–41.

Barbour AD (1985) The importance of age and water contact patterns in relation to *Schistosoma haematobium* infection. *Trans R Soc Trop Med Hyg* **79**:151–153.

Barbour AG, Nichols CR and Fukushima T (1976) An outbreak of giardiasis in a group of campers. *Am J Trop Med Hyg* **25**:384–389.

Barcina I, Gonzalez JM, Iriberri J and Egea L (1989) Effect of visible light on progressive dormancy of *Escherichia coli* cells during the survival process in natural freshwater. *Appl Environ Microbiol* **55**:246–251.

Barer MR and Wright AE (1990) *Cryptosporidium* and water. *Lett Appl Microbiol* **11**:271–277.

Barker DJP (1973) Epidemiology of *Mycobacterium ulcerans* infection. *Trans R Soc Trop Med Hyg* **67**:43–47.

Barker DJP and Carswell JW (1973) *Mycobacterium ulcerans* infection among tsetse control workers in Uganda. *Int J Epidemiol* **2**:161–165.

Baron RC, Murphy FD, Greenberg HB, Davis CE, Bregman DJ, Gary GW, Hughes JM and Schonberger LB (1982) An outbreak associated with swimming in a recreational lake and secondary person-to-person transmission. *Am J Epidemiol* **115**:163–172.

Barreto ML (1991) Geographical and socioeconomic factors relating to the distribution of *Schistosoma mansoni* infection in an urban area of north-east Brazil. *Bull World Health Organ* **69**:93–102.

Bates MN, Smith AH and Cantor KP (1995) Case-control study of bladder cancer and arsenic in drinking water. *Am J Epidemiol* **141**:523–530.

Bates MN, Smith AH and Hopenhayn-Rich C (1992) Arsenic ingestion and internal cancers: a review. *Am J Epidemiol* **135**:462–476.

Baum SG. (1995) Adenovirus. In: Mandell GL, Douglas RG and Bennett JE (eds) *Principles and Practice of Infectious Diseases*, 4th edn. Churchill Livingstone, New York, pp 1382–1387.

Bean JA, Isacson P, Hahne RMA and Kohler J (1982a) Drinking water and cancer incidence in Iowa. II. Radioactivity in drinking water. *Am J Epidemiol* **116**:924–932.

Bean JA, Isacson P, Hausler WJ Jr and Kohler J (1982b) Drinking water and cancer incidence in Iowa. I. Trends and incidence by source of drinking water and size of municipality. *Am J Epidemiol* **116**:912–923.

Bej AK, McCarty SC and Atlas RM (1991a) Detection of coliform bacteria and *Escherichia coli* by multiplex chain reaction: comparison with defined substrate and plating methods for water quality monitoring. *Appl Environ Microbiol* **57**:2429–2432.

Bej AK, DiCesare JL, Haff L and Atlas RM (1991) Detection of *Escherichia coli* and *Shigella* spp. in water by using the polymerase chain reaction and gene probes for *uid*. *Appl Environ Microbiol* **57**:1013–1017.

Belabbes H, Bouguermouh A, Benatallah A and Illoul G (1985) Epidemic non-A, non-B viral hepatitis in Algeria: strong evidence for its spread by water. *J Med Virol* **16**:257–263.

Belcher DW, Wurapa FK, Ward WB and Lourie IM (1975) Guinea worm in southern Ghana: its epidemiology and impact on agricultural productivity. *Am J Trop Med Hyg* **24**:243–249.

Bell A, Guasparini R, Meeds D, Mathias RG and Farley JD (1993) A swimming pool-associated outbreak of cryptosporidiosis in British Columbia. *Can J Public Health* **84**:334–337.

Benton C, Forbes GI, Paterson GM, Sharp JCM and Wilson TS (1989) The incidence of waterborne and water-associated disease in Scotland from 1945 to 1987. *Water Sci Technol* **21**:125–129.

Beresford SAA (1983) Cancer incidence and reuse of drinking water. *Am J Epidemiol* **117**:258–268.

Beresford SAA (1985) Is nitrate in the drinking water associated with the risk of cancer in the urban UK? *Int J Epidemiol* **14**:57–63.

Bergeisen GH, Hinds MW and Skaggs JW (1985) A waterborne outbreak of hepatitis A in Meade County, Kentucky. *Am J Public Health* **75**:161–164.

Bernardi D, Dini FL, Azzarelli A, Giaconi A, Volterrani C and Lunardi M (1995) Sudden cardiac death rate in an area characterized by high incidence of coronary artery disease and low hardness of drinking water. *Angiology* **46**:145–149.

Bernagozzi M, Bianucci F, Scerre E and Sacchetti R (1994) Assessment of some selective media for the recovery of *Aeromonas hydrophila* from surface waters. *Zentralb Hyg Umweltmed* **195**:121–134.

Best M, Yu VL, Stout J, Goetz A, Muder RR and Taylor F (1983) Legionellaceae in the hospital water-supply. Epidemiological link with disease and evaluation of a method for control of nosocomial Legionnaires' disease and Pittsburgh pneumonia. *Lancet* **ii**:307–310.

Bierenbau ML, Fleischman AI, Dunn J and Arnold J (1975) Possible toxic water factor in coronary heart disease. *Lancet* **i**:1008–1010.

Bifulco JM and Schaefer FW 3rd (1993) Antibody-magnetite method for selective concentration of *Giardia lamblia* cysts from water samples. *Appl Environ Microbiol* **59**:772–776.

Bile K, Isse A, Mohamud O, Allebeck P, Nilsson L, Norder H, Mushahwar IS and Magnius LO (1994) Contrasting roles of rivers and wells as sources of drinking water on attack and fatality rates in a hepatitis E epidemic in Somalia. *Am J Trop Med Hyg* **51**:466–474.

Billings WH (1981) Water associated human illness in Northeast Pennsylvania and its suspected association with blue-green algal blooms. In: Carmichael WW (ed.) *Algal Toxins and Health*. Plenum Press, New York, pp 243–255.

Birkhead G and Vogt RL (1989) Epidemiological surveillance for endemic *Giardia lamblia* infection in Vermont: the roles of waterborne and person to person transmission. *Am J Epidemiol* **129**:762–768.

Birkhead G, Janoff EN, Vogt RL and Smith PD (1989) Elevated levels of immunoglobulin A to *Giardia lamblia* during a waterborne outbreak of gastroenteritis. *J Clin Microbiol* **27**:1707–1710.

Blake PA, Ramos S, MacDonald KL, Rassi V, Tardelli-Gomes TA, Ivey C, Bean NH and Trabulsi LR (1993) Pathogen-specific risk factors and protective factors for acute diarrheal disease in urban Brazilian infants. *J Infect Dis* **167**:627–632.

Blake PA, Rosenberg ML, Costa JB, Ferreira PS, Guimaraes CL and Gangarosa EJ (1977a) Cholera in Portugal, 1974, I. Modes of transmission. *Am J Epidemiol* **105**:337–343.

Blake PA, Rosenberg ML, Costa JB, Ferreira PS, Guimaraes CL and Gangarosa EJ (1977b) Cholera in Portugal, 1974, II. Transmission by bottled mineral water. *Am J Epidemiol* **105**:344–348.

Blaser MJ and Cody HJ (1986) Methods for isolating *Campylobacter jejuni* from low-turbidity water. *Appl Environ Microbiol* **51**:312–315.

Bloch AB, Stramer SL, Smith JD, Margolis HS, Fields HA, McKinley TW, Gerba CP, Maynard JE and Sikes RK (1990) Recovery of hepatitis A virus from a water supply responsible for a common source outbreak of hepatitis A. *Am J Public Health* **80**:428–430.

Blostein J (1991) Shigellosis from swimming in a park pond in Michigan. *Public Health Rep* **106**:317–322.

Bockemuhl J, Roch K, Wohlers B, Aleksic V, Aleksic S and Wokatsch R (1986) Seasonal distribution of facultatively enteropathogenic vibrios (*Vibrio cholerae, Vibrio mimicus, Vibrio parahaemolyticus*) in the freshwater of the Elbe River at Hamburg. *J Appl Bacteriol* **60**:435–442.

Bolaños B (1991) Dermatophyte feet infection among students enrolled in swimming courses at a university pool. *Bol Asoc Med P R* **83**:181–184.

Bolton FJ, Coates D, Hutchinson DN and Godfree AF (1987) A study of thermophilic campylobacters in a river system. *J Appl Bacteriol* **62**:167–176.

Bora D, Prakash C, Bhattacharjee J and Datta KK (1993) Epidemiology of a jaundice outbreak in Rairangpur Town in Orissa. *J Commun Dis* **25**:1–5.

Borgoño JM, Vicent P, Venturino H and Infante A (1977) Arsenic in the drinking water of the city of Antofagasta: epidemiological and clinical study before and after the installation of a treatment plant. *Environ Health Perspect* **19**:103–105.

Bornstein N, Marmet D, Surgot M, Nowicki M, Arslan A, Esteve J and Fleurette J (1989) Exposure to Legionellaceae at a hot spring spa: a prospective clinical and epidemiological study. *Epidemiol Infect* **102**:31–36.

Botting BJ (1994) Limb reduction defects and coastal areas. *Lancet* **343**:1033–1034.

Bound JP, Harvey PW, Brookes DM and Sayers BMcA (1981) The incidence of anencephalus in the Fylde peninsula 1956–76 and changes in water hardness. *J Epidemiol Community Health* **35**:102–105.

Bourke ATC, Hawes RB, Neilson A and Stallman ND (1983) An outbreak of hepato-enteritis (the Palm Island mystery disease) possibly caused by algal intoxication. *Toxicon Suppl* **3**:45–48.

Bove FJ, Fulcomer MC, Klotz JB, Esmart J, Dufficy EM and Savrin JE (1995) Public drinking water contamination and birth outcomes. *Am J Epidemiol* **141**:850–862.

Bowen GS and McCarthy MA (1983) Hepatitis A associated with a hardware store water fountain and a contaminated well in Lancaster County, Pennsylvania, 1980. *Am J Epidemiol* **117**:695–705.

Boyce JM, Hughes JM, Alim ARMA, Khan M, Aziz KMA, Wells JG and Curlin GT (1982) Patterns of *Shigella* infection in families in rural Bangladesh. *Am J Trop Med Hyg* **31**:1015–1020.

Bradford-Hill A (1965) The environment and disease: association or causation? *Proc R Soc Med* **58**:295–300.

Brady PG and Wolfe JC (1974) Waterborne giardiasis. *Ann Intern Med* **81**:498–499.

Breiman RF, Cozen W, Fields BS, Mastro TD, Carr SJ, Spika JS and Mascola L (1990) Role of air-sampling in an investigation of an outbreak of Legionnaires' disease associated with exposure to aerosols from an evaporative condenser. *J Infect Dis* **161**:1257–1261.

Brennhovd O, Kapperud G and Langeland G (1992) Survey of thermotolerant *Campylobacter* spp. and *Yersinia* spp. in three surface water sources in Norway. *Int J Food Microbiol* **15**:327–338.

Brenniman GR, Namekata T, Kojola WH, Carnow BW and Levy PS (1979) Cardiovascular disease rates in communities with elevated levels of barium in drinking water. *Environ Res* **20**:318–324.

Brenniman GR, Kojola WH, Levy PS, Carnow BW and Namekata T (1981) High barium levels in public drinking water and its association with elevated blood pressure. *Arch Environ Health* **36**:28–32.

Bridgman SA, Robertson RMP, Syed Q, Speed N, Andrews N and Hunter PR

(1995) Outbreak of cryptosporidiosis associated with a disinfected ground-water supply. *Epidemiol Infect* **115**:555–566.

Brieseman MA (1987) Town water supply as the cause of an outbreak of campylobacter infection. *N Z Med J* **100**:212–213.

Brinkmann UK, Korte R and Schmidt-Ehry B (1988) The distribution and spread of schistosomiasis in relation to water resources management in Mali. *Trop Med Parasitol* **39**:182–185.

Broczyk A, Thompson S, Smith D and Lior H (1987) Water-borne outbreak of *Campylobacter laridis*-associated gastroenteritis. *Lancet* **i**:164–165.

Brouwer ID, Dirks OB, De-Bruin A and Hautvast JG (1988) Unsuitability of World Health Organization guidelines for fluoride concentrations in drinking water in Senegal. *Lancet* **i**:223–225.

Browne K (1982) Re: Asbestos in drinking water and cancer incidence in the San Francisco Bay area. *Am J Epidemiol* **115**:142–143.

Brussow H, Rahim H and Freire W (1992) Epidemiological analysis of sero-logically determined rotavirus and enterotoxigenic *Escherichia coli* infections in Ecuadorian children. *J Clin Microbiol* **30**:1585–1587.

Bryan JA, Lehmann JD, Setiady IF and Hatch MH (1974) An outbreak of hepatitis-A associated with recreational lake water. *Am J Epidemiol* **99**:145–154.

Burke V, Robinson J, Gracey M, Peterson D and Pertridge K (1984) Isolation of *Aeromonas hydrophila* from a metropolitan water supply: seasonal correlation with clinical isolates. *Appl Environ Microbiol* **48**:361–366.

Burns DN, Wallace RJ Jr, Schultz ME, Zhang Y, Zubairi SQ, Pang Y, Gilbert CL, Brown BA, Noel ES and Gordin FM (1991) Nosocomial outbreak of respiratory tract colonization with *Mycobacterial fortuitum*: demonstration of the usefulness of pulsed-filed gel electrophoresis in an epidemiological investigation. *Am Rev Respir Dis* **144**:1153–1159.

Byers VS, Levin AS, Ozonoff DM and Baldwin RW (1988) Association between clinical symptoms and lymphocyte abnormalities in a population with chronic domestic exposure to industrial solvent-contaminated domestic water supply and a high incidence of leukaemia. *Cancer Immunol Immunother* **27**:77–81.

Byskov J, Wouters JSM, Sathekge TJ and Swanepoel R (1989) An outbreak of suspected waterborne epidemic non-A, non-B hepatitis in northern Botswana with a high prevalence of hepatitis B carriers and hepatitis delta markers among patients. *Trans R Soc Trop Med Hyg* **83**:110–116.

Byth S (1980) Palm Island mystery disease. *Med J Aust* **2**:40–42.

Cabelli VJ, Dufour AP, Levin MA, McCabe LJ and Haberman PW (1979) Relationship of microbial indicators to health effects at marine bathing beaches. *Am J Public Health* **69**:690–696.

Cabelli VJ, Dufour AP, McCabe LJ and Levin MA (1982) Swimming-associated gastroenteritis and water quality. *Am J Epidemiol* **115**:606–616.

Cacciapuoti B, Ciceroni L, Maffei C, di Stanislao F, Strusi P, Calegari L,

Lupidi R, Scalise G, Cagnoni G and Renga G (1987) A waterborne outbreak of leptospirosis *Am J Epidemiol* **126**:535–545.

Cafferkey MT, Sloane A, McCrae S and O'Morain CA (1993) *Yersinia frederiksenii* infection and colonization in hospital staff. *J Hosp Infect* **24**:109–115.

Cain ARR, Wiley PF, Brownell B and Warhurst DC (1981) Primary amoebic meningoencephalitis. *Arch Dis Childhood* **56**:140–143.

Cairncross S and Feachem R (1993) *Environmental Health Engineering in the Tropics*. John Wiley and Sons, Chichester.

Calabrese EJ and Tuthill RW (1981) The influence of elevated levels of sodium in drinking water on elementary and high school students in Massachusetts. *Sci Total Environ* **18**:117–133.

Caldas EM and Sampaio MB (1979) Leptospirosis in the city of Salvador, Bahia, Brazil. *Int J Zoonoses* **6**:85–96.

Calderon RL, Wood EW and Dufour AP (1991) Health effects of swimmers and nonpoint sources of contaminated water. *Int J Environ Health Res* **1**:21–31.

Caldwell GC, Lindsey NJ, Wulff H, Donnelly DD and Bohl FN (1974) Epidemic of adenovirus type 7 conjunctivitis in swimmers. *Am J Epidemiol* **99**:230–234.

Cambria K and Alonso E (1995) Blood lead levels in 2- to 3-year-old children in the Greater Bilbao area (Basque Country, Spain): relation to dust and water lead levels. *Arch Environ Health* **50**:362–366.

Cannon RO, Poliner JR, Hirschhorn RB, Rodeheaver DC, Silverman PR, Brown EA, Talbot GH, Stine SE, Monroe SS, Dennis DT and Glass RI (1991) A multistate outbreak of Norwalk virus gastroenteritis associated with consumption of commercial ice. *J Infect Dis* **164**:860–863.

Cantor KP (1982) Epidemiological evidence of carcinogenicity of chlorinated organics in drinking water. *Environ Health Perspect* **46**:187–195.

Cantor KP, Hoover R, Hartge P, Mason TJ, Silverman DT, Altman R, Austin DF, Child MA, Key CR, Marrett LD, Myers MH, Narayana AS, Levin LI, Sullivan JW, Swanson GM, Thomas DB and West DW (1987) Bladder cancer, drinking water source and tap water consumption: a case-control study. *J Natl Cancer Inst* **79**:1269–1279.

Cardenas V, Saad C, Varona M and Linero M (1993) Waterborne cholera in Riohacha, Columbia 1992. *Bull Pan Am Health Organ* **27**:313–330.

Carmichael WW (1992) Cyanobacteria secondary metabolites – the cyanotoxins. *J Appl Bacteriol* **72**:445–459.

Carmichael WW, Jones CLA, Mahmood NA and Theiss WC (1985) Algal toxins and water-based diseases. *CRC Crit Rev Environ Contr* **15**:275–313.

Carmichael WW, Yu M-J, He Z-R, He JW and Yu J-L (1988) Occurrence of the toxic cyanobacterium (blue-green alga) *Microcystis aeruginosa* in central China. *Arch Hydrobiol* **114**:21–30.

Carpenter LM and Beresford SAA (1986) Cancer mortality and type of water source: findings from a study in the UK. *Int J Epidemiol* **15**:312–320.

Carson LA, Petersen NJ, Favero MS and Aguero SM (1978) Growth characteristics of atypical mycobacteria in water and their comparative resistance to disinfectants. *Appl Environ Microbiol* **36**:839–846.

Carter AM, Pacha RE, Clark GW and Williams EA (1987) Seasonal occurrence of *Campylobacter* spp. in surface waters and their correlation with standard indicator bacteria. *Appl Environ Microbiol* **53**:523–526.

Castilla EE and da Graça Dutra M (1994) Limb reduction defects and coastal areas. *Lancet* **343**:1034.

Catalan V, Moreno C, Dasi MA, Munoz C and Apraiz D (1994) Nested polymerase chain reaction for detection of *Legionella pneumophila* in water. *Res Microbiol* **145**:603–610.

Cebrián ME, Albores A, Aguilar M and Blakey E (1983) Chronic arsenic poisoning in the North of Mexico. *Human Toxicol* **2**:121–133.

Cech I, Holguin AH, Littell AS, Henry JP and O'Connell J (1987) Health significance of chlorination byproducts in drinking water: the Houston experience. *Int J Epidemiol* **16**:198–207.

Chakraborty AK and Saha KC (1987) Arsenical dermatosis from tubewell water in West Bengal. *Indian J Med Res* **85**:326–334.

Chakraborty S, Datta M, Pasha ST and Kumar S (1982) Non-A, non-B viral hepatitis: a common-source outbreak traced to sewage contamination of drinking water. *J Commun Dis* **14**:41–46.

Chan OY, Chia SE, Nadarajah N and Sng EH (1987) Leptospirosis risk in public cleansing and sewer workers. *Ann Acad Med* **16**:586–590.

Chandiwana SK and Woolhouse MEJ (1991) Heterogeneities in water contact patterns and the epidemiology of *S. haematobium*. *Parasitology* **103**:363–370.

Chandiwana SK, Woolhouse MEJ and Bradley M (1991) Factors affecting the intensity of reinfection with *S. haematobium* following treatment with praziquantel. *Parasitology* **103**:363–370.

Chandra S, Sharma R, Thergaonkar VP and Chaturvedi SK (1980) Determination of optimal fluoride concentration in drinking water in an area in India with dental fluorosis. *Community Dent Oral Epidemiol* **8**:92–96.

Chang HR, Loo LH, Kuah BG and Heng BH (1995) Comparison of multiplex PCR and culture for detection of legionellae in cooling tower water samples. *Southeast Asian J Trop Med Public Health* **26**:258–262.

Chapman JA and Collocott LP (1985) Cholera in children at Eshowe hospital. *S Afr Med J* **68**:249–253.

Chapman L (1976) Hepatitis attributed to polluted stream. *J Environ Health* **38**:238–241.

Cheesmond AK and Fenwick A (1981) Human excretion behaviour in a schistosomiasis endemic area of the Geizira, Sudan. *J Trop Med Hyg* **84**:101–107.

Chen CJ, Hsueh Y-M, Lai M-S, Shyu M-P, Chen S-Y, Wu M-M, Kuo T-L and Tai T-Y (1995) Increased prevalence of hypertension and long-term arsenic exposure. *Hypertension* **25**:53–60.

Chen C-J, Wu M-M, Lee S-S, Wang J-D, Cheng S-H and Wu H-Y (1988) Artherogenicity and carcinogenicity of high-arsenic artesian well water. Multiple risk factors and related malignant neoplasms of Blackfoot disease. *Arteriosclerosis* **8**:452–460.

Chen K, Lin C, QI, Zen N, Zhen G, Chen G, Yijun X, Yiejie L and Zhuang S (1991) The epidemiology of diarrhoeal disease in southeastern China. *J Diarrhoeal Dis Res* **9**:94–99.

Chen W, Xu R, Chen G, Zao J and Chen T (1993) Changes in the prevalence of endemic fluorosis after changing water souces in two villages in Guangdong, China. *Bull Environ Contamination Toxicol* **51**:479–482.

Cheung WHS, Chang KCK, Hung RPS and Kleevens JWL (1990) Health effects of beach water pollution in Hong Kong. *Epidemiol Infect* **105**:139–162.

Chongsuvivatwong V, Mo-suwam L, Chompikul J, Vitsupakorn K and McNeil D (1994) Effects of piped water supply on the incidence of diarrheal diseases in children in southern Thailand. *Southeast Asian J Trop Med Public Health* **25**:628–632.

Chuang Y-C, Yuan C-Y, Liu C-Y, Lan C-K and Huang AH-M (1992) *Vibrio vulnificus* infection in Taiwan: report of 28 cases and review of clinical manifestations and treatment. *Clin Infect Dis* **15**:271–276.

Clark CS, Meyer CR, Gartside PS, Majeti VA, Specker B, Balistreri WF and Elia VJ (1982) An environmental health survey of drinking water contamination by leachate from a pesticide waste dump in Hardeman County, Tennessee. *Arch Environ Health* **37**:9–18.

Claudon DG, Thompson DI, Christenson EH, Lawton GW and Dick EC (1971) Prolonged *Salmonella* contamination of a recreational lake by runoff waters. *Appl Microbiol* **21**:875–877.

Codd GA and Beattie KA (1991) Cyanobacteria (blue-green algae) and their toxins: awarenes and action in the United Kingdom. *PHLS Microbiol Digest* **8**:82–86.

Codd GA and Bell SG (1985) Eutrophication and toxic cyanobacteria. *J Water Pollut Contr* **34**:225–232.

Codd GA, Bell SG and Brooks WP (1989b) Cyanobacterial toxins in water. *Water Sci Technol* **21**(3):1–13.

Codd GA, Brooks WP, Priestley IM, Poon GK and Bell SG (1989a) Production detection, and quantification of cyanobacterial toxins. *Toxicity Assessment* **4**:499–511.

Coggon D (1991) Camelford revisited. *Brit Med J* **303**:1280–1281.

Cohen MT, Robertson J, Shlim DR, Fabian P and Rajah R (1991) Outbreaks of diarrheal illness associated with cyanobacteria (blue-green algae)-like bodies – Chicago and Nepal, 1989 and 1990. *MMWR* **40**:325–327.

Collins CH, Lyne PM and Grange JM (1995) *Microbiological Methods.* Oxford, Butterworth–Heinemann.

Collins CH, Grange JM, Noble WC and Yates MD (1985) *Mycobacterium marinum* infections in man. *J Hyg, Camb* **94**:135–149.

Collins M (1979) Possible link between water supply and high birth defect rate. In: *Proceedings of the American Water Works Association 1978 Annual Conference*, Part II, Atlantic City, NJ. AWWA, Denver, Colorado. Paper 24–5.

Collins MD, Gowans CS, Garro F, Estervig D, Swanson T (1981) Temporal association between an algal bloom and mutagenicity in a water reservoir. In: Carmichael WW (ed.) *Algal Toxins and Health.* Plenum Press, New York, pp 271–284.

Collman GW, Loomis DP and Sandler DP (1991) Childhood cancer mortality and radon concentration in drinking water in North Carolina. *Brit J Cancer* **63**:626–629.

Colquhoun KO, Timms S and Fricker CR (1995) Detection of *Escherichia coli* in potable water using direct impedance technology. *J Appl Bacteriol* **79**:635–639.

Comstock GW (1979) Water hardness and cardiovascular diseases. *Am J Epidemiol* **110**:375–400.

Comstock GW, Cauthen GM and Helsing KJ (1980) Water hardness at home and deaths from arteriosclerotic heart disease in Washington County, Maryland. *Am J Epidemiol* **112**:209–216.

Conforti PM (1983) Effect of population density on the results of the study of water supplies in five California Counties. *Environ Health Perspect* **53**:69–78.

Conforti PM, Kanarek MS, Jackson LA, Cooper RC and Murchio JC (1981) Asbestos in drinking water and cancer in the San Francisco Bay area: 1969–1974. *J Chronic Dis* **34**:211–224.

Cook GC (ed.) (1996) *Manson's Tropical Diseases*, 20th edn. WB Saunders, London.

Coppo A, Colombo M, Pazzani C, Bruni R, Mohamud KA, Omar KH, Mastrandrea S, Salvia AM, Rotigliano G and Maimone F (1995) *Vibrio cholerae* in the Horn of Africa: epidemiology, plasmids, tetracycline resistance gene amplification, and comparison between O1 and non-O1 strains. *Am J Trop Med Hyg* **53**:351–359.

Corbett SJ, Rubin GL, Curry GK, Kleinbaum DG and the Sydney Beach Users Study Advisory Group (1993) The health effects of swimming at Sydney Beaches. *Am J Public Health* **83**:1701–1706.

Cordes LG, Weisenthal AM, Gorman GW, Phair JP, Sommers HM, Brown A, Yu VL, Magnussen MH, Meyer RD, Wolf JS, Shands KN and Fraser DW (1981) Isolation of *Legionella pneumophila* from hospital shower heads. *Ann Intern Med* **94**:195–197.

Corwin A, Ryan A, Bloys W, Thomas R, Deniega B and Watts D (1990) A waterborne outbreak of leptospirosis among United States military personnel in Okinawa, Japan. *Int J Epidemiol* **19**:743–748.

Corwin A, Jarot K, Lubis I, Nasution K, Suparmawo S, Sumardiati A, Widodo S, Wilodo S, Nazir S, Orndorff G, Choi Y, Tan R, Sie A, Wignall S, Graham R and Hyams K (1995) Two years' investigation of epidemic hepatitis E virus transmission in West Kalimantan (Borneo), Indonesia. *Trans R Soc Trop Med Hyg* **89**:262–265.

Coura-Filho P, Rocha RS, Farah MW, da Silva GC and Katz N (1994) Identification of factors and groups at risk of infection with *Schistosoma mansoni*: a strategy for the implementation of control measures? *Rev Inst Med Trop Sao Paulo* **36**:245–253.

Craun GF (1988) Surface water supplies and health. *J Am Water Works Assoc* **80**:40–52.

Craun GF (1992) Waterborne disease outbreaks in the United States of America: causes and prevention. *World Health Stat Q* **45**:192–199.

Craun GF, Greathouse DG and Gunderson DH (1981) Methaemoglobin levels in young children consuming high nitrate well water in the United States. *Int J Epidemiol* **10**:309–317.

Crombie IK, Kenicer MB, Smith WC and Tunstall-Pedoe HD (1989) Unemployment, socioeconomic factors, and coronary heart disease in Scotland. *Brit Heart J* **61**:172–177.

Crowcroft NS (1994) Cholera: current epidemiology. *Commun Dis Rep Rev* **4**:R157–R164.

Cuello C, Correa P, Haenszel W, Gordillo G, Brown C, Archer M and Tannenbaum S (1976) Gastric cancer in Columbia. I. Cancer risk and suspect environmental agents. *J Natl Cancer Inst* **57**:1015–1020.

Cunliffe DA and Adcock P (1989) Isolation of *Aeromonas* spp. from water by using anaerobic incubation. *Appl Environ Microbiol* **55**:2138–2140.

Curtis V, Kanki B, Mertens T, Traoré, E, Diallo I, Tall F and Cousens S (1995) Potties, pits and pipes: explaining hygiene behaviour in Burkino Faso. *Soc Sci Med* **41**:383–393.

D'Alessio DJ, Minor TE, Allen CI, Tsiatis AA and Nelson DB (1981) A study of the proportions of swimmers among well controls and children with enterovirus-like illness shedding or not shedding an enterovirus. *Am J Epidemiol* **113**:533–541.

Dalton PR and Pole D (1978) Water-contact patterns in relation to *Schistosoma haematobium* infection. *Bull World Health Organ* **56**:417–426.

Dance DAB (1991) Medioidosis: the tip of the iceberg? *Clin Microbiol Rev* **4**:52–60.

D'Angelo LJ, Hierholzer JC, Keenlyside RA, Anderson LJ and Martone WJ (1979) Pharyngoconjunctival fever caused by adenovirus type 4: report of a swimming pool-related outbreak with recovery of virus from pool water. *J Infect Dis* **140**:42–47.

D'Antonio RG, Winn RE, Taylor JP, Gustafson TL, Current WL, Rhodes

MM, Gary GW and Zajac RA (1985) A waterborne outbreak of crypto-sporidiosis in normal hosts. *Ann Intern Med* **103**:886–888.

Dascalopoulos GA, Loukas S and Constantopoulos SH (1995) Wide geographic variations of sensitivity to MOTT sensitins in Greece. *Eur Respir J* **5**:715–717.

Davies DJ, Thornton I, Watt JM, Culbard EB, Harvey PG, Delves HT, Sherlock JC, Smart GA, Thomas JF and Quinn MJ (1990) Lead intake and blood lead in two-year-old UK urban children. *Sci Total Environ* **90**:13–29.

Davies JW, Cox KG, Simon WR, Bowmer EJ and Mallory A (1972) Typhoid at sea: epidemic aboard an ocean liner. *Can Med Assoc J* **106**:877–883.

de Vicente A, Borrego JJ, Arrabal F and Romero P (1986) Comparative study of selective media for enumeration of *Pseudomonas aeruginosa* from water by membrane filtration. *Appl Environ Microbiol* **51**:832–840.

Dean AG and Jones TC (1972) Seasonal gastroenteritis and malabsorption at an American military base in the Philippines I. Clinical and epidemiological investigations of the acute illness. *Am J Epidemiol* **95**:111–127.

Deane M, Swan SH, Harris JA, Epstein DM and Neutra RR (1989) Adverse pregnancy outcomes in relation to water contamination, Santa Clara County, California 1980–1981. *Am J Epidemiol* **129**:894–904.

Deane M, Swan SH, Harris JA, Epstein DM and Neutra RR (1992) Adverse pregnancy outcomes in relation to water consumption: a re-analysis of data from the original Santa Clara County study, California 1980–1981. *Epidemiology* **3**:94–97.

de Mondino SS, Nunes MP and Ricciardi ID (1995) Occurrence of *Plesiomonas shigelloides* in water environments of Rio de Janeiro city. *Mem Inst Oswaldo Cruz* **90**:1–4.

Dennis DT, Smith RP, Welch JJ, Chute CG, Anderson B, Herndon JL and von Reyn CF (1993). Endemic giardiasis in New Hampshire: a case-control study of environmental risks. *J Infect Dis* **167**:1391–1395.

Derry CW, Bourne DE and Sayed AR (1990) The relationship between the hardness of treated water and cardiovascular disease mortality in South African urban areas. *S Afr Med J* **77**:522–524.

Desmonts C, Minet J, Colwell R and Cormier M (1990) Fluorescent-antibody method useful for detecting viable but nonculturable *Salmonella* spp. in chlorinated wastewater. *Appl Environ Microbiol* **56**:1448–1452.

Dev VJ, Main M and Gould I (1991) Waterborne outbreak of *Escherichia coli* O157. *Lancet* **337**:1412.

Dewailly E, Poirer C and Meyer FM (1986) Health hazards associated with windsurfing on polluted water. *Am J Public Health* **76**:690–691.

Dhamabutra N, Kamol-Rathanakul P and Pienthaweechai K (1992) Isolation of campylobacters from the canals of Bangkok metropolitan area. *J Med Assoc Thai* **75**:350–364.

Divizia M, Gnesivo C, Bonapasta RA, Morace G, Pisani G and Pana A (1993)

Hepatitis A virus identification in an outbreak by enzymatic amplification. *Eur J Epidemiol* **9**:203–208.

Donovan TJ and van Netten P (1995) Culture media for the isolation and enumeration of pathogenic *Vibrio* species in foods and environmental samples. *Int J Food Microbiol* **26**:77–91.

Dorsch MM, Scragg RKR, McMichael AJ, Baghurst PA and Dyer KF (1984) Congenital malformation and maternal drinking water supply in rural South Australia: a case-control study. *Am J Epidemiol* **119**:473–486.

Dreisbach RH and Robertson WO (1987) *Handbook of Poisoning*. Appleton and Lange, Norwalk, CT.

du Moulin GC, Sherman IH, Hoaglin DC and Stottmeier KD (1985) *Mycobacterium avium* complex, an emerging pathogen in Massachusetts. *J Clin Microbiol* **22**:9–12.

du Moulin GC, Stottmeier KD, Pelletier PA, Tsang AY and Hedley-Whyte J (1988) Concentration of *Mycobacterium avium* by hospital hot water systems. *JAMA* **260**:1599–1601.

du Plessis JB, van Rooyen JJ, Naude DA and van der Merwe CA (1995) Water fluoridation in South Africa: will it be effective? *J Dent Assoc S Afr* **50**:545–549.

Duma RJ, Shumaker JB and Callicott JH (1971) Primary amebic meningo-encephalitis: a survey in Virginia. *Arch Environ Health* **23**:43–47.

DuPont HL, Levine MM, Hornick RB and Formal SB (1989) Inoculum size in shigellosis and implications for expected mode of transmission. *J Infect Dis* **159**:1126–1128.

DuPont HL, Chappell CL, Sterling CR, Okhuysen PC, Rose JB and Jakubowski W (1995) The infectivity of *Cryptosporidium parvum* in healthy volunteers. *N Engl J Med* **332**:855–859.

Dykes AC, Juranek DD, Lorenz RA, Sinclair S, Jakubowski W and Davies R (1980) Municipal waterborne giardiasis: an epidemiological investigation. *Ann Intern Med* **92**:165–170.

Eastcott HR (1988) Swimmers's itch, a surfacing problem? *Commun Dis Rep* **88**(12):3–4.

Eastwood JB, Levin GE, Pazianas M, Taylor AP, Denton J and Freemont AJ (1990) Aluminium deposition in bone after contamination of drinking water supply. *Lancet* **336**:462–464.

Eaton T, Falkinham JO, Aisu TO and Daniel TM (1995) Isolation and characteristics of *Mycobacterium avium* complex from water and soil samples in Uganda. *Tubercle Lung Dis* **76**:570–574.

Echeverria P, Seriwatana J, Leksomboon U, Tirapat C, Chaicumpa W and Rowe B (1984) Identification by DNA hybridisation of enterotoxigenic *Escherichia coli* in homes of children with diarrhoea. *Lancet* **i**:63–66.

Edberg SC, Allen MJ and Smith DB (1988) National field evaluation of a defined substrate method for the simultaneous enumeration of total coliforms and *Escherichia coli* from drinking water: comparison with the standard multiple tube fermentation method. *Appl Environ Microbiol* **54**:1595–1601.

Edberg SC, Allen MJ and Smith DB (1989) National field evaluation of a defined substrate method for the simultaneous detection of total coliforms and *Escherichia coli* from drinking water: comparison with presence–absence techniques. *Appl Environ Microbiol* **55**:1003–1008.

Edberg SC, Allen MJ, Smith DB and Kriz NJ (1990) Enumeration of total coliforms and *Escherichia coli* from source water by the defined substrate technology. *Appl Environ Microbiol* **56**:366–369.

Eden KV, Rosenberg ML, Stoopler M, Wood BT, Highsmith AK, Skaliy P, Wells JG and Feeley JC (1977) Waterborne gastrointestinal illness at a ski resort. *Public Health Rep* **92**:245–250.

Edwards C, Lawton LA and Codd GA (1994) Detection of cyanobacterial (blue-green algal) peptide toxins by protein phosphatase inhibition. In: Codd GA, Jefferies TM, Keevil CW and Potter E (eds) *Detection Methods for Cyanobacterial Toxins*. Royal Society of Chemistry, Cambridge, pp 175–180.

Egoz N, Shihab S, Leitner L and Lucian M (1988) An outbreak of typhoid fever due to contamination of the municipal water supply in Northern Israel. *Isr J Med Sci* **24**:640–643.

Egoz N, Shmilovitz M, Kretzer B, Lucian M, Porat V and Raz R (1991) An outbreak of *Shigella sonnei* infection due to contamination of a municipal water supply in Northern Israel. *J Infect* **22**:87–93.

El Saadi O and Cameron AS (1993) Illness associated with blue-green algae. *Med J Aust* **158**:792–793.

El Saadi O, Esterman AJ, Cameron S and Roder DM (1995) Murray River water, raised cyanobacterial cell counts, and gastrointestinal and dermatological symptoms. *Med J Aust* **162**:122–125.

El-Hawey AM, Abdel-Rahman AH, Agina AA, Amer MM, Hashem YA, Gomaa AA, Abou el-Dahab MO and Tolba MA (1995) Prevalence and morbidity of schistosomiasis among rural fishermen at two Egyptian villages (Gharbia Governorate). *J Egypt Soc Parasitol* **25**:649–657.

El-Sharkwai F, El-Attar L, Gawad AA and Molazem S (1989) Some environmental factors affecting survival of faecal pathogens and indicator organisms in seawater. *Water Sci Technol* **21**:115–120.

Elwood JM (1977) Anencephalus and drinking water composition. *Am J Epidemiol* **105**:460–467.

Elwood JM (1979) Comment on: anencephalus, drinking water, geomagnetism and cosmic radiation. *Am J Epidemiol* **109**:98–99.

Elwood JM and Coldman AJ (1981) Water composition in the etiology of anencephalus. *Am J Epidemiol* **113**:681–690.

el-Zimaity DMT, Hyams KC, Imam IZE, Watts DM, Bassily S, Naffea EK, Sultan Y, Emara K, Burans J, Purdy MA, Bradley DW and Carl M (1993)

Acute sporadic hepatitis E in an Egyptian pediatric population. *Am J Trop Med Hyg* **48**:372–376.

Engel RR and Smith AH (1994) Arsenic in drinking water and mortality from vascular disease: an ecologic analysis in 30 counties in the United States. *Arch Environ Health* **49**:418–427.

Engel RR, Hopenhayn-Rich C, Receveur O and Smith AH (1994) Vascular effects of chronic arsenic exposure: a review. *Epidemiol Rev* **16**:184–209.

Enroth H and Engstrand L (1995) Immunomagnetic separation and PCR for detection of *Helicobacter pylori* in water and stool samples. *J Clin Microbiol* **33**:2162–2165.

Epstein PR (1993) Algal blooms and the spread and persistence of cholera. *Biosystems* **31**:209–221.

Escudero ME, Velazquez L, De Cortinez YM, Di Genaro MS and de Guzman AM (1994) *Yersinia* ssp. in surface water in San Luis, Argentina. *Folia Microbiol* **39**:459–462.

Esrey SA, Habicht J-P, Latham MC, Sisler DG and Casella G (1988) Drinking water source, diarrheal morbidity, and child growth in villages with both traditional and improved water supplies in rural Lesotho, southern Africa. *Am J Public Health* **78**:1451–1455.

Esrey SA, Collett J, Miliotis MD, Koornhof HJ and Makhale P (1989) The risk of infection from *Giardia lamblia* due to drinking water supply, use of water, and latrines among preschool children in rural Lesotho. *Int J Epidemiol* **18**:248–253.

Esrey SA, Potash JB, Roberts L and Shiff C (1991) Effects of improved water supply and sanitation on ascaris, diarrhoea dracunculiasis, hookworm infection, schistosomiasis, and trachoma. *Bull World Health Organ* **69**:609–621.

Etard J-F, Audibert M and Dabo A (1995) Age-acquired resistance and predisposition to reinfection with *Schistosoma haematobium* after treatment with praziquantel in Mali. *Am J Trop Med* **52**:549–558.

Evans AC, Martin DJ and Ginsburg BD (1991) Katayama fever in scuba divers. *S Afr Med J* **79**:271–274.

Everard COR, Hayes RJ and Edwards CN (1989) Leptospiral infection in school-children from Trinidad and Barbados. *Epidemiol Infect* **103**:143–156.

Fagliano J, Berry M, Bove F and Burke T (1990) Drinking water contamination and the incidence of leukaemia: an ecologic study. *Am J Public Health* **80**:1209–1212.

Falconer IR and Buckley TH (1989) Tumour promotion by *Microcystis* sp, a blue-green alga occurring in water supplies. *Med J Aust* **150**:351.

Falconer IR, Beresford AM and Runnegar MTC (1983) Evidence of liver damage by toxin from a bloom of the blue-green alga, *Microcystis aeruginosa*. *Med J Aust* **i**:511–514.

Farthing MJG, Cevallos A-M and Kelly P (1996) Intestinal protozoa. In: Cook GC (ed.) *Manson's Tropical Diseases* 12th edn. WB Saunders Co, London.

Fattal B, Margalith M, Shuval HI, Wax Y and Morag A (1987) Viral antibodies in agricultural populations exposed to aerosols from wastewater irrigation during a viral disease outbreak. *Am J Epidemiol* **125**:899–906.

Faust SH (1982) Effects of drinking water and total sodium intake on blood pressure. *Am J Clin Nutr* **35**:1459–1467.

Fawell JK (1993) The impact of inorganic chemicals on water quality and health. *Ann Ist Super Sanita* **29**:293–303.

Feldman RE, Baine WB, Nitzkin JL, Saslaw MS and Pollard RA (1974) Epidemiology of *Salmonella typhi* infection in a migrant labor camp in Dade County, Florida. *J Infect Dis* **130**:334–342.

Ferley JP, Zmirou D, Collin JF and Charrel M (1986) Etude longitudinale des risques liés à la consommation d'eaux non conformes aux normes bactériologiques. *Rev Epidemiol Sante Publique* **34**:89–99.

Ferley JP, Zmirou D, Balducci F, Baleux B, Fera P, Larbaigt G, Jacq E, Moissonnier B, Blineau A and Boudot J (1989) Epidemiological significance of microbiological pollution criteria for river recreational waters. *Int J Epidemiol* **18**:198–205.

Fernando V (1996) *Water Supply*. Intermediate Technology Publications, London.

Fewtrell L, Godfree AF, Jones F, Kay D, Salmon RL and Wyer MD (1992) Health effects of white-water canoeing. *Lancet* **339**:1587–1589.

Fewtrell L, Godfree A, Jones F, Kay D and Merrett H (1994) *Pathogenic Microorganisms in Temperate Environmental Waters*. Samara Publishing, Cardigan, Dyfed.

Fiedorek SC, Malaty HM, Evans DL, Pumphrey CL, Casteel HB, Evans DJ Jr and Graham DY (1991) Factors influencing the epidemiology of *Helicobacter pylori* infection in children. *Pediatrics* **88**:578–582.

Fielding DW and Smithells RW (1971) Anencephalus and water hardness in South-West Lancashire. *Brit J Prevent Soc Med* **25**:217–219.

Finch GR, Black EK, Labatiuk CW, Gyurek L and Belosevic M (1993) Comparison of *Giardia lamblia* and *Giardia muris* cyst inactivation by ozone. *Appl Environ Microbiol* **59**:3674–3680.

Finkelstein MM (1994) Radium in drinking water and the risk of death from bone cancer among Ontario youths. *Can Med Assoc J* **151**:565–571.

Flaten TP (1990) Geographical associations between aluminium in drinking water and death rates with dementia (including Alzheimer's disease), Parkinson's disease and amyotrophic lateral sclerosis in Norway. *Environ Geochem Health* **12**:152–167.

Fleisher JM, Jones F, Kay D, Stanwell-Smith R, Wyer M and Morano R (1993) Water and non-water risk factors for gastroenteritis among bathers exposed to sewage-contaminated marine waters. *Int J Epidemiol* **22**:698–708.

Flint KP (1987) The long term survival of *Escherichia coli* in river water. *J Appl Bacteriol* **63**:261–270.

Forbes WF and McAiney CA (1992) Aluminium and dementia. *Lancet* **340**:1668–1669.

Forbes WF, Hayward LM and Agwani N (1991) Dementia, aluminium and fluoride. *Lancet* **338**:1592–1593.

Forster DP, Newens AJ, Kay DWK and Edwardson JA (1995) Risk factors in clinically diagnosed presenile dementia of the Alzheimer type: a case-control study in northern England. *J Epidemiol Community Health* **49**:253–258.

Foy HM, Tarmapai S, Eamchan P and Metdilogkul O (1992–93) Chronic arsenic poisoning from well water in a mining area in Thailand. *Asia Pac J Public Health* **6**:150–152.

Franzblau A and Lilis R (1989) Acute arsenic intoxication from environmental arsenic exposure. *Arch Environ Health* **44**:385–389.

Fraser DW, Tsai TR, Orenstein W, Parkin WE, Beecham HJ, Sharrar RG, Harris J, Mallison GF, Martin SM, McDade JE, Shepard CC, Brachman PS and the field investigation team (1977) Legionnaires' disease: description of an epidemic of pneumonia. *N Engl J Med* **297**:1189–1197.

Fraser GG and Cooke KR (1991) Endemic giardiasis and municipal water supply. *Am J Public Health* **81**:760–762.

Frecker MF (1991) Dementia in Newfoundland: identification of a geographical isolate? *J Epidemiol Community Health* **45**:307–311.

Frerichs RR, Sloss EM and Satin KP (1982) Epidemiologic impact of water reuse in Los Angeles County. *Environ Res* **29**:109–122.

Fricker EJ and Fricker CR (1994) Application of the polymerase chain reaction to the identification of *Escherichia coli* and coliforms in water. *Lett Appl Bacteriol* **19**:44–46.

Fukushima H, Gomyoda M, Tsubokura M and Aleksic S (1995) Isolation of *Yersinia pseudotuberculosis* from river waters in Japan and Germany using direct KOH and HeLa cell treatments. *Int J Med Microbiol Virol Parasitol Infect Dis* **282**:40–49.

Fukushima H, Hoshina K and Gomyoda M (1994) Selective isolation from HeLa cell lines of *Yersinia pseudotuberculosis*, pathogenic *Y. enterocolitica* and enteroinvasive *Escherichia coli*. *Int J Med Microbiol Virol Parasitol Infect Dis* **280**:332–337.

Fuortes L, McNutt LA and Lynch C (1990) Leukemia incidence and radio-activity in drinking water in 59 Iowa towns. *Am J Public Health* **80**:1261–1262.

Furtado C, Stuart JM, Adak GK, Evans HS, Knerer G, Casemore DP (1996) Waterborne outbreaks of gastroenteritis in England and Wales: a four year review. In: *PHLS 21st Annual Scientific Conference*, University of Warwick. PHLS, London, poster no. 22.

Galbraith NS (1994) A historical review of microbial disease spread by water in England and Wales. In: Golding AMB, Noah N and Stanwell-Smith R (eds) *Water and Public Health*. Smith-Gordon & Co, London, pp 15–37.

Galbraith NS, Barrett NJ and Stanwell-Smith R (1987) Water and disease after

Croydon: a review of water-borne and water-associated disease in the UK 1937–86. *J Inst Water Environ Manag* **1**:7–21.

Gale P and Broberg PJ (1994) Use of a commercial gene probe assay kit for rapid MPN enumeration of *Escherichia coli* in drinking water. *Lett Appl Microbiol* **18**:346–348.

Gallaher MM, Herndon JL, Nims LJ, Sterling CR, Grabowski DJ and Hull HF (1989) Cryptosporidiosis and surface water. *Am J Public Health* **79**:39–42.

Garcia-Villanova RB, Cueto EA and Bolanos CMJ (1987) A comparative study of strains of salmonella isolated from irrigation waters, vegetables and human infections. *Epidemiol Infect* **98**:271–276.

Garin D, Fuchs F, Crance JM, Rouby Y, Chapalain JC, Lamarque D, Gounot AM and Aymard M (1994) Exposure to enteroviruses and hepatitis A virus among divers in environmental waters in France, first biological and serological survey of a controlled cohort. *Epidemiol Infect* **113**:541–549.

Gavan DT and Nutt JW (1970) An epidemic of waterborne infectious hepatitis in France. *Arch Environ Health* **20**:523–532.

Gentles JC and Evans EGV (1973) Foot infections in swimming baths. *Brit Med J* **ii**:260–262.

Georges-Courbot MC, Cassel-Beraud AM, Gouandjika I, Monges J and Georges AJ (1990) A cohort study of enteric campylobacter infection in children from birth to two years in Bangui (Central African Republic). *Trans R Soc Trop Med Hyg* **84**:122–125.

Gessner BD, Beller M, Middaugh JP and Whitford GM (1994) Acute fluoride poisoning from a public water system. *N Engl J Med* **330**:95–99.

Gilgen M, Wegmuller B, Burkhalter P, Buhler HP, Muller U, Luthy J and Candrian U (1995) Reverse transcription PCR to detect enteroviruses in surface waters. *Appl Environ Microbiol* **61**:1226–1231.

Gilli G, Corrao G and Favilli S (1984) Concentrations of nitrates in drinking water and incidence of gastric carcinomas: first descriptive study of the Piemonte region, Italy. *Sci Total Environ* **34**:35–48.

Glass RI, Alim ARMA, Eusof A, Snyder JD, Jusuf B, Anwar S, Bakri Z, Helmi C and Winardi B (1984) Cholera in Indonesia: epidemiologic studies of transmission in Aceh Province. *Am J Trop Med Hyg* **33**:933–939.

Glass RI, Claeson M, Blake PA, Waldman RJ and Pierce NF (1991) Cholera in Africa: lessons on transmission and control for Latin America. *Lancet* **338**:791–795.

Glick TH, Gregg MB, Berman B, Mallison G, Rhodes WW Jr and Kassanoff I (1978) Pontiac fever. An epidemic of unknown etiology in a health department: I. Clinical and epidemiological aspects. *Am J Epidemiol* **107**:149–160.

Goldberg DJ, Wrench JG, Collier PW, Emslie JA, Fallon RJ, Forbes GI, McKay TM, Macpherson AC, Marwick TA and Reid D (1989) Lochgoilhead fever: outbreak of non-pneumonic legionellosis due to *Legionella micdadei*. *Lancet* **i**:316–318.

Goldberg SJ, Lebowitz MD, Graver EJ and Hicks S (1990) An association of human congenital cardiac malformations and drinking water contaminants. *J Am Coll Cardiol* **16**:155–164.

Golding J, Rowland A, Greenwood R and Lunt P (1991) Aluminium sulphate in water in north Cornwall and outcome of pregnancy. *Brit Med J* **302**:1175–1177.

Goma Epidemiology Group (1995) Public health impact of Rwandan refugee crisis: what happened in Goma, Zaire, in July, 1994. *Lancet* **345**:339–344.

Gonzalez-Cortes A, Bessudo D, Sanchez-Leyva R, Fragoso R, Hinojosa M and Becerril P (1973) Water-borne transmission of chloramphenicol-resistant *Salmonella typhi* in Mexico. *Lancet* **ii**:605–607.

Goodman KJ and Correa P (1995) The transmission of *Helicobacter pylori*. A critical review of the evidence. *Int J Epidemiol* **24**:875–887.

Goodman KJ, Correa P, Aux HJT, Ramírez H, DeLany JP, Pepinosa OG, Quiñones ML and Parra TC (1996) *Helicobacter pylori* infection in the Columbian Andes: a population-based study of transmission pathways. *Am J Epidemiol* **144**:290–299.

Goodman RA, Buehler JW, Greenberg HB, McKinley TW and Smith JD (1982) Norwalk gastroenteritis associated with a water system in a rural Georgia community. *Arch Environ Health* **37**:358–360.

Gorter AC, Sandiford P, Smith GD and Pauw JP (1991) Water supply, sanitation and diarrhoel disease in Nicaragua: results from a case-control study. *Int J Epidemiol* **20**:527–533.

Gottlieb MS, and Carr JK (1982) Case-control cancer mortality study and chlorination of drinking water in Louisiana. *Environ Health Perspect* **46**:169–177.

Gottlieb MS, Carr JK and Clarkson JR (1982) Drinking water and cancer in Louisiana: a retrospective case-control study. *Am J Epidemiol* **116**:652–667.

Gottlieb MS, Carr JK and Morris DT (1981) Cancer and drinking water in Louisiana: colon and rectum. *Int J Epidemiol* **10**:117–125.

Grabow WOK, Favorov MO, Khudyakova NS, Taylor MB and Fields HA (1994) Hepatitis E seroprevalence in selected individuals in South Africa. *J Med Virol* **44**:384–388.

Grant RS (1981) Well water nitrate poisoning review: a survey in Nebraska 1973 to 1978. *Nebr Med J* **66**:197–200.

Gray NF (1994) *Drinking Water Quality, Problems and Solutions.* John Wiley and Sons, Chichester.

Gray SF, Gunnell DJ and Peters TJ (1994) Risk factors for giardiasis: a case-control study in Avon and Somerset. *Epidemiol Infect* **113**:95–102.

Greathouse DG and Osborne RH (1980) Preliminary report on nationwide study of drinking water and cardiovascular diseases. *J Environ Pathol Toxicol* **4**:65–76.

Greco D, Allegrini G, Tizzi T, Ninu E, Lamanna A and Luzi S (1987) A waterborne tularemia outbreak. *Eur J Epidemiol* **3**:35–38.

Green E, Warhust D, Williams J, Dickens T and Miles M (1990) Application of a capture enzyme immunoassay in an outbreak of waterborne giardiasis in the United Kingdom. *Eur J Clin Microbiol Infect Dis* **9**:424–428.

Greenberg AE and Ongerth HJ (1966) Salmonellosis in Riverside, Calif. *J Am Water Works Assoc* **58**:1145–1150.

Greensmith CT, Stanwick RS, Elliot BE and Fast MV (1988) Giardiasis associated with a water slide. *Pediatr Infect Dis J* **7**:91–94.

Griffith J, Riggan WB, Duncan RC and Pellom AC (1989) Cancer mortality in US counties with hazardous waste sites and ground water pollution. *Arch Environ Health* **44**:69–74.

Grimaldo M, Borja-Aburto VH, Ramírez AL, Ponce M, Rosas M and Díaz-Barriga F (1995) Endemic fluorosis in San Luis Potosi, Mexico. *Environ Res* **68**:25–30.

Grobe S, Wingender J and Truper HG (1995) Characterization of mucoid *Pseudomonas aeruginosa* strains isolated from technical water systems. *J Appl Bacteriol* **79**:94–102.

Gross R, Schell B, Molina MCB, Leão MAC and Strack U (1989) The impact of improvement of water supply and sanitation facilities on diarrhea and intestinal parasites: a Brazilian experience with children in two low-income urban communities. *Rev Saude Publica* **23**:214–220.

Grundmann H, Kropec A, Hartung D, Berner R and Daschner F (1993) *Pseudomonas aeruginosa* in a neonatal intensive care unit: reservoirs and ecology of the nosocomial pathogen. *J Infect Dis* **168**:943–947.

Gupta SK, Gupta RC, Seth AK and Chaturvedi CS (1995) Increased incidence of spina bifida occulta in fluorosis prone areas. *Acta Paediatr Jpn* **37**:503–506.

Guttman-Bass N, Tchorsh Y and Marva E (1987) Comparison of methods for rotavirus detection in water and results of a survey of Jerusalem wastewater. *Appl Environ Microbiol* **53**:761–767.

Gyllerup S, Lanke J, Lindholm LH and Schersten B (1991) Water hardness does not contribute substantially to the high coronary mortality in cold regions of Sweden. *J Intern Med* **230**:487–492.

Haimanot RT, Fekadu A and Bushra B (1987) Endemic fluorosis in the Ethiopian Rift Valley. *Trop Geogr Med* **39**:209–217.

Hale TL, Oaks V and Formal SB (1985) Identification and antigenic characterization of virulence-associated plasmid-coded proteins of *Shigella* spp. and enteroinvasive *Escherichia coli*. *Infect Immun* **50**:620–629.

Hallenbeck WH, Brenniman GR and Anderson RJ (1981) High sodium in drinking water and its effect on blood pressure. *Am J Epidemiol* **114**:817–826.

Hänninen M-L and Siitonen A (1995) Distribution of *Aeromonas* phenospecies and genospecies among strains isolated from water, foods or from human clinical samples. *Epidemiol Infect* **115**:39–50.

Harrington JM, Baker EL Jr, Folland DS, Saucier JW and Sandifer SH

(1978b) Chlordane contamination of a municipal water system. *Environ Res* **15**:155–159.

Harrington JM, Middaugh JP, Morse DL and Housworth J (1978a) A survey of a population exposed to high concentrations of arsenic in well water in Fairbanks, Alaska. *Am J Epidemiol* **108**:377–385.

Hart AS, Ridinger MT, Soundarajan R, Peters CS, Swaito AL and Kocka FE (1990) Novel organism associated with chronic diarrhoea in AIDS. *Lancet* **335**:169–170.

Harter L, Frost F, Grunenfelder G, Perkins-Jones K and Libby J (1984) Giardiasis in an infant and toddler swim class. *Am J Public Health* **74**:155–156.

Hatch DL, Waldman RJ, Lungu GW and Piri C (1994) Epidemic cholera during refugee resettlement in Malawi. *Int J Epidemiol* **23**:1292–1299.

Havelaar AH, Bosman M and Borst J (1983) Otitis externa by *Pseudomonas aeruginosa* associated with whirlpools. *J Hyg, Camb* **90**:489–498.

Havelaar AH, During M and Versteegh JF (1987) Ampicillin-dextrin agar medium for the enumeration of *Aeromonas* species in water by membrane filtration. *J Appl Bacteriol* **62**:279–287.

Havelaar AH, Schets FM, van Silfhout A, Jansen WH, Wieten G and van der Kooij D (1992) Typing of *Aeromonas* strains from patients with diarrhoea and from drinking water. *J Appl Bacteriol* **72**:435–444.

Hawkins PR, Runnegar MTC, Jackson ARB and Falconer IR (1985) Severe hepatotoxicity caused by the tropical cyanobacterium (blue-green alga) *Cylindrospermopsis raciborskii* (Woloszynska) Seenaya and Subba Raju isolated from a domestic water supply reservoir. *Appl Environ Microbiol* **50**:1292–1295.

Hawley HB, Morin DP, Geraghty ME, Tomkow J and Phillips CA (1973) Coxsackievirus B epidemic at a boys' summer camp. Isolation of virus from swimming water. *JAMA* **226**:33–36.

Hayes EB, Matte TD, O'Brien TR, McKinley TW, Logsdon GS, Rose JB, Ungar BLP, Word DM, Pinsky PF, Cummings ML, Wilson MA, Long EG, Hurwitz ES and Juranek DD (1989) Large community outbreak of cryptosporidiosis due to contamination of a filtered public water supply. *N Engl J Med* **320**:1372–1376.

Hayman J (1991) Postulated epidemiology of *Mycobacterium ulcerans* infection. *Int J Epidemiol* **20**:1093–1098.

Hector JSR, Pang Y, Mazurek GH, Zhang Y, Brown BA and Wallace RJ Jr (1992) Large restriction fragment patterns of genomic *Mycobacterium fortuitum* DNA as strain-specific markers and their use in epidemiologic investigation of four nosocomial outbreaks. *J Clin Microbiol* **30**:1250–1255.

Henderson PL, Fontaine RE and Kyeyune G (1988) Guinea worm disease in Northern Uganda: a major public health problem controllable through an effective water programme. *Int J Epidemiol* **17**:434–439.

Hennekens, CH and Buring, JE (1987) *Epidemiology in Medicine*. Little, Brown and Co., Boston, MA.

Hertz-Picciotto I, Swan SH, Neutra RR and Samuels SJ (1989) Spontaneous abortions in relation to consumption of tap water: an application of methods from survival analysis to a pregnancy follow-up study. *Am J Epidemiol* 130:79–93.

Herwaldt BL, Craun GF, Stokes SL and Juranek DD (1991) Waterborne-disease outbreaks, 1989–1990. *MMWR* 40(SS-3):1–21.

Higgins ITT (1981) Re: Asbestos in drinking water and cancer incidence in the San Francisco Bay area. *Am J Epidemiol* 114:161–162.

Highsmith AK, Feeley JC, Skaliy P, Wells JG and Wood BT (1977) Isolation of *Yersinia enterocolitica* from well water and growth in distilled water. *Appl Environ Microbiol* 34:745–750.

Hildebrand JM, Maguire HC, Holliman RE Kangesu E (1996). An outbreak of *Escherichia coli* O157 infection linked to paddling pools. *Commun Dis Rep Rev* 6:R33–R36.

Hindman SH, Favero MS, Carson LA, Petersen NJ, Schonberger LB and Solano JT (1975) Pyogenic reactions during haemodialysis caused by extramural endotoxin. *Lancet* ii:732–734.

HMSO (1989) Isolation and identification of *Giardia* cysts, *Cryptosporidium* oocysts and freeliving pathogenic amoebae in water etc. In: *Methods for the Examination of Waters and Associated Materials*. HMSO, London.

HMSO (1994) *The Microbiology of Water 1994*, Part 1, *Drinking Water*. HMSO, London.

Hoadley AW and Knight DE (1975) External otitis among swimmers and nonswimmers. *Arch Environ Health* 30:445–448.

Hoffman AH, Crusberg TC and Savilonis BJ (1979) Viral hepatitis and hydraulic parameters: an alternative hypothesis. *Arch Environ Health* 34:87–91.

Hoffman CJ (1988) Does the sodium level in drinking water affect blood pressure levels? *J Am Diet Assoc* 88:1432–1435.

Hoffman W, Kranefeld A and Schmitz-Feuerhake I (1993) Radium-226–contaminated drinking water: hypothesis on an exposure pathway in a population with elevated childhood leukemia. *Environ Health Perspect*, Suppl 101(3):113–115.

Hoffman R, Mann J, Calderone J, Trumbull J and Burkhart M (1980) Acute fluoride poisoning in a New Mexico elementary school. *Pediatrics* 65:897–900.

Hofman A, Valkenburg HA and Vaandrager GJ (1980) Increased blood pressure in schoolchildren related to high sodium levels in drinking water. *J Epidemiol Community Health* 34:179–181.

Hoge CW and Breiman RF (1991) Advances in the epidemiology and control of *Legionella* infections. *Epidemiol Rev* 13:329–340.

Hoge CW, Shlim DR, Rajah R, Triplett J, Shear M, Rabold JG and

Echeverria P (1993) Epidemiology of diarrhoeal illness associated with coccidian-like organism among travellers and foreign residents in Nepal. *Lancet* **341**:1175–1179.

Hollyoak V, Allison D and Summers J (1995a) *Pseudomonas aeruginosa* wound infection associated with a nursing home's whirlpool bath. *Commun Dis Rep Rev* **5**:R100–R102.

Hollyoak V, Boyd P and Freeman R (1995) Whirlpool baths in nursing homes: use, maintenance, and contamination with *Pseudomonas aeruginosa*. *Commun Dis Rep Rev* **5**:R102–R104.

Holmberg SD, Schell WL, Fanning GR, Wachsmuth IK, Hickman-Brenner FW, Blake PA, Brenner DJ and Farmer JJ 3rd (1986) Aeromonas intestinal infections in the United States. *Ann Intern Med* **105**:683–689.

Hooper RS (1970) The recovery of *Salmonella dublin* from rivers in Anglesey. *Vet Rec* **87**:583–587.

Hopkins RS and Juranek DD (1991) Acute giardiasis: an improved clinical case definition for epidemiological studies. *Am J Epidemiol* **133**:402–407.

Hopkins RS, Olmsted R and Istre GR (1984) Endemic *Campylobacter jejuni* infection in Colorado: identified risk factors. *Am J Public Health* **74**:249–250.

Hopkins RS, Gaspard GB, Williams FP, Karlin RJ, Cukor G and Blacklow NR (1984) A community waterborne gastroenteritis outbreak: evidence for rotavirus as the agent. *Am J Public Health* **74**:263–265.

Horák Z, Poláková H and Králová M (1986) Water-borne *Mycobacterium xenopi* – a possible cause of pulmonary mycobacteriosis in man. *J Hyg Epidemiol Microbiol Immunol* **30**:405–409.

Horsburgh CR Jr, Chin DP, Yajko DM, Hopewell PC, Nasssos PS, Elkin EP, Hadley WK, Stone EN, Simon EM, Gonzalez P, Ostroff S and Reingold AL (1994) Environmental risk factors for acquisition of *Mycobacterium avium* complex in persons with human immunodeficiency virus infection. *J Infect Dis* **170**:362–367.

Howe HL, Wolfgang PE, Burnett WS, Nasca PC and Youngblood L (1989) Cancer incidence following exposure to drinking water with asbestos leachate. *Public Health Rep* **104**:251–255.

Hrudey SE, Soskolne CL, Berkel J and Fincham S (1990) Drinking water fluoridation and osteosarcoma. *Can J Public Health* **81**:415–416.

Hughes JM, Boyce JM, Levine RJ, Khan M, Aziz KMA, Huq MI and Curlin GT (1982) Epidemiology of eltor cholera in rural Bangladesh: importance of surface water in transmission. *Bull World Health Organ* **60**:395–404.

Hughes MS, Coyle PV and Connolly JH (1992) Enteroviruses in recreational waters of Northern Ireland. *Epidemiol Infect* **108**:529–536.

Hulten K, Han SW, Enroth H, Klein PD, Opekun AR, Evans DG, Engstrand L, Graham DY and El-Zaatari FA (1996) *Helicobacter pylori* in the drinking water in Peru. *Gastroenterology* **110**:1031–1035.

Humphrey TJ (1986) Techniques for the optimum recovery of cold injured *Campylobacter jejuni* from milk or water. *J Appl Bacteriol* **61**:125–132.

Humphrey TJ (1989) An appraisal of the efficacy of pre-enrichment for the isolation of *Campylobacter jejuni* from water and food. *J Appl Bacteriol* **66**:119–126.

Humphry T, Sherman K, Strickland W, Thibeau M, Anderson P, Grodhaus G and Werner SB (1982) Cercarial dermatitis among bathers in California. *MMWR* **31**:435–436.

Hung T, Chen G, Wang C, Yao H, Fang Z, Chao T, Chou Z, Ye W, Chang X, Den S, Liong X and Chang W (1984) Waterborne outbreak of rotavirus diarrhoea in adults in China caused by a novel rotavirus. *Lancet* **i**:1139–1142.

Hunter PR (1991) Human illness associated with freshwater cyanobacteria (blue-green algae). *PHLS Microbiology Digest* **8**:96–100.

Hunter PR (1993) A review: the microbiology of bottled natural mineral waters. *J Appl Bacteriol* **74**:345–353.

Hunter PR (1994) An epidemiological critique of reports of human illness associated with cyanobacteria. In: Codd GA, Jefferies TM, Keevil CW and Potter E (eds.) *Detection Methods for Cyanobacterial Toxins*. Cambridge, Royal Society of Chemistry, pp 11–18.

Hurst CJ (1991) Presence of enteric viruses in freshwater and their removal by the conventional drinking water treatment process. *Bull World Health Organ* **69**:113–119.

Huttly SRA (1990) The impact of inadequate sanitary conditions on health in developing countries. *World Health Stat Q* **43**:118–126.

Ijsselmuiden CB, Gaydos C, Feighner B, Novakoski WL, Serwadda D, Caris LH, Vlahov D and Comstock GW (1992) Cancer of the pancreas and drinking water: a population-based case-control study in Washington County, Maryland. *Am J Epidemiol* **136**:836–842.

Ikeda RM, Kondracki SF, Drabkin PD, Birkhead GS and Morse DL (1993) Pleurodynia among football players at a high school: an outbreak associated with coxsackievirus B1. *JAMA* **270**:2205–2206.

Ikram R, Chambers S, Mitchell P, Brieseman MA and Ikram OH (1994) A case control study to determine risk factors for campylobacter infection in Christchurch in the summer of 1992–3. *N Z Med J* **107**:430–432.

Imwidthaya P, Suthiravitayavaniz K and Phongpanich S (1989) Mycobacterium other than tubercle bacilli in various environments in Bangkok. *J Med Assoc Thai* **72**:317–320.

Inoue M, Nakashima H, Ishida T and Tsubokura M (1988) Three outbreaks of *Yersinia pseudotuberculosis* infection. *Zentralb Bakteriol Mikrobiol Hyg (B)* **186**:504–511.

Insler MS and Gore H (1986) Pseudomonas keratitis and folliculitis from whirlpool exposure. *Am J Ophthalmol* **101**:41–43.

Iqbal M, Ahmed A, Qamar A, Dixon K, Duncan JF, Islam NU, Rauf A,

Bryan JP, Malik IA and Legters LJ (1989) An outbreak of enterically transmitted non-A, non-B hepatitis in Pakistan. *Am J Trop Med Hyg* **40**:438–443.

Iredell J, Whitby M and Blacklock Z (1992) *Mycobacterium marinum* infection: epidemiology and presentation in Queensland 1971–1990. *Med J Aust* **157**:596–598.

Isa AR, Othman WM, Ishak A (1990) Cholera outbreak in Tumpat Kelantan. *Med J Malaya* **45**:187–193.

Isaac-Renton JL and Philon JJ (1992) Factors associated with acquiring giardiasis in British Columbia residents. *Can J Public Health* **83**:155–158.

Isaac-Renton JL, Cordeiro C, Sarafis K and Shahriari H (1993) Characterization of *Giardia duodenalis* isolates from a waterborne outbreak. *J Infect Dis* **167**:431–440.

Isaac-Renton JL, Lewis LF, Ong CSL and Nulsen MF (1994) A second community outbreak of waterborne giardiasis in Canada and serological investigation of patients. *Trans R Soc Trop Med Hyg* **88**:395–399.

Isaacson M, Canter PH, Effler P, Arntzen L, Bomans P and Heenan R (1993) Haemorrhagic colitis epidemic in Africa. *Lancet* **341**:961.

Isacson P, Bean JA, Splinter R, Olson DB and Kohler J (1985) Drinking water and cancer incidence in Iowa. III. Association of cancer with indices of contamination. *Am J Epidemiol* **121**:856–869.

Islam MS, Alam MJ and Khan SI (1991) Distribution of *Plesiomonas shigelloides* in various components of pond ecosystems in Dhaka, Bangladesh. *Microbiol Immunol* **35**:927–932.

Islam MS, Drasar BS and Sack RB (1994) Probable role of blue-green algae in maintaining endemicity and seasonality of cholera in Bangladesh: a hypothesis. *J Diarrhoeal Dis Res* **12**:245–256.

Islam MS, Hasan MK, Miah MA, Sur GC, Felsenstein A, Venkatesan M, Sack RB and Albert MJ (1993) Use of the polymerase chain reaction and fluorescent-antibody methods for detecting viable but nonculturable *Shigella dysenteriae* type 1. *Appl Environ Microbiol* **59**:536–540.

Istre GR, Dunlop TS, Gaspard B and Hopkins RS (1984) Waterborne giardiasis at a mountain resort: evidence for acquired immunity. *Am J Public Health* **74**:602–604.

Jackson LA, Kaufmann AF, Adams WG, Phelps MB, Andreasen C, Langkop CW, Francis BJ and Wenger JD (1993) Outbreak of leptospirosis associated with swimming. *Pediatr Infect Dis J* **12**:48–54.

Jacqmin H, Commenges D, Letenneur L, Barberger-Gateau P and Dartigues J-F (1994) Components of drinking water and risk of cognitive impairment in the elderly. *Am J Epidemiol* **139**:48–57.

Jacob J and Stelzer W (1992) Comparison of two media for the isolation of thermophilic campylobacters from waste waters of different quality. *Zentralb Mikrobiol* **147**:41–44.

James A (1994) Marine pollution and limb reduction defects. *Lancet* **343**:990–991.

Jarvis SN, Straube RC, Williams ALJ and Bartlett CLR (1985) Illness associated with contamination of drinking water supplies with phenol. *Brit Med J* **290**:1800–1802.

Jeans AK and Schwellnus MP (1994) The risk of schistosomiasis in Zimbabwean triathletes. *S Afr Med J* **84**:756–758.

Jehl-Pietri C, Hugues B, Andre M, Diez JM and Bosch A (1993) Comparison of immunological and molecular hybridization detection methods for the detection of hepatitis A virus in sewage. *Lett Appl Microbiol* **17**:162–166.

Jephcott AE, Begg NT and Baker IA (1986) Outbreak of giardiasis associated with mains water in the United Kingdom. *Lancet* **i**:730–732.

Jessop EG, Horsley SD and Wood L (1985) Recreational use of inland water and health: are Windermere and Coniston Water a Health Hazard? *Public Health* **99**:338–342.

Jiang X, Estes MK, Metcalf T and Melnick J (1986) Detection of hepatitis A virus in seeded estuarine samples by hybridisation with cDNA probes. *Appl Environ Microbiol* **52**:711–717.

Jiménez-Jiménez FJ, Mateo D and Giménez-Roldán S (1992) Exposure to well water and pesticides in Parkinson's disease: a case-control study in the Madrid area. *Mov Disord* **7**:149–152.

Jin A, Hertzman C, Peck SH and Lockitch G (1995) Blood lead levels in children aged 24 to 36 months in Vancouver. *Can Med Assoc J* **152**:1077–1086.

Joce RE, Bruce J, Kiely D, Noah ND, Dempster WB, Staker R, Gumsley P, Chapman PA, Norman P, Watkins J, Smith HV, Price TJ and Watts D (1991) An outbreak of cryptosporidiosis associated with a swimming pool. *Epidemiol Infect* **107**:497–508.

Johnson CJ and Kross BC (1990) Continuing importance of nitrate contamination of groundwater and wells in rural areas. *Am J Ind Med* **18**:449–456.

Johnson CJ, Bonrud PA, Dosch TL, Kilness AW, Senger KA, Busch DC and Meyer MR (1987) Fatal outcome of methemoglobinemia in an infant. *JAMA* **257**:2796–2797.

Johnson DW, Pieniazek NJ, Griffin DW, Misener L and Rose JB (1995) Development of a PCR protocol for sensitive detection of *Cryptosporidium* oocysts in water samples. *Appl Environ Microbiol* **61**:3849–3855.

Johnson S and Joshi V (1982) Dracontiasis in Rajasthan. VI. Epidemiology of dracontiasis in Barmer District Western Rajasthan, India. *Int J Epidemiol* **11**:26–30.

Johnston JM, Becker SF and McFarland LM (1985) *Vibrio vulnificus*. Man and the sea. *JAMA* **253**:2850–2853.

Jolley RL, Brungs WA and Cummings RB (1985) *Water Chlorination: Chemistry, Environmental Impact, and Health Effects.* Lewis, Chelsea, MI.

Jones DM, Sutcliffe EM and Curry A (1991) Recovery of viable but non-culturable *Campylobacter jejuni*. *J Gen Microbiol* **137**:2477–2482.

Jones K, Betaieb M and Telford DR (1990) Seasonal variation of thermophilic campylobacters in sewage sludge. *J Appl Bacteriol* **69**:185–189.

Jordan P, Bartholomew RK, Unrau GO, Upatham ES, Grist E and Christie JD (1978) Further observations from St Lucia on control of *Schistosoma mansoni* transmission by provision of domestic water supplies. *Bull World Health Organ* **56**:965–973.

Joseph C, Hamilton G, O'Connor M, Nicholas S, Marshall R, Stanwell-Smith R, Sims R, Ndawula E, Casemore D, Gallagher P and Harnett P (1991) Cryptosporidiosis in the Isle of Thanet: an outbreak associated with local drinking water. *Epidemiol Infect* **107**:509–519.

Josephson KL, Gerba CP and Pepper IL (1993) Polymerase chain reaction detection of nonviable bacterial pathogens. *Appl Environ Microbiol* **59**:3513–3515.

Jothikumar N, Aparna K, Kamatchiammal S, Paulmurugan R, Saravanadevi S and Khanna P (1993) Detection of hepatitis E virus in raw and treated wastewater with polymerase chain reaction. *Appl Environ Microbiol* **59**:2558–2562.

Jothikumar N, Khanna P, Paulmurugan R, Kamatchiammal S and Padmanabhan P (1995) A simple device for the concentration and detection of enterovirus, hepatitis E virus and rotavirus from water samples by reverse transcription-polymerase chain reaction. *J Virol Methods* **55**:401–415.

Juuti M and Heinonen OP (1980) Incidence of urolithiasis and composition of household water in southern Finland. *Scand J Urol Nephrol* **14**:181–187.

Kain KC and Kelly MT (1989) Clinical features, epidemiology, and treatment of *Plesiomonas shigelloides* diarrhea. *J Clin Microbiol* **27**:998–1001.

Kale OO (1977) The clinico-epidemiological profile of guinea worm in the Ibadan district of Nigeria. *Am J Trop Med Hyg* **26**:208–214.

Kalil K, Lindblom GB, Mazhar K and Kaijser B (1994) Flies and water as reservoirs for bacterial enteropathogens in urban and rural areas in and around Lahore Pakistan. *Epidemiol Infect* **113**:435–444.

Kamili MA, Ali G, Shah MY, Rashid S, Khan S and Allaqaband GQ (1993) Multiple drug resistant typhoid fever outbreak in Kashmir Valley. *Indian J Med Sci* **47**:147–151.

Kanai K and Dejsirilert S (1988) *Pseudomonas pseudomallei* and *melioidosis*, with special reference to the status in Thailand. *Jpn J Med Sci Biol* **41**:123–157.

Kanarek MS and Young TB (1982) Drinking water treatment and risk of cancer death in Wisconsin. *Environ Health Perspect* **46**:179–186.

Kanarek MS, Conforti PM, Jackson LA, Cooper RC and Murchio JC (1980) Asbestos in drinking water and cancer incidence in the San Francisco Bay area. *Am J Epidemiol* **112**:54–72.

Kaper JB, Lockman H, Colwell RR and Joseph SW (1981) *Aeromonas hydrophila*: ecology and toxigenicity of isolates from an estuary. *J Appl Bacteriol* **50**:359–377.

Kaplan JE, Goodman RA, Schonberger LB, Lippy EC and Gary GW (1982) Gastroenteritis due to Norwalk virus: an outbreak associated with a municipal water system. *J Infect Dis* **146**:190–197.

Kapperud G, Vardund T, Skjerve E, Hornes E and Michaelsen TE (1993) Detection of pathogenic *Yersinia enterocolitica* in foods and water by immunomagnetic separation, nested polymerase chain reactions, and colorimetric detection of amplified DNA. *Appl Environ Microbiol* **59**:2938–2944.

Kappus KD, Marks JS, Holman RC, Bryant JK, Baker C, Gary GW and Greenberg HB (1982) An outbreak of Norwalk gastroenteritis associated with swimming in a pool and secondary person-to-person transmission. *Am J Epidemiol* **116**:834–839.

Kapuscinski RB and Mitchell R (1981) Solar radiation induces sublethal injury in *Escherichia coli* in seawater. *Appl Environ Microbiol* **41**:670–674.

Kaspar CW and Tamplin ML (1993) Effects of temperature and salinity on the survival of *Vibrio vulnificus* in seawater and shellfish. *Appl Environ Microbiol* **59**:2425–2429.

Katila M-L, Iivanainen E, Torkko P, Kauppinen J, Martikainen P and Väänänen P (1995) Isolation of potentially pathogenic mycobacteria in the Finnish environment. *Scand J Infect Dis*, Suppl **98**:9–11.

Katz AR, Manea SJ and Sasaki DM (1991) Leptospirosis on Kauai: investigation of a common source waterborne outbreak. *Am J Public Health* **81**:1310–1312.

Kaysner CA, Abeyta C Jr, Wekell MM, DePoala A Jr, Stott RF and Leitch JM (1987) Virulent strains of *Vibrio vulnificus* isolated from estuaries on the United States West Coast. *Appl Environ Microbiol* **53**:1349–1351.

Kee F, McElroy G, Stewart D, Coyle P and Watson J (1994) A community outbreak of echovirus infection associated with an outdoor swimming pool. *J Public Health Med* **16**:145–148.

Keene WE, McAnulty JM, Hoesly FC, Williams LP, Hedberg K, Oxman GL, Barrett TJ, Pfaller MA and Fleming DW (1994) A swimming-associated outbreak of hemorrhagic colitis caused by *Escherichia coli* O157:H7 and *Shigella sonnei*. *N Engl J Med* **331**:579–584.

Kelly KA, Koehler JM and Ashdown LR (1993) Spectrum of extraintestinal disease due to *Aeromonas* species in tropical Queensland, Australia. *Clin Infect Dis* **16**:574–579.

Kent JP, Greenspan JR, Herndon JL, Mofenson LM, Harris J-AS, Eng TR and Waskin HA (1988) Epidemic giardiasis caused by a contaminated public water supply. *Am J Public Health* **78**:139–143.

Keswick BH, Gerba CP and Goyal SM (1981) Occurrence of enteroviruses in community swimming pools. *Am J Public Health* **71**:1026–1030.

Khalil K, Lindblom G-B, Mazhar K and Kaijser B (1994) Flies and water as reservoirs for bacterial enteropathogens in urban and rural areas around Lahore, Pakistan. *Epidemiol Infect* **113**:435–444.

Khan AA and Cerniglia CE (1994) Detection of *Pseudomonas aeruginosa* from clinical and environmental samples by amplification of the exotoxin A gene using PCR. *Appl Environ Microbiol* **60**:3739–3745.

Khan AS, Moe CL, Glass RI, Monroe SS, Estes MK, Chapman LE, Jiang X, Humphrey C, Pon E, Iskander JK and Schonberger LB (1994) Norwalk virus-associated gastroenteritis traced to ice consumption aboard a cruise ship in Hawaii: comparison and application of molecular method-based assays. *J Clin Microbiol* **32**:318–322.

Khan MU and Munshi MH (1983) Clinical illnesses and causes of death in a Burmese refugee camp in Bangladesh. *Int J Epidemiol* **12**:460–464.

Khan MU and Shahidullah M (1980) Contrasting epidemiology of *Shigella dysenteriae* and *Shigella flexneri*, Dacca. *Trans R Soc Trop Med Hyg* **74**:528–533.

Khan M, Curlin GT and Huq I (1979) Epidemiology of *Shigella dysenteriae* type 1 infections in Dacca Urban Area. *Trop Geogr Med* **31**:213–223.

Khan MU, Roy NC, Islam MR, Huq MI and Stoll B (1985) Fourteen years of shigellosis in Dhaka: an epidemiological analysis. *Int J Epidemiol* **14**:607–613.

Khuroo MS (1980) Study of an epidemic of non-A, non-B hepatitis, possibility of another human hepatitis virus distinct from post-transfusion non-A, non-B type. *Am J Med* **68**:818–824.

Kilburn KH and Warshaw RH (1992) Prevalence of symptoms of systemic lupus erythematosus (SLE) and of fluorescent antinuclear antibodies associated with chronic exposure to trichloroethylene and other chemicals in well water. *Environ Res* **57**:1–9.

Kilburn KH and Warshaw RH (1993) Effects of neurobehavioral performance of chronic exposure to chemically contaminated well water. *Toxicol Ind Health* **9**:391–404.

Kim-Farley RJ, Rutherford G, Lichfield P, Hsu S-T, Orenstein WA, Schonberger LB, Bart KJ, Lui K-J and Lin C-C (1984) Outbreak of paralytic poliomyelitis, Taiwan. *Lancet* **ii**:1322–1324.

King C-C, Chen C-J, You S-L, Chuang Y-C, Huang H-H and Tsai W-C (1989) Community-wide epidemiological investigation of a typhoid outbreak in a rural township in Taiwan, Republic of China. *Int J Epidemiol* **18**:254–260.

Kirk R and Rowe MT (1994) A PCR assay for the detection of *Campylobacter jejuni* and *Campylobacter coli* in water. *Lett Appl Microbiol* **19**:301–303.

Kirpenko YA, Sirenko LA and Kirpenko NI (1981) Some aspects concerning remote after-effects of blue-green algal toxin impact on warm-blooded animals. In: Carmichael WW (ed.) *The Water Environment, Algal Toxins and Health*. Plenum Press, New York, pp 257–269.

Kirschenbaum MB (1979) Swimmer's itch: a review and case report. *Cutis* **23**:212–218.

Kirschner RA Jr, Parker BC and Falkinham JO 3rd (1992) Epidemiology of infection by nontuberculous mycobacteria. *Mycobacterium avium, Mycobacterium intracellulare,*and *Mycobacterium scrofulaceum* in acid, brown-water swamps of the southeastern United States and their association with environmental variables. *Am Rev Resp Dis* **145**:271–275.

Klein PD, Gastrointestinal physiology working group, Graham DY, Gaillour A, Opekun AR and O'Brian Smith E (1991) Water source as risk factor for *Helicobacter pylori* infection in Peruvian children. *Lancet* **337**:1503–1506.

Klenner MF and Weber G (1979) Hydrotherapy pools, microbiological and chemical results. *Zentralb Bakteriol Mikrobiol Hyg (B)* **169**:271–281.

Klontz KC, Lieb S, Schreiber M, Janowski HT, Baldy LM and Gunn RA (1988) Syndromes of *Vibrio vulnificus* infections. Clinical and epidemiological features in Florida cases, 1981–1987. *Ann Intern Med* **109**:318–323.

Kloos H, Higashi GI, Schinski VD, Mansour NS, Murrell KD and Miller FD (1990) Water contact and *Schistosoma haematobium* infection: a case study from an Upper Egyptian village. *Int J Epidemiol* **19**:749–758.

Knobeloch L, Krenz K, Anderson H and Hovell C (1993) Methemoglobinemia in an infant – Wisconsin, 1992. *MMWR* **42**:217–218.

Ko YC (1986) A critical review of epidemiologic studies on black-foot disease. *Sangyo Ika Daigaku Zasshi* **8**:339–353.

Koide M, Saito A, Kusano N and Higa F (1993) Detection of *Legionella* spp. in cooling tower water by the polymerase chain reaction method. *Appl Environ Microbiol* **59**:1943–1946.

Koivusalo M, Jaakkola JJK, Vartiainen T, Hakulinen T, Karjalainen S, Pukkala E and Tuomisto J (1994) Drinking water mutagenicity and gastrointestinal and urinary tract cancers: an ecological study in Finland. *Am J Public Health* **84**:1223–1228.

Koivusalo M, Pukkal E, Vartiained T, Jaakkola JJK and Hakulinen T (1995) Drinking water mutagenicity and leukemia, lymphomas, cancer of the liver pancreas, and soft tissue. *Arch Environ Health* **50**:269–276.

Kolarova L, Gottwaldova V, Cechova D and Sevcova M (1989) The occurrence of cercarial dermatitis in central Bohemia. *Zentralb Hyg Umweltmed* **189**:1–13.

Koopman JS, Eckert EA, Greenberg HB, Strohm BC, Isaacson RE and Monto AS (1982) Norwalk virus enteric illness acquired by swimming exposure. *Am J Epidemiol* **115**:173–177.

Kopecka H, Dubrou S, Prevot J, Marechal J and Lopez-Pila JM (1993) Detection of naturally occurring enteroviruses in waters by reverse transcription, polymerase chain reaction, and hybridization. *Appl Environ Microbiol* **59**:1213–1219.

Koplan JP, Deen DR, Swanston WH and Tota B (1978) Contaminated roof-collected rainwater as a possible cause of an outbreak of salmonellosis. *J Hyg, Camb* **81**:303–309.

Korhonen LK and Martikainen PJ (1990) Comparison of some enrichment broths and growth media for the isolation of thermophilic campylobacters from surface water samples. *J Appl Bacteriol* **68**:593–599.

Kosatsky T and Kleeman J (1985) Superficial and systemic illness related to a hot tub. *Am J Med* **79**:10–12.

Kostraba JN, Gay EC, Rewers M and Hamman RF (1992) Nitrate levels in community drinking waters and risk of IDDM: An ecological analysis. *Diabetes Care* **15**:1505–1508.

Kramer MD, Lynch CF, Isacson P and Hanson JW (1992) The association of waterborne chloroform with intrauterine growth retardation. *Epidemiology* **3**:407–413.

Kramer MH, Herwaldt BL, Craun GF, Calderon RL and Juranek DD (1996) Surveillance for waterborne-disease outbreaks – United States, 1993–1994. *MMWR* **45(SS-1)**:1–33.

Krasovskii GN, Vasukovich LY and Chariev OG (1979) Experimental study of biological effects of lead and aluminium following oral administration. *Environ Health Perspect* **30**:47–51.

Kraus AS and Forbes WF (1992) Aluminium fluoride and the prevention of Alzheimer's disease. *Can J Public Health* **83**:97–100.

Kross BC, Hallberg GR, Bruner DR, Cherryholmes K and Johnson JK (1993) The nitrate contamination of private well water in Iowa. *Am J Public Health* **83**:270–272.

Kubalek I and Komenda S (1995) Seasonal variations in the occurrence of environmental mycobacteria in potable water. *APMIS* **103**:327–330.

Kubalek I, Komenda S and Mysak J (1995) The spring–fall variations in the prevalence of environmental mycobacteria in drinking water supply system. *Cent Eur J Public Health* **3**:146–148.

Kuberski T, Flood T, Tera T and the New Zealand cholera relief team (1979) Cholera in the Gilbert Islands: I epidemiological features. *Am J Trop Med Hyg* **28**:677–684.

Kueh CS and Grohmann GS (1989) Recovery of viruses and bacteria in waters off Bondi beach: a pilot study. *Med J Aust* **151**:632–638.

Kuijper EJ, Bol P, Peeters MF, Steigerwalt AG, Zanen HC and Brenner DJ (1989) Clinical and epidemiological aspects of members of *Aeromonas* hybridization groups isolated from human feces. *J Clin Microbiol* **27**:1531–1537.

Kullavanijaya P and Wongwaisayawan H (1983) Outbreak of cercarial dermatitis in Thailand. *Int J Dermatol* **32**:113–115.

Kuritsky JN, Bullen MG, Broome CV, Silcox VA, Good RC and Wallace RJ Jr (1983) Sternal wound infections and endocarditis due to organisms of the *Mycobacterium fortuitum* complex. *Ann Intern Med* **98**:938–939.

Kush BJ and Hoadley AW (1980) A preliminary survey of the association of

Pseudomonas aeruginosa with commercial whirlpool bath waters. *Am J Public Health* **70**:279–281.

Kusnetsov JM, Jousimies-Somer HR, Nevalainen AI and Martikainen PJ (1994) Isolation of *Legionella* from water samples using various culture methods. *J Appl Bacteriol* **76**:155–162.

Kustner HGV, Gibson IHN, Carmichael TR, Van Zyl L, Chouler CA, Hyde JP and du Plessis JN (1981) The spread of cholera in South Africa. *S Afr Med J* **60**:87–90.

Kwaga JKP, Adesiyun AA, Bello CS and Abdullahi SU (1988) Occurrence of *Plesiomonas shigelloides* in humans and water in Zaria, Nigeria. *Microbiologica* **11**:165–167.

Lackland DT, Weinrich M, Wheeler FC and Shepard DM (1985) Sodium in drinking water in South Carolina. *Am J Public Health* **75**:772–774.

Lagarde E, Joussemet M, Lataillade J-J and Fabre G (1995) Risk factors for hepatitis A infection in France: drinking tap water may be of importance. *Eur J Epidemiol* **11**:145–148.

Lai M-S, Hsueh Y-M, Chen C-J, Shyu M-P, Chen S-Y, Kuo T-L, Wu M-M and Tai, T-Y (1994) Ingested inorganic arsenic and prevalence of diabetes mellitus. *Am J Epidemiol* **139**:484–492.

Lampi P, Hakulinen T, Luostarinen T, Pukkala E and Teppo L (1992) Cancer incidence following chlorophenol exposure in a community in southern Finland. *Arch Environ Health* **47**:167–175.

Landrigan PJ, Stein GF, Kominsky JR, Ruhe RL and Watanabe AS (1987) Common-source community and industrial exposure to trichloroethylene. *Arch Environ Health* **42**:327–332.

Lares-Villa F, de Jonckheere JF, de Moura H, Rechi-Iruretagoyena A, Ferreira-Guerrero E, Fernandez-Quintanilla G, Ruiz-Matus C and Visvesvara GS (1993) Five cases of primary amebic meningoencephalitis in Mexicali Mexico: study of the isolates. *J Clin Microbiol* **31**:685–688.

Larsen RA (1989) *Biohazards of Drinking Water Treatment*. Lewis, Chelsea, MI.

Laursen E, Mygind O, Rasmussen B and Rønne T (1994) Gastroenteritis: a waterborne outbreak affecting 1600 people in a small Danish town. *J Epidemiol Community Health* **48**:453–458.

Lavy A, Rusu R and Mates A (1992) *Mycobacterium xenopi*, a potential human pathogen. *Isr J Med Sci* **28**:772–775.

Lawson HW, Braun MM, Glass RIM, Stine SE, Monroe SS, Atrash HK, Lee LE and Englender SJ (1991) Waterborne outbreak of Norwalk virus gastroenteritis at a southwest US resort: role of geological formations in contamination of well water. *Lancet* **337**:1200–1204.

Lawson R (1991) Camelford revisited. *Brit Med J* **303**:1480.

Lawton LA, Campbell DL, Beattie KA and Codd GA (1990) Use of a rapid bioluminescence assay for detecting cyanobacterial microcystin toxicity. *Lett Appl Microbiol* **11**:205–207.

LeChevallier MW, Norton WD and Lee RG (1991a) Occurrence of *Giardia* and *Cryptosporidium* spp. in surface water supplies. *Appl Environ Microbiol* **57**:2610–2616.

LeChevallier MW, Norton WD and Lee RG (1991b) *Giardia* and *Cryptosporidium* spp. in filtered drinking water supplies. *Appl Environ Microbiol* **57**:2617–2621.

LeChevallier MW, Norton WD, Siegel JE and Abbaszadegan M (1995) Evaluation of the immunofluorescence procedure for detection of *Giardia* cysts and *Cryptosporidium* oocysts in water. *Appl Environ Microbiol* **61**:690–697.

Leelarasamee A and Bovornkitti S (1989) Medioidosis: review and update. *Rev Infect Dis* **11**:413–425.

Lenaway DD, Brockmann R, Dolan GJ and Cruz-Uribe F (1989) An outbreak of an enterovirus-like illness at a community wading pool: implications for public health inspection programs. *Am J Public Health* **79**:889–890.

Leoni V, Fabiani L and Ticchiarelli L (1985) Water hardness and cardiovascular mortality rate in Abruzzo, Italy. *Arch Environ Health* **40**:274–278.

Levine MM and Levine OS (1994) Changes in human ecology and behavior in relation to the emergence of diarrheal diseases, including cholera. *Proc Natl Acad Sci USA* **91**:2390–2394.

Levine MM, Ferreccio C, Prado V, Cayazzo M, Abrego P, Martinez J, Maggi L, Baldini MM, Martin W, Maneval D, Kay B, Guers L, Lior H, Wasserman SS and Nataro JP (1993) Epidemiological studies of *Escherichia coli* diarrheal infections in a low socioeconomic level peri-urban community in Santiago Chile. *Am J Epidemiol* **138**:849–869.

Levine RJ, Khan MR, D'Souza S and Nalin DR (1976a) Failure of sanitary wells to protect against cholera and other diarrhoeas in Bangladesh. *Lancet* **ii**:86–89.

Levine RJ, Khan MR, D'Souza S and Nalin DR (1976b) Cholera transmission near a cholera hospital. *Lancet* **ii**:84–86.

Levine WC, Stephenson WT and Craun GF (1990) Waterborne disease outbreaks, 1986–88. *MMWR* **39**(SS-1):1–13.

Levine WC, Griffin PM and the Gulf Coast *Vibrio* Working Group (1993) *Vibrio* infections on the Gulf Coast: results of first year of regional surveillance. *J Infect Dis* **167**:479–483.

Lewis CM and Mak JL (1989) Comparison of membrane filtration and Autoanalysis Colilert presence–absence techniques for analysis of total coliforms and *Escherichia coli* in drinking water samples. *Appl Environ Microbiol* **55**:3091–3094.

Lewis DW and Banting DW (1994) Water fluoridation: current effectiveness and dental fluorosis. *Community Dent Oral Epidemiol* **22**:153–158.

Li Y (1993) Fluoride: safety issues. *J Indiana Dent Assoc* **72**:22–26.

Lima e Costa MFF, Rocha RS, Leite MLC, Carneiro RG, Colley D, Gazzinelli G and Katz N (1991) A multivariate analysis of sociodemographic factors, water contact patterns and *Schistosoma mansoni* infection in an endemic area in Brazil. *Rev Inst Med Trop Sao Paulo* **33**:58–63.

Lin SD (1985) *Giardia lamblia* and water supply. *J Am Water Works Assoc* **77**:40–47.

Lindberg AA and Pal T (1993) Strategies for development of potential candidate *Shigella* vaccines. *Vaccine* **11**:168–179.

Lippy EC and Erb J (1976) Gastrointestinal illness at Sewickley, Pa. *J Am Water Works Assoc* **76**:60–70.

Ljungstrom I and Castor B (1992) Immune response to *Giardia lamblia* in a water-borne outbreak of giardiasis in Sweden. *J Med Microbiol* **36**:347–352.

Lockwood WW, Friedman C, Bus N, Pierson C and Gaynes R (1989) An outbreak of *Mycobacterium terrae* in clinical specimens associated with a hospital potable water supply. *Am Rev Respir Dis* **140**:1614–1617.

Logue JN, Stroman RM, Reid D, Hayes CW and Sivarajah K (1985) Investigation of potential health effects associated with well water chemical contamination in Londonderry Township, Pennsylvania, USA. *Arch Environ Health* **40**:155–160.

Lombin LH, Adesiyun AA, Haruna M, Kwaga JK and Agbonlahor DE (1986) A survey for *Yersinia enterocolitica* in water from ponds, streams and wells in Northern Nigeria. *Microbiologica* **9**:95–100.

Long EG, Ebrahimzadeh A, White EH, Swisher B and Callaway CS (1990) Alga associated with diarrhea in patients with acquired immunodeficiency syndrome and in travelers. *J Clin Microbiol* **28**:1101–1104.

Lopez CE, Juranek DD, Sinclair SP and Schultz MG (1978) Giardiasis in American travellers to Madeira Island, Portugal. *Am J Trop Med Hyg* **27**:1128–1132.

Lopez CE, Dykes AC, Juranek DD, Sinclair SP, Conn JM, Christie RW, Lippy EC, Schultz MG and Mires MH (1980) Waterborne giardiasis: a communitywide outbreak of disease and a high rate of asymptomatic infection. *Am J Epidemiol* **112**:495–507.

Lowe CR, Roberts CJ and Lloyd S (1971) Malformations of central nervous system and softness of local water supplies. *Brit Med J* **i**:357–363.

Lowermoor Incident Health Advisory Group (1989) *Water Pollution at Lowermoor, North Cornwall.* Cornwall and Isles of Scilly District Health Authority, Truro.

Lowermoor Incident Health Advisory Group (1991) *Water Pollution at Lowermoor, North Cornwall*, 2nd edn. HMSO, London.

Lupidi R, Cinco M, Balanzin D, Delprete E and Varaldo PE (1991) Serological follow-up of patients involved in a localized outbreak of leptospirosis. *J Clin Microbiol* **29**:805–809.

Lyman GH, Lyman CG and Johnson W (1985) Association of leukemia with radium groundwater contamination. *JAMA* **254**:621–626.

Ma JF, Gerba CP and Pepper IL (1995) Increased sensitivity of poliovirus detection in tap water concentrates by reverse transcriptase-polymerase chain reaction. *J Virol Methods* **55**:295–302.

MacKenzie WR, Hoxie NJ, Proctor ME, Gradus MS, Blair KA, Peterson DE, Kazmierczak JJ, Addiss DG, Fox KR, Rose JB and Davis JP (1994) A massive outbreak in Milwaukee of cryptosporidium infection transmitted through the public water supply. *N Engl J Med* **331**:161–167.

MacKenzie WR, Kazmierczak JJ and Davis JP (1995) An outbreak of cryptosporidiosis associated with a resort swimming pool. *Epidemiol Infect* **115**:545–553.

MacKintosh RW, Dalby KN, Campbell DG, Cohen PT, Cohen P and MacKintosh C (1995) The cyanobacterial toxin microcystin binds covalently to cysteine-273 on protein phosphatase 1. *FEBS Lett* **371**:236–240.

Maguire HC, Holmes E, Hollyer J, Strangeways JEM, Foster P, Holliman RE and Stanwell-Smith R (1995) An outbreak of cryptosporidiosis in South London: what value the *p* value? *Epidemiol Infect* **115**:279–287.

Mahalanabis D, Alam AN, Rahman N and Hasnat A (1991) Prognostic indicators and risk factors for increased duration of acute diarrhoea and for persistent diarrhoea in children. *Int J Epidemiol* **20**:1064–1072.

Mahmud MA, Chappell C, Hossain MM, Habib M and Dupont HL (1995) Risk factors for development of first symptomatic *Giardia* infection among infants of a birth cohort in rural Egypt. *Am J Trop Med Hyg* **53**:84–88.

Mahoney FJ, Farley TA, Kelso KY, Wilson SA, Horan JM and McFarland LM (1992) An outbreak of hepatitis A associated with swimming in a public pool. *J Infect Dis* **165**:613–618.

Maiwald M, Kissal K, von Knebel Doeberitz M and Sonntag HG (1994) Comparison of polymerase chain reaction and conventional culture for the detection of legionellas in hospital water samples. *J Appl Bacteriol* **76**:216–215.

Makintubee S, Mallonee J and Istre GR (1987) Shigellosis outbreak associated with swimming. *Am J Public Health* **77**:166–168.

Malaty HM, Kim JG, Kim SD and Graham DY (1996) Prevalence of *Helicobacter pylori* infection in Korean children: inverse relation to socioeconomic status despite a uniformly high prevalence in adults. *Am J Epidemiol* **143**:257–262.

Mallin K (1990) Investigation of a bladder cancer cluster in Northwestern Illinois. *Am J Epidemiol,* Suppl **132**(1):S96–S106.

Mandell GL, Douglas RG and Bennett JE (1995) *Principles and Practice of Infectious Diseases,* 4th edn. Churchill Livingstone, New York.

Mangione EJ, Remis RS, Tait KA, McGee HB, Gorman GW, Wentworth BB, Baron PA, Hightower AW, Barbaree JM and Broome CV (1985) An outbreak of Pontiac fever related to whirlpool use, Michigan 1982. *JAMA* **253**:535–539.

Manji F, Baelum V and Fejerskov O (1986) Dental fluorosis in an area of Kenya with 2 ppm fluoride in the drinking water. *J Dent Res* **65**:659–662.

Marcal O Jr, Hotta LK, Patucci RM, Glasser CM, Dias LC (1993) *Schisto-somiasis mansoni* in an area of low transmission. II. Risk factors for infection. *Rev Inst Med Trop Sao Paulo* **35**:331–335.

Marcus WL (1986) Lead health effects in drinking water. *Toxicol Ind Health* **2**:363–407.

Marrie T, Green P, Burbridge S, Bezanson G, Neale S, Hoffman PS and Haldane D (1994) Legionellaceae in the potable water of Nova Scotia and Halifax residences. *Epidemiol Infect* **112**:143–150.

Marshall BJ and Warren JR (1984) Unidentified curved bacilli in the stomach of patients with gastritis and peptic ulceration. *Lancet* **i**:1311–1313.

Marston BJ, Diallo MO, Horsburgh CR Jr, Diomande I, Saki MZ, Kanga J-M, Patrice G, Lipman HB, Ostroff SM and Good RC (1995) Emergence of Buruli ulcer disease in the Daloa region of cote D'Ivoire. *Am J Trop Med Hyg* **52**:219–224.

Martin-Prevel Y, Berteau F, Bouyssou M, Ripert C and Pinder M (1992) An epidemiological study of a *Schistosoma intercalatum* focus in south-east Gabon. *Trans R Soc Trop Med Hyg* **86**:401–405.

Martone WJ, Hierholzer JC, Keenlyside RA, Fraser DW, D'Angelo LJ and Winkler WG (1980) An outbreak of adenovirus type 3 disease at a private recreation centre swimming pool. *Am J Epidemiol* **111**:229–237.

Martyn CN, Barker DJP, Osmond C, Harris EC, Edwardson JA and Lacey RF (1989) Geographical relation between Alzheimer's disease and aluminium in drinking water. *Lancet* **i**:59–62.

Masironi R and Shaper AG (1981) Epidemiological studies of health effects of water from different sources. *Ann Rev Nutr* **1**:375–400.

Massa S, Cesaroni D, Poda G and Trovatelli LD (1988) Isolation of *Yersinia enterocolitica* and related species from river water. *Zentralb Mikrobiol* **143**:575–581.

Mastroiacovo P, Botto L, Fusco D, Rosano A and Scarano G (1994) Limb reduction defects and coastal areas. *Lancet* **343**:1034–1035.

Mates A (1992) The significance of testing for *Pseudomonas aeruginosa* in recreational seawater beaches. *Microbios* **71**: 89–93.

Mathan VI, Bhat P, Kapadia CR, Ponniah J and Baker SJ (1984) Epidemic dysentery caused by the shiga bacillus in a southern Indian village. *J Diarrhoeal Dis Res* **2**:27–32.

Mathias RG, Riben PD and Osei WD (1992) Lack of an association between endemic giardiasis and a drinking water source. *Can J Public Health* **83**:382–384.

Mayon-White RT and Frankenberg RA (1989) "Boil the water". *Lancet* **ii**:216.

McAnulty JM, Fleming DW and Gonzalez AH (1994) A community-wide outbreak of cryptosporidiosis associated with swimming at a wave pool. *JAMA* **272**:1597–1600.

McAnulty JM, Rubin GL, Carvan CT, Huntley EJ, Grohmann G and Hunter R (1993) An outbreak of Norwalk-like gastroenteritis associated with contaminated drinking water at a caravan park. *Aust J Public Health* **17**:36–41.

McCarthy SA and Khambaty FM (1994) International dissemination of epidemic *Vibrio cholerae* by cargo ship ballast and other non-potable waters. *Appl Environ Microbiol* **60**:2597–2601.

McEvoy MB, Bartlett C, Emslie J, MacIntyre AB (1984) Outbreak of illness associated with holiday in Soviet Central Asia. *Commun Dis Scotland* **18**(19):vii–x.

Medema G and Schets C (1993) Occurrence of *Plesiomonas shigelloides* in surface water: relationship with faecal pollution and trophic state. *Zentralb Hyg Umweltmed* **194**:398–404.

Megraud F and Serceau R (1990) Search for *Campylobacter* species in the public water supply of a large urban community. *Zentralb Hyg Umweltmed* **189**:536–542.

Mehnert DU and Stewien KE (1993) Detection and distribution of rotavirus in raw sewage and creeks in São Paulo, Brazil. *Appl Environ Microbiol* **59**:140–143.

Melby K, Dahl OP, Crisp L and Penner JL (1990) Clinical and serological manifestations in patients during a waterborne epidemic due to *Campylobacter jejuni. J Infect* **21**:309–316.

Melby K, Gondrosen B, Gregusson S, Ribe H and Dahl OP (1991) Waterborne campylobacteriosis in northern Norway. *Int J Food Microbiol* **12**:151–156.

Mentzing L-O (1981) Waterborne outbreaks of campylobacter enteritis in central Sweden. *Lancet* **ii**:352–354.

Merson MH, Tenny JH, Meyers JD, Wood BT, Wells JG, Rymzo W, Cline B, De Witt WE, Skaliy P and Mallison F (1975) Shigellosis at sea: an outbreak aboard a passenger cruise ship. *Am J Epidemiol* **101**:165–175.

Metcalf TG and Jiang X (1988) Detection of hepatitis A virus in estuarine samples by gene probe assay. *Microbiol Sci* **5**:296–300.

Mignani E, Palmieri F, Fontana M and Marigo S (1988) Italian epidemic of waterborne tularaemia. *Lancet* **ii**:1423.

Miller CJ, Drasar BS and Feachem RG (1982) Cholera and estuarine salinity in Calcutta and London. *Lancet* **i**:1216–1218.

Millette JR, Craun GF, Stober JA, Kraemer DF, Tousignant HG, Hildago E, Duboise RL and Benedict J (1983) Epidemiology study of the use of asbestos-cement pipe for the distribution of drinking water in Escambia County, Florida. *Environ Health Perspect* **53**:91–98.

Millson M, Bokhout M, Carlson J, Spielberg L, Aldis R, Borczyk A and Lior H (1991) An outbreak of *Campylobacter jejuni* gastroenteritis linked to meltwater contamination of a municipal well. *Can J Public Health* **82**:27–31.

Mintz ED, Reiff FM and Tauxe RV (1995) Safe water treatment and storage in the home: a practical new strategy to prevent waterborne disease. *JAMA* **273**:948–953.

Mitchell HM, Li YY, Hu PJ, Liu Q, Chen M, Du GG, Wang ZJ, Lee A and Hazell SL (1992) Epidemiology of *Helicobacter pylori* in southern China: identification of early childhood as the critical period for acquisition. *J Infect Dis* **166**:149–153.

Mitchell P, Graham P and Brieseman MA (1993) Giardiasis in Canterbury: the first nine months reported. *N Z Med J* **106**:350–352.

Mitscherlich E and Marth EH (1984) *Microbial Survival in the Environment.* Springer Verlag, New York, pp 449–460.

Miyamura K, Yamashita K, Yamadera S, Kato N, Akatsuka M, Hara M, Inouye S and Yamazaki S (1992) Poliovirus surveillance: isolation of polioviruses in Japan, 1980–1991. A report of the National Epidemiological Surveillance of Infectious Agents in Japan. *Jpn J Med Sci Biol* **45**:203–214.

Moe CL, Sobsey MD, Samsa GP and Mesolo V (1991) Bacterial indicators of risk of diarrhoeal disease from drinking-water in the Philippines. *Bull World Health Organ* **69**:305–317.

Moiraghi A, Castellani-Pastoris M, Barral C, Carle F, Sciacovelli A, Passarino G and Marforio P (1987) Nosocomial legionellosis associated with use of oxygen bubble humidifiers and underwater chest drains. *J Hosp Infect* **10**:47–50.

Molbak K, Hojlyng N and Gaarslev K (1988) High prevalence of campylobacter excretors among Liberian children related to environmental conditions. *Epidemiol Infect* **100**:227–237.

Momas I, Brette F, Spinasse A, Squinazi F, Dab W and Festy B (1993) Health affects of attending a public swimming pool: follow up of a cohort of pupils in Paris. *J Epidemiol Community Health* **47**:464–468.

Monceyron C and Grinde B (1994) Detection of hepatitis A virus in clinical and environmental samples by immunomagnetic separation and PCR. *J Virol Methods* **46**:157–166.

Moore AC, Herwaldt BL, Craun GF, Calderon RL, Highsmith AK and Juranek DD (1993) Surveillance for waterborne disease outbreaks – United States, 1991–1992. *MMWR* **42**(SS-5):1–22.

Moore NJ and Margolin AB (1993) Evaluation of radioactive and nonradioactive gene probes and cell culture for detection of poliovirus in water samples. *Appl Environ Microbiol* **59**:3145–3146.

Moorehead WP, Guasparini R, Donovan CA, Mathias RG, Cottle R and Baytalan G (1990) Giardiasis outbreak from a community water supply. *Can J Public Health* **81**:358–362.

Morace G, Pisani G, Divizia M and Pana A (1993) Detection of hepatitis A virus in concentrated river water by polymerase chain reaction. *Zentralb Hyg Umweltmed* **193**:521–527.

Morales-Suarez-Varela MM, Llopis-Gonzalez A and Tejerizo-Perez ML (1995) Impact of nitrates in drinking water on cancer mortality in Valencia, Spain. *Eur J Epidemiol* **11**:15–21.

Morales-Suarez-Varela MM, Llopis-Gonzalez A, Tejerizo-Perez ML and

Ferrer-Caraco E (1994) Chlorination of drinking water and cancer incidence. *J Environ Pathol Toxicol Oncol* **13**:39–41.

Morano A, Jiménez-Jiménez FJ, Molina JA and Antolín MA (1994) Risk-factors for Parkinson's disease: case-control study in the province of Cáceres, Spain. *Acta Neurol Scand* **89**:164–170.

Moren A, Stefanaggi S, Antona D, Bitar D, Etchegorry MG, Tchatchioka M and Lungu G (1991) Practical field epidemiology to investigate a cholera outbreak in a Mozambican refugee camp in Malawi 1988. *J Trop Med Hyg* **94**:1–7.

Morgan D, Allaby M, Crook S, Casemore D, Healing TD, Soltanpoor N, Hill S and Hooper W (1995) Waterborne cryptosporidiosis associated with a borehole supply. *Commun Dis Rep Rev* **5**:R93–R97.

Morin MM, Sharrett AR, Bailey KR and Fabsitz RR (1985) Drinking water source and mortality in US cities. *Int J Epidemiol* **14**:254–264.

Morinigo MA, Munoz MA, Martinez-Manzanares E, Sanchez JM and Borrego JJ (1993) Laboratory study of several enrichment broths for the detection of *Salmonell* spp. particularly in relation to water samples. *J Appl Bacteriol* **74**:330–335.

Morris RD and Levin R (1995) Estimating the incidence of waterborne infectious disease related to drinking water in the United States. In: Reichard EG and Zapponi GA (eds.) *Assessing and Managing Health Risks from Drinking Water Contamination: Approaches and Applications.* IAHS Press, Wallingford, Oxfordshire, pp. 75–88.

Morris RD, Audet A-M, Angelillo IF, Chalmers TC and Mosteller F (1992) Chlorination, chlorination by-products and cancer: a meta-analysis. *Am J Public Health* **82**:955–963.

Morrissey AB, Aisu TO, Falkinham JO 3rd, Eriki PP, Ellner JJ and Daniel TM (1992) Absence of *Mycobacterium avium* complex disease in patients with AIDS in Uganda. *J Acquir Immune Defic Syndr* **5**:477–478.

Morse LJ, Bryan JA, Hurley JP, Murphy JF, O'Brien TF and Wacker WEC (1972) The Holy Cross College football team hepatitis outbreak. *JAMA* **219**:706–708.

Morton W, Starr G, Pohl D, Stoner J, Wagner S and Weswig P (1976) Skin cancer and water arsenic in Lane County, Oregon. *Cancer* **37**:2523–2532.

Mujica OJ, Quick RE, Palacios AM, Beingolea L, Vargas R, Moreno D, Barrett TJ, Bean NH, Seminario L and Tauxe RV (1994) Epidemic cholera in the Amazon: the role of produce in disease risk and prevention. *J Infect Dis* **169**:1381–1384.

Mulder YM, Drijver, M and Kreis IA (1994) Case-control study on the association between a cluster of childhood haemopoietic malignancies and local environmental factors in Aalsmeer, The Netherlands. *J Epidemiol Community Health* **48**:161–165.

Muntzel M and Drueke T (1992) A comprehensive review of the salt and blood pressure relationship. *Am J Hypertens* **5**:1S–42S.

Murphy AM, Grohmann GS and Sexton MFH (1983) Infectious gastroenteritis in Norfolk Island and recovery of viruses from drinking water. *J Hyg, Camb* **91**:139–146.

Murray JJ (1993) Efficacy of preventative agents for dental caries. Systemic fluorides: water fluoridation. *Caries Res* **27**, suppl 1:2–8.

Murray PR, Baron EJ, Pfaller MA, Tenover FC and Yolken RH (eds) (1995) *Manual of Clinical Microbiology*, 6th edn. ASM Press, Washington, DC.

Mushak P and Crocetti AF (1989) Determination of numbers of lead-exposed American children as a function of lead source: integrated summary of a report to the US Congress on childhood lead poisoning. *Environ Res* **50**:210–229.

Musial CE, Arrowood MJ, Sterling CR and Gerba CP (1987) Detection of *Cryptosporidium* in water by using polypropylene cartridge filters. *Appl Environ Microbiol* **53**:687–692.

Myatt DC and Davis GH (1989) Isolation of medically significant *Vibrio* species from riverine sources in south east Queensland. *Microbios* **60**:111–123.

Nail SR, Aggarwal R, Salunke PN and Mehrotra NN (1992) A large waterborne viral hepatitis E epidemic in Kanpur, India. *Bull World Health Organ* **70**:597–604.

Nakano H, Kameyama T, Venkateswaran K, Kawakami H and Hashimoto H (1990) Distribution and characterisation of hemolytic, and enteropathogenic motile *Aeromonas* in aquatic environment. *Microbiol Immunol* **34**:447–458.

Nasser AM and Metcalf TG (1987) An A-ELISA to detect hepatitis A virus in estuarine samples. *Appl Environ Microbiol* **53**:1192–1195.

National Cryptosporidium Survey Group (1992) A survey of *Cryptosporidium* oocysts in surface and groundwaters in the UK. *J Inst Water Environ Manag* **6**:697–703.

Navin TR, Juranek DD, Ford M, Minedew DJ, Lippy EC and Pollard RA (1985) Case-control study of waterborne giardiasis in Reno, Nevada. *Am J Epidemiol* **112**:269–275.

Ndamba J, Chidimu MG, Zimba M, Gomo E and Munjoma M (1994) An investigation of the schistosomiasis transmission status in Harare. *Centr Afr J Med* **40**:337–342.

Needleman HL and Gatsonis C (1990) Low level lead exposure and the IQ of children. *JAMA* **263**:673–678.

Needleman HL, Gunnoe C, Leviton A, Reed R, Peresis H, Maher C and Barrett P (1979) Deficits in psychological and classroom performance of children with elevated dentine lead levels. *N Engl J Med* **300**:689–695.

Neill MA, Agosti J and Rosen H (1985) Hemorrhagic colitis with *Escherichia coli* O157:H7 preceding adult hemolytic uremic syndrome. *Arch Intern Med* **145**:2215–2217.

Nelson KE, Ager EA, Galton MM, Gillespie RWH and Sulzer CR (1973) An outbreak of leptospirosis in Washington State. *Am J Epidemiol* **98**:336–347.

Nerbrand C, Svardsudd K, Ek J and Tibblin G (1992) Cardiovascular mortality and morbidity in seven counties in Sweden in relation to water hardness and geological settings. The project: myocardial infarction in mid-Sweden. *Eur Heart J* **13**:721–727.

Neri LC and Hewitt D (1991) Aluminium Alzheimer's disease, and drinking water. *Lancet* **338**:390.

Neringer R, Andersson Y and Eitrem R (1987) A water-borne outbreak of giardiasis in Sweden. *Scand J Infect Dis* **19**:85–90.

Newman RD, Wuhib T, Lima AAM, Guerrant RL and Sears CL (1993) Environmental sources of *Cryptosporidium* in an urban slum in northeastern Brazil. *Am J Trop Med Hyg* **49**:270–275.

Niizeki K, Kano O and Kondo Y (1984) An epidemic study of molluscum contagiosum: relationship to swimming. *Dermatologica* **169**:197–198.

Nimri LF and Batchoun R (1994) Prevalence of *Cryptosporidium* species in elementary school children. *J Clin Microbiol* **32**:1040–1042.

Nishiwaki-Matsushima R, Ohta T, Nishiwaki S, Sugawama M, Kohyama K, Ishikawa T, Carmichael WW and Fujiki H (1992) Liver cancer promoted by the cyanobacterial cyclic peptide toxin microcystin LR. *J Cancer Res Clin Oncol* **118**:420–424.

Nouasria B, Larouze B, Dazza MC, Gaudebout C, Saimot AG, Aouati A (1984) Direct evidence that non-A, non-B hepatitis is a waterborne disease. *Lancet* **ii**:94.

O'Brien AAJ, Moore DP and Keogh JAB (1990) Acute epidemic aluminium osteomalacia secondary to water supply contamination. *Ir J Med Sci* **159**:71–73.

O'Brien TR, Decouflé P and Rhodes PH (1987) Leukemia and radium groundwater contamination. *JAMA* **257**:317.

Oliver JD (1995) The viable but non-culturable state in the human pathogen *Vibrio vulnificus*. *FEMS Microbiol Lett* **133**:203–208.

Olson BH, Clark DL, Milner BB, Stewart MH and Wolfe RL (1991) Total coliform detection in drinking water: comparison of membrane filtration with Colilert and Coliquik. *Appl Environ Microbiol* **57**:1535–1539.

Olusanya O and Taiwo O (1989) Rotavirus as an aetiological agent of acute childhood diarrhoea in Ile-Ife, Nigeria. *East Afr Med J* **66**:100–104.

Oluwasanmi JO, Solanke TF, Olurin EO, Itayemi SO, Alabi GO and Lucas AO (1976) *M. ulcerans* (Buruli) skin ulceration in Nigeria. *Am J Trop Med Hyg* **25**:122–128.

O'Mahony MC, Noah ND, Evans B, Harper D, Rowe B, Lowes JA, Pearson A and Goode B (1986) An outbreak of gastroenteritis on a passenger cruise ship. *J Hyg, Camb* **97**:229–236.

O'Neill KR, Jones SH and Grimes DJ (1992) Seasonal incidence of *Vibrio vulnificus* in the Great Bay estuary of New Hampshire and Maine. *Appl Environ Microbiol* **58**:3257–3262.

Ongerth JE and Stibbs HH (1987) Identification of *Cryptosporidium* oocysts in river water. *Appl Environ Microbiol* 53:672–676.

Oreberg M, Jonsson GG, West K, Eberhard-Grahn M, Rastam, L and Melander A (1992) Large intercommunity difference in cardiovascular drug consumption: relation to mortality risk factors and socioeconomic differences. *Eur J Clin Pharmacol* 43:449–454.

Ostroff SM, Kapperud G, Hutwagner LC, Nesbakken T, Bean NH, Lassen J and Tauxe RV (1994) Sources of sporadic *Yersinia enterocolitica* infections in Norway: a prospective case-control study. *Epidemiol Infect* 112:133–141.

Owen PJ and Miles DPB (1995) A review of hospital discharge rates in a population around Camelford in North Cornwall up to the fifth anniversary of an episode of aluminium sulphate absorption. *J Public Health Med* 17:200–204.

Pöyry T, Stenvik M and Hovi T (1988) Viruses in sewage waters during and after a poliomyelitis outbreak and subsequent nationwide oral poliovirus vaccination campaign in Finland. *Appl Environ Microbiol* 54:371–374.

Pain GC, Chakraborty AK and Choudry NR (1983) Outbreak of non-A, non-B type viral hepatitis in a Calcutta slum. *J Indian Med Assoc* 80:125–128.

Palmer SR (1989) Epidemiology in search of infectious diseases: methods in outbreak investigation. *J Epidemiol Community Health* 43:311–314.

Palmer SR, Gully PR, White KM, Pearson AD, Suckling WG, Jones DM, Rawes JCL and Penner JL (1983) Water-borne outbreak of campylobacter gastroenteritis. *Lancet* i:287–290.

Palmer CJ, Tsai YL, Lang AL and Sangermano LR (1993a) Evaluation of colilert-marine water for detection of total coliforms and *Escherichia coli* in the marine environment. *Appl Environ Microbiol* 59:786–790.

Palmer CJ, Tsai YL, Paszko-Kolva C, Mayer C and Sangermano LR (1993b) Detection of *Legionella* species in sewage and ocean water by polymerase chain reaction, direct fluorescent-antibody and plate culture methods. *Appl Environ Microbiol* 59:3618–3624.

Pana A, Divizia M, de Filippis P and di Napoli A (1987) Isolation of hepatitis A virus from polluted river water on FRP/3 cells. *Lancet* ii:1328.

Panda SK, Datta R, Kaur J, Zuckerman AJ and Nayak NC (1989) Enterically transmitted non-A, non-B hepatitis: recovery of virus-like particles from an epidemic in South Delhi and transmission studies in rhesus monkeys. *Hepatology* 10:466–472.

Panwalker AP and Fuhse E (1986) Nosocomial *Mycobacterium gordonae* pseudoinfection from contaminated ice machines. *Infect Control* 7:67–70.

Papapetropoulou M, Iliopoulou J, Rodopoulou G, Detorakis J and Paniara O (1994) Occurrence and antibiotic-resistance of *Pseudomonas* species isolated from drinking water in southern Greece. *J Chemother* 6:111–116.

Papapetropoulou M, Rodopoulou G and Giannoulaki E (1995) Improved glutamate-starch-penicillin agar for the isolation and enumeration of

Aeromonas hydrophila from seawater by membrane filtration. *Pathol Biol* **43**:622–627.

Parker MT and Duerden BI (eds) (1990) *Topley and Wilson's Principles of Bacteriology, Virology and Immunity*, 8th edn, vol 2. Edward Arnold, London.

Parkinson IS, Feest TG, Ward MK, Fawcett RWP and Kerr DNS (1979) Fracturing dialysis osteodystrophy and dialysis encephalopathy: an epidemiological study. *Lancet* **i**:406–409.

Parveen S, Islam MS and Huq A (1995) Abundance of *Aeromonas* spp. in lake waters in and around Dhaka, Bangladesh. *J Diarrhoeal Dis Res* **13**:183–186.

Payment P, Franco E and Fout GS (1994) Incidence of Norwalk virus infections during a prospective epidemiological study of drinking water related gastrointestinal illness. *Can J Microbiol* **40**:805–809.

Payment P, Franco E, Richardson L and Siemiatycki J (1991a) Gastrointestinal health effects associated with the consumption of drinking water produced by point-of-use domestic reverse-osmosis filtration units. *Appl Environ Microbiol* **57**:945–948.

Payment P, Richardson L, Siemiatycki J, Dewar R, Edwards M and Franco E (1991b) A randomized trial to evaluate the risk of gastrointestinal disease due to consumption of drinking water meeting currently accepted microbiological standards. *Am J Public Health* **81**:703–708.

Pazzaglia G, Bourgeois AL, Araby I, Mikhail I, Podgore JK, Mourad A, Riad S, Gaffar T and Ramadan AM (1993) *Campylobacter*-associated diarrhoea in Egyptian infants: epidemiology and clinical manifestation of disease and high frequency of concomitant infections. *J Diarrhoeal Dis Res* **11**:6–13.

Pelletier PA, du Moulin GC and Stottmeier KD (1988) Mycobacteria in public water supplies: comparative resistance to chlorine. *Microbiol Sci* **5**:147–148.

Penman AD, Lanier DC Jr, Avara WT 3rd, Canant KE, DeGroote JW, Brackin BT, Currier MM and Hotchkiss RL (1995) *Vibrio vulnificus* wound infections from the Mississippi Gulf coastal waters: June to August 1993. *South Med J* **88**:531–533.

Penn C and Kain KC (1990) Pseudomonas folliculitis: an outbreak associated with bromine-based disinfectants, British Columbia. *Can Dis Weekly Rep* **16**:31–33.

Penny PT (1991) Hydrotherapy pools of the future – the avoidance of health problems. *J Hosp Infect Suppl* **18**(A): 535–542.

Perry HM, Kopp SY, Erlanger MW and Perry EF (1983) Cardiovascular effect of chronic barium ingestion. *Trace Subst Environ Health* **16**:155–164.

Peters M, Muller C, Rusch-Gerdes S, Seidel C, Gobel U, Pohle HD and Ruf B (1995) Isolation of atypical mycobacteria from tap water in hospitals and homes: is this a possible source of disseminated MAC infection in AIDS patients? *J Infect* **31**:39–44.

Petersen LR, Denis D, Brown D, Hadler JL and Helgerson SD (1988)

Community health effects of a municipal water supply hyperfluoridation accident. *Am J Public Health* **78**:711–713.

Philipp R, Evans EJ, Hughes AO, Grisdale SK, Enticott RG and Jephcott AE (1985) Health risks of snorkel swimming in untreated water. *Int J Epidemiol* **14**:624–627.

Philippines Cholera Committee (1970) Study on the transmission of el tor cholera during an outbreak in Can-Itom Community in the Philippines. *Bull World Health Organ* **43**:413–419.

Philpot J, Tarr J, Hopkins R and Dean G (1992) Katayama syndrome among travelers to Ethiopia. *MMWR* **31**:436–437.

Picard B and Goullet Ph. (1987) Season prevalence of nosocomial *Aeromonas hydrophila* infection related to aeromonas in hospital water. *J Hosp Infect* **10**:152–155.

Pilotto L and Gorski J (1992) Progress towards the eradication of dracunculiasis. *J R Soc Health* **112**:78–83.

Pocock SJ, Smith M and Baghurst P (1994) Environmental lead and children's intelligence: a systematic review of the epidemiological evidence. *Brit Med J* **309**:1189–1197.

Pocock SJ, Shaper AG, Cook DG, Packham RF, Lacey RF, Powell P and Russell PF (1980) British Regional Heart Study: geographic variations in cardiovascular mortality, and the role of water quality. *Brit Med J* **i**:1243–1248.

Polissar L, Severson RK, and Boatman ES (1983) Cancer risk from asbestos in drinking water: summary of a case-control study in western Washington. *Environ Health Perspect* **53**:57–60.

Polissar L, Severson RK and Boatman ES (1984) A case-control study of asbestos in drinking water and cancer risk. *Am J Epidemiol* **119**:456–471.

Polissar L, Severson RK, Boatman ES and Thomas DB (1982) Cancer incidence in relation to asbestos in drinking water in the Puget Sound region. *Am J Epidemiol* **116**:314–328.

Pomrehn PR, Clarke WR, Sowers MF, Wallace RB and Lauer RM (1983) Community differences in blood pressure levels and drinking water sodium. *Am J Epidemiol* **118**:60–71.

Popovitch GG and Bondarenko VI (1982) *Shigella* and *Salmonella* viability in river water at varying temperatures. *Biol Abstr* **74**:42094.

Porter JD, Ragazzoni HP, Buchanon JD, Wakin HA, Juranek DD and Parkin WE (1988) *Giardia* transmission in a swimming pool. *Am J Public Health* **78**:659–662.

Powell JJ, Greenfield SM, Thompson RPH, Cargnello JA, Kendall MD, Landsberg JP, Watt F, Delves HT and House I (1995) Assessment of toxic metal exposure following the Camelford water pollution incident: evidence of acute mobilization of lead into drinking water. *Analyst* **120**:793–798.

Power C, Barker DJ and Blacklock NJ (1987) Incidence of renal stones in 18 British towns. A collaborative study. *Brit J Urol* **59**:105–110.

Price D and Ahearn DG (1988) Incidence and persistence of *Pseudomonas aeruginosa* in whirlpools. *J Clin Microbiol* **26**:1650–1654.

Prociv P (1987) Palm Island reconsidered. Was it copper poisoning? *Aust N Z J Med* **17**:345–349.

Puig M, Jofre J, Lucena F, Allard A, Wadell G and Girones R (1994) Detection of adenoviruses and enteroviruses in polluted waters by nested PCR amplification. *Appl Environ Microbiol* **60**:2963–2970.

Punsar S, Erametsa O, Karvonen MJ, Ryhanen A, Hilska P and Vornamo H (1975) Coronary heart disease and drinking water. A search in two Finnish male cohorts for epidemiological evidence of a water factor. *J Chronic Dis* **28**:259–287.

Pyle BH, Broadaway SC and McFeters GA (1995) A rapid, direct method for enumerating respiring enterohemorrhagic *Escherichia coli* O157:H7 in water. *Appl Environ Microbiol* **61**:2614–2619.

Quick RE, Thompson BL, Zuniga A, Dominguez G, de Brizuela EL, de Palma O, Almeida S, Valencia A, Reis AA, Bean NH and Blake PA (1995) Epidemic cholera in rural El Salvador: risk factors in a region covered by a cholera prevention campaign. *Epidemiol Infect* **114**:249–255.

Quigley C (1996) Legionnaires' disease. *Microbiol Eur* **4**(3):10–14.

Quraishi MS, Ahmad M, Rashid H, Mushtaq S and Ahmed SA (1988) Hepatitis non-A, non-B – report of a water-borne outbreak. *J Pak Med Assoc* **38**:203–205.

Rabold JG, Hoge CW, Shlim DR, Kefford C, Rajah R and Echeverria P (1994) Cyclospora outbreak associated with chlorinated drinking water. *Lancet* **344**:1360–1361.

Rademacher JJ, Young TB and Kanarek MS (1992) Gastric cancer mortality and nitrate levels in Wisconsin drinking water. *Arch Environ Health* **47**:292–294.

Rahaman MM, Khan MM, Aziz KM, Islam MS and Kibriya AK (1975) An outbreak of dysentery caused by *Shigella dysenteriae* type 1 on a coral island in the Bay of Bengal. *J Infect Dis* **132**:15–19.

Rajasekaran P, Dutt PR and Pisharoti KA (1977) Impact of water supply on the incidence of diarrhoea and shigellosis among children in rural communities in Madurai. *Indian J Med Res* **66**:189–199.

Rajput AH, Stern W, Christ A and Laverty W (1984) Etiology of Parkinson's disease: environmental factor(s). *Neurology*, Suppl **34**(1):207.

Rajput AH, Uitti RJ, Stern W and Laverty W (1986) Early onset Parkinson's disease in Saskatchewan – environmental considerations for etiology. *Can J Neurol Sci* **13**:312–316.

Rajput AH, Uitti RJ, Stern W, Laverty W, O'Donnell K, O'Donnell D, Yuen WK and Dua A (1987) Geography, drinking water chemistry, pesticides and herbicides and the etiology of Parkinson's disease. *Can J Neurol Sci*, Suppl **14**(3):414–418.

Ramlow JM (1995) Cancer risk and tetrachloroethylene-contaminated drinking water in Massachusetts. *Arch Environ Health* **50**:170–171.

Ramsay CN and Marsh J (1990) Giardiasis due to deliberate contamination of a water supply. *Lancet* **336**:880–881.

Ratnam S, Hogan K, March SB and Butler RW (1986) Whirlpool-associated folliculitis caused by *Pseudomonas aeruginosa*: report of an outbreak and review. *J Clin Microbiol* **23**:655–659.

Rautelin H, Koota K, von Essen R, Jahkola M, Siitonen A and Kosunen TU (1990) Waterborne *Campylobacter jejuni* epidemic in a Finnish hospital for rheumatic diseases. *Scand J Infect Dis* **22**:321–326.

Regua AH, Bravo VLR, Leal MC and Lobo-Leite MEL (1990) Epidemiological survey of the enteropathogenic *Escherichia coli* isolated from children with diarrhoea. *J Trop Paediatr* **36**:176–179.

Reid TMS and Porter IA (1981) An outbreak of otitis externa in competitive swimmers due to *Pseudomonas aeruginosa*. *J Hyg, Camb* **86**:357–362.

Reinthaler FF, Sattler J, Schaffler-Dullnig K, Weinmayr B and Marth E (1993) Comparative study of procedures for isolation and cultivation of *Legionella pneumophila* from tap water in hospitals. *J Clin Microbiol* **31**:1213–1216.

Rennie TF (1970) Infectious hepatitis: report of an outbreak, apparently waterborne, in an institution. *Med J Aust* **ii**:135–136.

Reynolds CS (1984) *The Ecology of Freshwater Phytoplankton*. Cambridge University Press, Cambridge .

Rhodes JB, Smith HL and Ogg JE (1986) Isolation of non-O1 *Vibrio cholerae* serovars from surface waters in Western Colarado. *Appl Environ Microbiol* **51**:1216–1219.

Ribas F, Araujo R, Frias J, Huguet JM, Ribas FR and Lucena F (1991) Comparison of different media for the identification and quantification of *Aeromonas* spp. in water. *Antonie Van Leeuwenhoek* **59**:225–228.

Richardson AJ, Frankenberg RA, Buck AC, Selkon JB, Colbourne JS, Parsons JW and Mayon-White RT (1991) An outbreak of waterborne cryptosporidiosis in Swindon and Oxfordshire. *Epidemiol Infect* **107**:485–495.

Ries AA, Vugia DJ, Beingolea L, Palacios AM, Vasquez E, Wells JG, Baca NG, Swerdlow DL, Pollack M, Bean NH, Seminario L and Tauxe RV (1992) Cholera in Piura, Peru: a modern urban epidemic. *J Infect Dis* **166**:1429–1433.

Ripa LW (1993) A half-century of community water fluoridation in the United States: review and commentary. *J Public Health Dent* **53**:17–44.

Rippka R, Deruelles J, Waterbury JB, Herdman M and Stanier RY (1979) Generic assignments, strain histories and properties of pure cultures of cyanobacteria. *J Gen Microbiol* **111**:1–61.

Risbud AR, Chadha MS, Kushwah SS, Arankalle VA, Rodrigues FM and Banerjee K (1992) Non A non B hepatitis epidemic in Rewa District of Madhya Pradesh. *J Assoc Physicians India* **40**:262–264.

Rivera SC, Hazen TC and Toranzos GA (1988) Isolation of fecal coliforms from pristine sites in a tropical rain forest. *Appl Environ Microbiol* **54**:513–517.

Roach PD, Olson ME, Whitley G and Wallis PM (1993) Waterborne giardia cysts and cryptosporidium oocysts in the Yukon, Canada. *Appl Environ Microbiol* **59**:67–73.

Roberts D (1992) Growth and survival of *Vibrio cholerae* in foods. *PHLS Microbiol Digest* **9**:24–31.

Robertson JS and Parker V (1978) Cot deaths and water-sodium. *Lancet* **ii**:1012–1014.

Robertson MH, Clarke IR, Coghlan JD and Gill ON (1981) Leptospirosis in trout farmers. *Lancet* **ii**:626–627.

Rogol M, Sechter I, Falk H, Shtark Y, Alfi S, Greenberg Z and Mizrachi R (1983) Waterborne outbreak of *Campylobacter* enteritis. *Eur J Clin Microbiol* **2**:588–590.

Rollins DM and Colwell RR (1986) Viable but non-culturable stage of *Campylobacter jejuni* and its role in survival in the natural aquatic environment. *Appl Environ Microbiol* **52**:531–538.

Rose HD, Franson TR, Sheth NK, Chusid MJ, Macher AM and Zeirdt CH (1983) *Pseudomonas* pneumonia associated with use of a home whirlpool spa. *JAMA* **250**:2027–2029.

Rose JB (1988) Occurrence and significance of cryptosporidium in water. *J Am Water Works Assoc* **88**(2):53–58.

Rosenberg ML, Koplan JP and Pollard RA (1980) The risk of acquiring hepatitis from sewage-contaminated water. *Am J Epidemiol* **112**:17–22.

Rosenberg ML, Hazlet KK, Schaefer J, Wells JG and Pruneda RC (1976) Shigellosis from swimming. *JAMA* **236**:1849–1852.

Rosenberg ML, Koplan JP, Wachsmuth IK, Wells JG, Gangarosa EJ, Guerrant RL and Sacks DA (1977) Epidemic diarrhea at Crater Lake from enterotoxigenic *Escherichia coli*. A large waterborne outbreak. *Ann Intern Med* **86**:714–718.

Rowland A, Grainger R, Stanwell-Smith R, Hicks N and Hughes A (1990) Water contamination in North Cornwall: a retrospective cohort study into the acute and short-term effects of the aluminium sulphate incident in July 1988. *J R Soc Health* **110**:166–172.

Rozas VV, Port PK and Easterling RE (1978) An outbreak of dialysis dementia due to aluminium in the dialysate. *J Dial* **2**:459–470.

Runnegar M, Berndt N and Kaplowitz N (1995) Microcystin uptake and inhibition of protein phosphatases: effects of chemoprotectants and self-inhibition in relation to known hepatic transporters. *Toxicol Appl Pharmacol* **134**:264–272.

Rush BA, Chapman PA and Ineson RW (1990) A probable waterborne outbreak of cryptosporidiosis in the Sheffield area. *J Med Microbiol* **32**:239–242.

Rycroft RJG and Penny PT (1983) Dermatoses associated with brominated swimming pools. *Brit Med J* **287**:462.

Rylander R, Bonevik H and Rubenowitz E (1991) Magnesium and calcium in drinking water and cardiovascular mortality. *Scand J Work Environ Health* **17**:91–94.

Sabater JF and Zaragoza JM (1993) A simple identification system for slowly growing mycobacteria. II. Identification of 25 strains isolated from surface water in Valencia (Spain). *Acta Microbiol Hung* **40**:343–349.

Sacks JJ, Lieb S, Baldy LM, Berta S, Patton CM, White MC, Bigler WJ and Witte JJ (1986) Epidemic campylobacteriosis associated with a community water supply. *Am J Public Health* **76**:424–429.

Sadler TD, Rom WN, Lyon JL and Mason JO (1984) The use of asbestos-cement pipe for public water supply and the incidence of cancer in selected communities in Utah. *J Community Health* **9**:285–293.

Sæbø, A, Kapperud G, Lassen J and Waage J (1994) Prevalence of antibodies to *Yersinia enterocolitica* O:3 among Norwegian military recruits: association with risk factors and clinical manifestations. *Eur J Epidemiol* **10**:749–755.

Salmen P, Dwyer DM, Vorse H and Kruse W (1983) Whirlpool-associated *Pseudomonas aeruginosa* urinary tract infections. *JAMA* **250**:2025–2026.

Sama MT and Ratard RC (1994) Water contact and schistosomiasis infection in Kumba, south-western Cameroon. *Ann Trop Med Parasitol* **88**:629–634.

Samonis G, Elting L, Skoulika E, Maraki S and Tselentis Y (1994) An outbreak of diarrhoeal disease attributed to *Shigella sonnei*. *Epidemiol Infect* **112**:235–245.

Sanden GN, Morrill WE, Fields BS, Breiman RF and Barbaree JM (1992) Incubation of water samples containing amoebae improves detection of legionellae by the culture method. *Appl Environ Microbiol* **58**:2001–2004.

Sasaki DM, Pang L, Minette HP, Wakida CK, Fujimoto WL, Manea SJ, Kunioka R and Middleton CR (1993) Active surveillance and risk factors for leptospirosis in Hawaii. *Am J Trop Med Hyg* **48**:35–43.

Sathe PV, Karandikar VN, Gupte MD, Niphadkar KB, Joshi BN, Polakhare JK, Jahagirdar PL and Deodhar NS (1983) Investigation report of an epidemic of typhoid fever. *Int J Epidemiol* **12**:215–219.

Savioli L, Dixon H, Kisumku UM and Mott KE (1989) Control of morbidity due to *Schistosoma haematobium* on Pemba island; selective population chemotherapy of school children with haematyria to identify high-risk localities. *Trans R Soc Trop Med Hyg* **83**:805–810.

Savitz DA, Andrews KW and Pastore LM (1995) Drinking water and pregnancy outcome in Central North Carolina: source, amount and trihalomethane levels. *Environ Health Perspect* **103**:592–596.

Schramel P, Müller-Höcker J, Meyer U, Weiß M and Eife R (1988) Nutritional copper intoxication in three German infants with severe liver cell damage (features of Indian childhood cirrhosis). *J Trace Elem Electrolytes Health Dis* **2**:85–89.

Schulze-Robbecke R and Buchholtz K (1992) Heat susceptibility of aquatic mycobacteria. *Appl Environ Microbiol* **58**:1869–1873.

Schulze-Robbecke R, Janning B and Fischeder R (1992) Occurrence of mycobacteria in biofilm samples. *Tubercle Lung Dis* **73**:141–144.

Sellwood J and Wyn-Jones P (1996) Viruses in water: present knowledge and future opportunities. *Microbiol Eur* **4**(6):10–16.

Semchuk KM and Love EJ (1995) Effects of agricultural work and other proxy-derived case-control data on Parkinson's disease risk estimates. *Am J Epidemiol* **141**:747–754.

Seyfried PL and Cook RJ (1984) Otitis externa infections related to *Pseudomonas aeruginosa* levels in five Ontario Lakes. *Can J Public Health* **75**:83–91.

Seyfried PL, Tobin RS, Brown NE and Ness PF (1985a) A prospective study of swimming-related illness. I. Swimming associated health risk. *Am J Public Health* **75**:1068–1070.

Seyfried PL, Tobin RS, Brown NE and Ness PF (1985b) A prospective study of swimming-related illness. II. Morbidity and the microbiological quality of water. *Am J Public Health* **75**:1071–1075.

Shadix LC and Rice EW (1991) Evaluation of beta-glucuronidase assay for the detection of *Escherichia coli* from environmental waters. *Can J Microbiol* **37**:908–911.

Shahamat M, Paszco-Kolva C, Yamamoto H *et al.* (1989a) Ecological studies of *Campylobacter pylori* (abstract). *Klin Wochenschr* **67**:62–63.

Shahamat M, Vives-Rego J, Paszco-Kolva C *et al.* (1989b) Survival of *Campylobacter pylori* in river water (abstract). *Klin Wochenschr* **67**:63.

Shannon M and Graef JW (1989) Lead intoxication from lead-contaminated water used to reconstitute infant formula. *Clin Pediatr* **28**:380–382.

Shannon M and Graef JW (1992) Lead intoxication in infancy. *Pediatrics* **89**:87–90.

Shaper AG (1994) Water-hardness and coronary heart disease. In: Golding AMB, Noah N and Stanwell-Smith R (eds) *Water and Public Health*. Smith-Gordon & Co, London, pp 155–170.

Shaw JH (1984) A retrospective comparison of the effectiveness of bromination and chlorination in controlling *Pseudomonas aeruginosa* in spas (whirlpools) in Alberta. *Can J Public Health* **75**:61–68.

Shaw JW (1987) The potential for unexpected disinfectant failures with bromine-based disinfectants in spas (whirlpools). *N Z Sports Med* **15**:59–62.

Shaw PK, Brodsky RE, Lyman DO, Wood BT, Hibler CP, Healy GR, Macleod KIE, Stahl W and Schultz MG (1977) A communitywide outbreak of giardiasis with evidence of transmission by a municipal water supply. *Ann Intern Med* **87**:426–432.

Shears P, Hussein MA, Chowdhury AH and Mamun KZ (1995) Water sources and environmental transmission of multiply resistant enteric bacteria in rural Bangladesh. *Ann Trop Med Parasitol* **89**:297–303.

Shieh YS, Baric RS, Sobsey MD, Ticehurst J, Miele TA, DeLeon R and Walter R (1991) Detection of hepatitis A virus and other enteroviruses in water by ssRNA probes. *J Virol Methods* **31**:119–136.

Shlim DR, Cohen MT, Eaton M, Rajah R, Long EG and Ungar BLP (1991) An alga-like organism associated with an outbreak of prolonged diarrhea among foreigners in Nepal. *Am J Trop Med Hyg* **45**:383–389.

Shuster J, Finlayson B, Scheaffer R, Sierakowski R, Zoltek J and Dzegede S (1982) Water hardness and urinary stone disease. *J Urol* **128**:422–425.

Sidhu KS, Nash DF and McBride DE (1995) Need to revise the national drinking water regulation for copper. *Regul Toxicol Pharmacol* **22**:95–100.

Sierakowski R, Finlayson B and Landes R (1979) Stone incidence as related to water hardness in different geographical regions of the United States. *Urol Res* **7**:157–160.

Silverman P, Hreha M, Brunwasser A, Tuttle A, Faller D, Vukotich C and Richards NM (1981) Chlordane contamination of a public water supply – Pittsburgh Pennsylvania. *MMWR* **30**:571–572, 577.

Simchen E, Franklin D and Shuval HI (1984) "Swimmer's ear" among children of kindergarten age and water quality of swimming pools in 11 Kibbutzim. *Isr J Med Sci* **20**:584–588.

Sinclair GS, Mphahlele M, Duvenhage H, Nichol R, Whitehorn A and Kustner HGV (1982) Determination of the mode of transmission of cholera in Lebowa. *S Afr Med J* **62**:753–755.

Singh J, Aggarwal NR, Bhattacharjee J, Prakash C, Bora D, Jain DC, Sharma RS and Datta KK (1995b) An outbreak of viral hepatitis E: role of community practices. *J Commun Dis* **27**:92–96.

Singh J, Bora D, Sharma RS, Khanna KK and Verghese T (1995a) Epidemiology of cholera in Delhi – 1992. *J Trop Paediatr* **41**:139–142.

Singh PP and Kiran R (1993) Are we overstressing water quality in urinary stone disease? *Int Urol Nephrol* **25**:29–36.

Singleton FL, Attwell RW, Jangi S and Colwell RR (1982) Influence of salinity and organic nutrient concentration on survival and growth of *Vibrio cholerae* in aquatic microcosms. *Appl Environ Microbiol* **43**:1080–1085.

Sitas F (1986) Some observations on a cholera outbreak at the Umvoti Mission Reserve, Natal. *S Afr Med J* **70**:215–218.

Skirrow MB (1977) *Campylobacter* enteritis: A "new" disease. *Brit Med J* **ii**:9–11.

Skirrow MB (1991) Epidemiology of campylobacter enteritis. *Int J Food Microbiol* **12**:9–16.

Skjerve E and Brennhovd O (1992) A multiple logistic model for predicting the occurrence of *Campylobacter jejuni* and *Campylobacter coli* in water. *J Appl Bacteriol* **73**:94–98.

Skulberg OM, Codd GA and Carmichael WW (1984) Toxic blue-green algal blooms in Europe: a growing problem. *Ambio* **12**:244–247.

Smith HV and Rose JB (1990) Waterborne cryptosporidiosis. *Parasitol Today* **6**:8–12.

Smith HV, Patterson WJ, Hardie R, Greene LA, Benton C, Tulloch W, Gilmour RA, Girdwood RWA, Sharp JCM and Forbes GI (1989) An outbreak of cryptosporidiosis caused by post-treatment contamination. *Epidemiol Infect* **103**:703–715.

Smith WC and Crombie IK (1987) Coronary heart disease and water hardness in Scotland – is there a relationship? *J Epidemiol Community Health* **41**:227–228.

Sniadack DH, Ostroff SM, Karlix MA, Smithwick RW, Schwartz B, Sprauer MA, Silcox VA and Good RC (1993) A nosocomial pseudo-outbreak of *Mycobacterium xenopi*: lessons in prevention. *Infect Control Hosp Epidemiol* **14**:636–641.

Šlosárek M, Kubín M and Jaréhová, M (1993) Water-borne household infections due to *Mycobacterium xenopi*. *Centr Eur J Public Health* **1**:78–80.

Soave R, Dubey JP, Ramos LJ and Tummings M (1986) A new intestinal pathogen? *Clin Res* **34**:533A.

Sontz E and Schwieger J (1995) The "green water" syndrome: copper-induced hemolysis and subsequent acute renal failure as consequence of a religious ritual. *Am J Med* **98**:311–315.

Soong FS, Maynard E, Kirke K and Luke C (1992) Illness associated with blue-green algae. *Med J Aust* **156**:67.

Sorvillo FJ, Waterman SH, Vogt JK and England B (1988) Shigellosis associated with recreational water contact in Los Angeles County. *Am J Trop Med Hyg* **38**:613–617.

Sorvillo FJ, Fujioka K, Nahlen B, Tormey MP, Kebabjian R and Mascola L (1992) Swimming-associated cryptosporidiosis. *Am J Public Health* **82**:742–744.

Sorvillo F, Lieb LE, Nahlen B, Miller J, Mascola L and Ash LR (1994) Municipal drinking water and cryptosporidiosis among persons with AIDS in Los Angeles County. *Epidemiol Infect* **113**:313–320.

Southgate VR (1996) Medical helminthology. In Cook GC (ed.) *Manson's Tropical Diseases*, 12th edn. WB Saunders Co, London, pp 1580–1649.

Spitalny KC, Brondum J, Vogt RL, Sargent HE and Kappel S (1984) Drinking-water-induced copper intoxication in a Vermont family. *Pediatrics* **74**:1103–1106.

Springer GL and Shapiro ED (1985) Fresh water swimming as a risk factor for otitis externa: a case-control study. *Arch Environ Health* **40**:202–206.

Šrámová H and Kovácová D (1984) Outbreaks of alimentary bacterial infections reported in CSR between 1979 and 1982. *J Hyg Epidemiol Microbiol Immunol* **28**:353–362.

Sreenivasan MA, Sehgal A, Prasad SR and Dhorje S (1984) A sero-epidemiological study of water-borne epidemic of viral hepatitis in Kolhapur City, India. *J Hyg, Camb* **93**:113–122.

St Louis ME (1988) Water-related disease outbreaks, 1985. *MMWR* **37**(SS-2):15–24.

Stanwell-Smith R (1994) Water and public health in the United Kingdom. Recent trends in the epidemiology of water-borne disease. In: Golding AMB, Noah N and Stanwell-Smith R (eds) *Water and Public Health*. Smith-Gordon & Co, London, pp 39–54.

Starko KM, Lippy EC, Dominguez LB, Haley CE and Fisher HJ (1986) Camper's diarrhea outbreak traced to water-sewage link. *Public Health Rep* **101**:527–531.

Stebbings JH, Lucas HF and Toohey RE (1986) Leukemia and radium groundwater contamination. *JAMA* **255**:901–902.

Stehr-Green JK, Nicholls C, McEwan S, Payne A and Mitchell P (1991) Waterborne outbreak of *Campylobacter jejuni* in Christchurch: the importance of a combined epidemiologic and microbiologic investigation. *N Z Med J* **104**:356–358.

Stelzer W, Mochmann H, Richter U and Dobberkau HJ (1989) A study of *Campylobacter jejuni* and *Campylobacter coli* in a river system. *Zentralb Hyg Umweltmed* **189**:20–28.

Stenström TA (1994) A review of waterborne outbreaks of gastroenteritis in Scandinavia. In: Golding AMB, Noah N and Stanwell-Smith R (eds) *Water and Public Health*. Smith-Gordon & Co, London, pp 137–143.

Stern M, Dulaney E, Gruber SB, Golbe L, Bergen M, Hurtig H, Gollomp S and Stolley P (1991) The epidemiology of Parkinson's disease. A case-control study of young-onset and old-onset patients. *Arch Neurol* **48**:903–907.

Still CN and Kelley P (1980) On the incidence of primary degenerative dementia vs. water fluoride content in South Carolina. *Neurotoxicology* **1**:125–131.

Stoll NR (1947) This wormy world. *J Parasitol* **32**:1–18.

Stout J, Yu VL, Vickers RM and Shonnard J (1982) Potable water supply as the hospital reservoir for Pittsburgh pneumonia agent. *Lancet* **i**:471–472.

Stout JE, Yu VL, Yee YC, Vaccarello S, Diven W and Lee TC (1992) *Legionella pneumophila* in residential water supplies: environmental surveillance with clinical assessment for Legionnaires' disease. *Epidemiol Infect* **109**:49–57.

Stroffolini T, Biagini W, Lorenzoni L, Palazzesi GP, Divizia M and Frongillo R (1990) An outbreak of hepatitis A in young adults in central Italy. *Eur J Epidemiol* **6**:156–159.

Stroffolini T, Manzillo G, de Sena R, Manzillo E, Pagliano P, Zaccarelli M, Russo M, Soscia M and Giusti G (1992) Typhoid fever in the Neapolitan area: a case-control study. *Eur J Epidemiol* **8**:539–542.

Suputtamongkol Y, Hall AJ, Dance DAB, Chaowagul W, Rajchanuvong A,

Smith MD and White NJ (1994) The epidemiology of melioidosis in Ubon Ratchatani, Northeast Thailand. *Int J Epidemiol* **23**:1082–1090.

Sutmoller F, Azeredo RS, Lacerda MD, Barth OM, Pereira HG, Hoffer E and Schatzmayr HG (1982) An outbreak of gastroenteritis caused by both rotavirus and *Shigella sonnei* in a private school in Rio de Janeiro. *J Hyg, Camb* **88**:285–293.

Sutmoller F, Gaspar AMC, Cynamon SE, Richa N, Mercadante LAC and Schatzmayr HG (1982) A water-borne hepatitis A outbreak in Rio de Janeiro. *Mem Inst Oswaldo Cruz* **77**:9–17.

Swaddiwudhipong W, Karintraratana S and Kavinum S (1995) A common-source outbreak of shigellosis involving a piped public water supply in northern Thai communities. *J Trop Med Hyg* **98**:145–150.

Swan SH, Shaw G, Harris JA and Neutra RR (1989) Congenital cardiac anomalies in relation to water contamination, Santa Clara County, California, 1981–1983. *Am J Epidemiol* **129**:885–893.

Swerdlow DL, Mintz ED, Rodriguez M, Tejada E, Ocampo C, Espejo L, Greene KD, Saldana W, Seminario L, Tauxe RV, Wells JG, Bean NH, Ries AA, Pollack M, Vertiz B and Blake PA (1992a) Waterborne transmission of epidemic cholera in Trujillo, Peru: lessons for a continent at risk. *Lancet* **340**:28–33.

Swerdlow DL, Woodruff BA, Brady RC, Griffin PM, Tippen S, Donnell HD Jr, Geldreich E, Payne BJ, Meyer A Jr, Wells JG, Greene KD, Bright M, Bean NH and Blake PA (1992b) A waterborne outbreak in Missouri of *Escherichia coli* O157:H7 associated with bloody diarrhoea and death. *Ann Intern Med* **117**:812–819.

Tacket CO, Barrett TJ, Mann JM, Roberts MA and Blake PA (1984) Wound infections caused by *Vibrio vulnificus*, a marine vibrio, in inland areas of the United States. *J Clin Microbiol* **19**:197–199.

Takács S (1987) Nitrate content of drinking water and tumours of the digestive organ. *Zentralb Bakteriol Mikrobiol Hyg (B)* **184**:269–279.

Tamanai-Shacoori Z, Jolivet-Gougeon A, Pommepuy M, Cormier M and Colwell RR (1994) Detection of enterotoxigenic *Escherichia coli* in water by polymerase chain reaction amplification and hybridization. *Can J Microbiol* **40**:243–249.

Tambini G, Andrus JK, Marques E, Boshell J, Pallansch M, de Quadros CA and Kew O (1993) Direct detection of wild poliovirus circulation by stool surveys of healthy children and analysis of community wastewater. *J Infect Dis* **168**:1510–1514.

Tani N, Dohi Y, Kurumatani N and Yonemasu K (1995) Seasonal distribution of adenoviruses, enteroviruses and reoviruses in urban river water. *Microbiol Immunol* **39**:577–580.

Tarter ME, Cooper RC and Freeman WR (1983) A graphical analysis of the interrelationships among waterborne asbestos, digestive system cancer and population density. *Environ Health Perspect* **53**:79–89.

Tauxe RV, Holmberg SD, Dodin A, Wells JV and Blake PA (1988) Epidemic cholera in Mali: high mortality and multiple routes of transmission in a famine area. *Epidemiol Infect* **100**:279–289.

Taylor DN, McDermott KT, Little JR, Wells JG and Blaser MJ (1983) Campylobacter enteritis from untreated water in the Rocky Mountains. *Ann Intern Med* **99**:38–40.

Taylor JW, Gary GW Jr and Greenberg HB (1981) Norwalk-related viral gastroenteritis due to contaminated drinking water. *Am J Epidemiol* **114**:584–592.

Taylor MB, Becker PJ, Van Rensburg EJ, Harris BN, Bailey IW and Grabow WOK (1995) A serosurvey of water-borne pathogens amongst canoeists in South Africa. *Epidemiol Infect* **115**:299–307.

Teh BH, Lin J-T, Pan W-H, Lin S-H, Wang L-Y, Lee T-K and Chen C-J (1994) Seroprevalence and associated risk factors of *Helicobacter pylori* infection in Taiwan. *Anticancer Res* **14**:1389–1392.

Teixeira MGLC, Costa MCN, de Carvalho VLP, Pereira MS and Hage E (1993) Gastroenteritis epidemic in the area of the Itaparica dam Bahia, Brazil. *Bull Pan Am Health Organ* **27**:244–253.

Thom S, Warhurst D and Drasar BS (1992) Association of *Vibrio cholerae* with freshwater amoebae. *J Med Microbiol* **36**:303–306.

Thomas DL, Mundy LM and Tucker PC (1993) Hot tub legionellosis. Legionnaires' disease and Pontiac fever after a point-source exposure to *Legionella pneumophila*. *Arch Intern Med* **153**:2597–2599.

Thompson JS and Gravel MJ (1986) Family outbreak of gastroenteritis due to *Yersinia enterocolitica* serotype 0:3 from well water. *Can J Microbiol* **32**:700–701.

Thornton L, Fogarty J, Hayes C, Laffoy M, O'Flanagan D, Corcoran R, Parry JV and Perry KR (1995) The risk of hepatitis A from sewage contamination of a water supply. *Commun Dis Rep Rev* **5**:R1–R4.

Tohani VK, McCann R, Fox M and Fulton R (1991) Skin rash associated with accidental addition of excess aluminium sulphate to the water supply. *Ulster Med J* **60**:108–110.

Trincher RC and Rissing JP (1983) Contamination of potable water by phenol from a solar water tank liner – Georgia. *MMWR* **32**:493–494.

Tsai YL, Palmer CJ and Sangermano LR (1993) Detection of *Escherichia coli* in sewage and sludge by polymerase chain reaction. *Appl Environ Microbiol* **59**:353–357.

Tsai YL, Tran B, Sangermano LR and Palmer CJ (1993) Detection of poliovirus, hepatitis A virus, and rotavirus from sewage and ocean water by triplex reverse transcriptase PCR. *Appl Environ Microbiol* **60**:2400–2407.

Tsai YL, Tran B, Sangermano LR and Palmer CJ (1994) Detection of poliovirus, hepatitis A virus, and rotavirus from sewage and ocean water by triplex reverse transcriptase PCR. *Appl Environ Microbiol* **60**:2400–2407.

Tsega E, Mengesha B, Bengt-Goran H, Lindberg J and Nordenfelt E (1986)

Hepatitis A, B and delta infection in Ethiopia: a serologic survey with demographic data. *Am J Epidemiol* **123**:344–351.

Tsega E, Krawczynski K, Hansson B-G, Nordenfelt E, Negusse Y, Alemu W and Bahru Y (1991) Outbreak of acute hepatitis E virus infection among military personnel in Northern Ethiopia. *J Med Virol* **34**:232–236.

Tseng C-H, Chong C-K, Chen C-J, Lin BJ and Tai T-Y (1995) Abnormal peripheral microcirculation in seemingly normal subjects living in blackfoot-disease-hyperendemic villages in Taiwan. *Int J Microcirc* **15**:21–27.

Tseng WP (1989) Blackfoot disease in Taiwan: a 30-year follow-up study. *Angiology* **40**:547–558.

Tsuda T, Babazono A, Yamamoto E, Kurumatani N, Mino Y, Ogawa T, Kishi Y and Hideyasu H (1995) Ingested arsenic and internal cancer: a historical cohort study followed for 33 years. *Am J Epidemiol* **141**:198–209.

Tsukamoto T, Kinoshita Y, Shimada T and Sakazaki R (1978) Two epidemics of diarrhoeal disease possibly caused by *Plesiomonas shigelloides*. *J Hyg, Camb* **80**:275–280.

Tulchinsky TH, Burla E, Halperin R, Bonn J and Ostroy P (1993) Water quality, waterborne disease and enteric disease in Israel 1976–92. *Isr J Med Sci* **29**:783–790.

Turner M, Istre GR, Beauchamp H, Baum M and Arnold S (1987) Community outbreak of adenovirus type 7a infections associated with a swimming pool. *South Med J* **80**:712–715.

Turner PC, Gammie AJ, Hollinrake K and Codd GA (1990) Pneumonia associated with contact with cyanobacteria. *Brit Med J* **300**:1440–1441.

Tuthill RW and Calabrese EJ (1979) Elevated sodium levels in the public drinking water as a contributor to elevated blood pressure levels in the community. *Arch Environ Health* **34**:197–203.

Tuthill RW, Giusti RA, Moore GS and Calabrese EJ (1982) Health effects among newborns after prenatal exposure to ClO_2-disinfected drinking water. *Environ Health Perspect* **46**:39–45.

Tuttle J, Ries AA, Chimba RM, Perera CU, Bean NH and Griffin PM (1995) Antimicrobial-resistant epidemic *Shigella dysenteriae* type 1 in Zambia: modes of transmission. *J Infect Dis* **171**:371–375.

Uganda Buruli Group (1971) Epidemiology of *Mycobacterium ulcerans* infection (Buruli ulcer) at Kinyara, Uganda. *Trans R Soc Trop Med Hyg* **65**:763–775.

Umoh JU, Adesiyun AA, Adekeye JO and Nadarajah M (1983) Epidemiological features of an outbreak of gastroenteritis/cholera in Katsina, Northern Nigeria. *J Hyg, Camb* **91**:101–111.

Van Asperen IA, de Rover CM, Schijven JF, Bambang Oetomo S, Schellekens JFP, van Leeuwen NJ, Collé C, Havelaar AH and Kromhout D (1995) Risk of otitis externa after swimming in recreational fresh water lakes containing *Pseudomonas aeruginosa*. *Brit Med J* **311**:1407–1410.

VanDerslice J and Briscoe J (1995) Environmental interventions in developing countries and their implications. *Am J Epidemiol* **141**:135–144.

VanDerslice J, Popkin B and Briscoe J (1994) Drinking-water quality, sanitation and breast-feeding: their interactive effects on infant health. *Bull World Health Organ* **72**:589–601.

Veenstra J, Rietra PJ, Coster JM, Slaats E and Dirks-Go S (1994) Seasonal variations in the occurrence of *Vibrio vulnificus* along the Dutch coast. *Epidemiol Infect* **112**:285–290.

Velazquez O, Stetler HC, Avila C, Ornelas G, Alvarez C, Hadler SC, Bradley DW, and Sepulveda J (1990) Epidemic transmission of enterically transmitted non-A, non-B hepatitis in Mexico, 1986–1987. *JAMA* **263**:3281–3285.

Vesey G, Slade JS, Byrne M, Sheperd K, Dennis PJ and Fricker CR (1993) Routine monitoring of *Cryptosporidium* oocysts in water using flow cytometry. *J Appl Bacteriol* **75**:87–90.

Vesey G, Hutton P, Champion A, Ashbolt N, Williams KL, Warton A and Veal D (1994) Application of flow cytometric methods for the routine detection of cryptosporidium and giardia in water. *Cytometry* **16**:1–6.

Vig BK, Figueroa ML, Cornforth MN and Kenkins SH (1984) Chromosome studies in human subjects chronically exposed to arsenic in drinking water. *Am J Ind Med* **6**:325–338.

Virtanen SM, Jaakkola L, Rasanen L, Ylonen K, Aro A, Lounamaa R, Akerblom HK and Tuomilehto J (1994) Nitrate and nitrite intake and the risk for type 1 diabetes in Finnish children. Childhood Diabetes in Finland Study Group. *Diabet Med* **11**:656–662.

Visser LG, Polderman AM and Stuiver PC (1995) Outbreak of schistosomiasis among travelers returning from Mali, West Africa. *Clin Infect Dis* **20**:280–285.

Visvesvara GS and Stehr-Green JK (1990) Epidemiology of free-living ameba infections. *J Protozool* **37**:25S–33S.

Vogt RL, Sours HE, Barrett T, Feldman RA, Dickinson RJ and Witherell L (1982a) Campylobacter enteritis associated with contaminated water. *Ann Intern Med* **96**:292–296.

Vogt RL, Witherell L, LaRue D and Klaucke L (1982b) Acute fluoride poisoning associated with an on-site fluoridator in a Vermont elementary school. *Am J Public Health* **72**:1168–1169.

Vogt RL, Little AA, Spitalny KC and Visvesvara G (1984) Investigation of a waterborne outbreak of giardiasis using serologic testing by IFA. *Am J Public Health* **74**:272.

Vogt RL, Hudson PJ, Orciari L, Heun EM and Woods TC (1987) Legionnaires' disease and a whirlpool-spa. *Ann Intern Med* **107**:596.

Von Mühlendahl K and Lange H (1994) Copper and childhood cirrhosis. *Lancet* **344**:1515–1516.

Von Reyn CF, Waddell RD, Eaton T, Arbeit RD, Maslow JN, Barber TW,

Brindle RJ, Gilks CF, Lumio J, Lähdevirta J, Ranki A, Dawson D and Falkinham JO 3rd (1993) Isolation of *Mycobacterium avium* complex from water in the United States, Finland, Zaire, and Kenya. *J Clin Microbiol* **31**:3227–3230.

Von Reyn CF, Maslow JN, Barber TW, O'Falkinham JO 3rd and Arbeit RD (1994) Persistent colonisation of potable water as a source of *Mycobacterium avium* infection in AIDS. *Lancet* **343**:1137–1141.

Von Schirnding YER, Kfir R, Cabelli V, Franklin L and Joubert G (1992). Morbidity among bathers exposed to polluted seawater: a prospective study. *S Afr Med J* **81**:543–546.

Voss LM, Rhodes KH and Johnson KA (1992) Musculoskeletal and soft tissue *Aeromonas* infection: an environmental disease. *Mayo Clin Proc* **67**:422–427.

Vrati S, Giri DK, Parida SK and Talwar GP (1992) An epidemic of non-A, non-B hepatitis in South Delhi: epidemiological studies and transmission of the disease to rhesus monkeys. *Arch Virol* **125**:319–326.

Wagner SL, Maliner JS, Morton WE and Braman RS (1979) Skin cancer and arsenical intoxication from well water. *Arch Dermatol* **115**:1205–1207.

Waldbott GL (1981) Mass intoxication from accidental overfluoridation of drinking water. *Clin Toxicol* **18**:531–541.

Walker JT, Sonesson A, Keevil CW and White DC (1993) Detection of *Legionella pneumophila* in biofilms containing a complex microbial consortium by gas chromatography-mass spectrometry analysis of genus-specific hydroxy fatty acids. *FEMS Microbiol Lett* **113**:139–144.

Wallace RJ Jr (1987) Nontuberculous mycobacteria and water: a love affair with increasing clinical importance. *Infect Dis Clin North Am* **1**:677–686.

Wang X, Liu X, Tan C, Liu R, Luo S, Yue X, Qin F, Bu Z, Tian X, Song D, Qing J and Luo K (1990) Epidemic non-A, non-B hepatitis in Xinjiang. *Chin Med J* **103**:890–898.

Ward MK, Feest TG, Ellis HA, Parkinson IS, Kerr DNS, Herrington J and Goode GL (1978) Osteomalacic dialysis osteodystrophy: evidence for a water-borne aetiological agent probably aluminium. *Lancet* **i**:841–845.

Warnakulasuriya KA, Balasuriya S, Perera PA and Peiris LC (1992) Determining optimal levels of fluoride in drinking water for hot dry climates – a case study in Sri Lanka. *Community Dent Oral Epidemiol* **20**:364–367.

Watts SJ (1986) Human behaviour and the transmission of dracunculiasis: a case study from the Ilorin area of Nigeria. *Int J Epidemiol* **15**:252–256.

Way JS, Josephson KL, Pillai SD, Abbaszadegan M, Gerba CP and Pepper IL (1993) Specific detection of *Salmonella* spp. by multiplex polymerase chain reaction. *Appl Environ Microbiol* **59**:1473–1479.

Weber JT, Mintz ED, Canizares R, Semiglia A, Gomez I, Sempertegui R, Davila A, Greene KD, Puhr ND, Cameron DN, Tenover FC, Barrett TJ, Bean NH, Ivey C, Tauxe RV and Blake PA (1994) Epidemic cholera in Ecuador: multidrug-resistance and transmission by water and sea-food. *Epidemiol Infect* **112**:1–11.

Wechsler LS, Checkoway H, Franklin GM and Costa LG (1991) A pilot study of occupational and environmental risk factors for Parkinson's disease. *Neurotoxicology* **12**:387–392.

Weinstein P, Macaitis M, Walker C and Cameron S (1993) Cryptosporidial diarrhoea in South Australia: an exploratory case-control study of risk factors for transmission. *Med J Aust* **158**:117–119.

Weisenburger DD (1993) Potential health consequences of ground-water contamination by nitrates in Nebraska. *Nebr Med J* **78**:7–10.

Weissman JB, Craun GF, Lawrence DN, Pollard RA, Saslaw MS and Gangarosa EJ (1976) An epidemic of gastroenteritis traced to a contaminated public water supply. *Am J Epidemiol* **103**:391–398.

Wellings FM, Amuso PT, Chang SL and Lewis AL (1977) Isolation and identification of pathogenic *Naegleria* from Florida lakes. *Appl Environ Microbiol* **34**:661–667.

Welty TK, Freni-Titulaer L, Zack MM, Weber P, Sippel J, Huete N, Justice J, Dever D and Murphy MA (1986) Effects of exposure to salty drinking water in an Arizona community. Cardiovascular mortality, hypertension prevalence, and relationships between blood pressure and sodium intake. *JAMA* **255**:622–626.

Weniger BG, Blaser MJ, Gedrose J, Lippy EC and Juranek DD (1983) An outbreak of waterborne giardiasis associated with heavy water runoff due to warm weather and volcanic ashfall. *Am J Public Health* **73**:868–872.

West PA (1989) The human pathogenic vibrios – a public health update with environmental perspectives. *Epidemiol Infect* **103**:1–34.

West PA, Millar MR and Tompkins DS (1992) Effects of physical environment on survival of *Helicobacter pylori*. *J Clin Pathol* **45**:228–231.

Wettstein A, Aeppli J, Gautschi K and Peters M (1991) Failure to find a relationship between mnestic skills of octogenarians and aluminium in drinking water. *Int Arch Occup Environ Health* **63**:97–103.

White FMM and Pedersen AT (1976) Epidemic shigellosis on a worktrain in Labrador. *Can Med Assoc J* **115**:647–649.

Whorton MD, Wong O, Morgan RW and Gordon N (1989) An epidemiologic investigation of birth outcomes in relation to dibromochloropropane contamination in drinking water in Fresno County, California, USA. *Int Arch Occup Environ Health* **61**:403–407.

Wigle DT, Mao Y, Semenciw R, Smith MH and Toft P (1986) Contaminants in drinking water and cancer risks in Canadian cities. *Can J Public Health* **77**:335–342.

Wiley R, Wolfe D, Flahart R, Konigsberg C and Silverman PR (1992) Cercarial dermatitis outbreak at a State Park – Delaware, 1991. *MMWR* **41**:225–228.

Wilkins JR 3rd and Comstock GW (1981) Source of drinking water at home and site-specific cancer incidence in Washington County, Maryland. *Am J Epidemiol* **114**:178–189.

Wilkins JR 3rd, Reiches NA and Krusé CW (1979) Organic chemical contaminants in drinking water and cancer. *Am J Epidemiol* **110**:420–448.

Williams LA and La Rock PA (1985) Temporal occurrence of *Vibrio* species and *monas hydrophila* estuarine sediments. *Appl Environ Microbiol* **50**:1490–1495.

Wilson R, Anderson LJ, Holman RC, Gary GW and Greenberg HB (1982) Waterborne gastroenteritis due to the Norwalk agent: clinical and epidemiological investigation. *Am J Public Health* **72**:72–74.

Wishart DL (1986) Leukemia and radium groundwater contamination. *JAMA* **255**:901–902.

Wolfe M, Parenti D, Pollner J, Kobrine A and Schwartz A (1993) Schistosomiasis in US peace corps volunteers – Malawi, 1992. *MMWR* **42**:565–570.

Wones RG, Stadler BL and Frohman LA (1990) Lack of effect of drinking water barium on cardiovascular risk factors. *Environ Health Perspect* **85**:355–359.

Wong O, Morgan RW, Whorton MD, Gordon N and Kheifets L (1989) Ecological analyses and case-control studies of gastric cancer and leukaemia in relation to DBCP in drinking water in Fresno County, California. *Brit J Ind Med* **46**:521–528.

Wood DJ, Cooper C, Stevens J and Edwardson J (1988) Bone mass and dementia in hip fracture patients from areas with different aluminium concentrations in water supplies. *Age Ageing* **17**:415–419.

World Health Organization (1984) *Guidelines for Drinking-Water Quality*, vol 2, *Health Criteria and Other Supporting Information*. World Health Organization, Geneva.

Wrensch M, Swan S, Lipscomb J, Epstein D, Fenster L, Claxton K, Murphy PJ, Shuster D and Neutra R (1990a) Pregnancy outcomes in women potentially exposed to solvent-contaminated drinking water in San Jose, California. *Am J Epidemiol* **131**:283–300.

Wrensch M, Swan S, Murphy PJ, Lipscomb J, Claxton K, Epstein D and Neutra R (1990b) Hydrogeological assessment of exposure to solvent-contaminated drinking water: pregnancy outcomes in relation to exposure. *Arch Environ Health* **45**:210–216.

Wrensch M, Swan SH, Lipscomb J, Epstein DM, Neutra RR and Fenster L (1992) Spontaneous abortions and birth defects related to tap and bottled water use, San Jose, California, 1980–1985. *Epidemiology* **3**:99–103.

Wright RA, Spencer HC, Brodsky RE and Vernon TM (1977) Giardiasis in Colorado: an epidemiological study. *Am J Epidemiol* **105**:330–336.

Wu M-M, Kuo T-L, Hwang Y-H and Chen C-J (1989) Dose–response relation between arsenic concentration in well water and mortality from cancers and vascular diseases. *Am J Epidemiol* **130**:1123–1132.

Wurtz RM, Kocka FE, Peters CS, Weldon-Linne CM, Kuritza A and Yungbluth P (1993) Clinical characteristics of seven cases of diarrhea associated with a novel acid-fast organism in the stool. *Clin Infect Dis* **16**:136–138.

Yajko DM, Chin DP, Gonzalez PC, Nassos PS, Hopewell PC, Reingold AL, Horsburgh CR Jr, Yakrus MA, Ostroff SM and Hadley WK (1995) *Mycobacterium avium* complex in water, food, and soil samples collected from the environment of HIV-infected individuals. *J Acquir Immune Defic Syndr Human Retrovirol* **9**:176–182.

Yamamoto H, Hashimoto Y and Ezaki T (1993) Comparison of detection methods for *Legionella* species in environmental water by colony isolation, fluorescent antibody staining and polymerase chain reaction. *Microbiol Immunol* **37**:617–622.

Yeh F-S (1989) Primary liver cancer in Guangxi. In: Tang Z-Y, Wu M-C and Xia S-S (eds.) *Primary Liver Cancer*. China Academic Publishers, Beijing, pp 223–236.

Yoshpe-Purer Y and Golderman S (1987) Occurrence of *Staphylococcus aureus* and *Pseudomonas aeruginosa* in Israeli coastal water. *Appl Environ Microbiol* **53**:1138–1141.

Young TB, Kanarek MS and Tsiatis AA (1981) Epidemiologic study of drinking water chlorination and Wisconsin female cancer mortality. *J Natl Cancer Inst* **67**:1191–1198.

Young TB, Wolf DA and Kanarek MS (1987) Case-control study of colon cancer and drinking water trihalomethanes in Wisconsin. *Int J Epidemiol* **16**:190–197.

Yu S-Z (1989) Drinking water and primary liver cancer. In: Tang Z-Y, Wu M-C and Xia S-S (eds.) *Primary Liver Cancer*. China Academic Publishers, Beijing, pp 30–37.

Yu Y, Taylor PR, Li J-Y, Dawsey SM, Wang G-Q, Guo W-D, Wang W, Liu B-Q, Blot WJ, Shen Q and Li B (1993) Retrospective cohort study of risk-factors for oesophageal cancer in Linxian, People's Republic of China. *Cancer Causes Control* **4**:195–202.

Zacheus OM and Martikainen PJ (1994) Occurrence of legionellae in hot water distribution systems of Finnish apartment buildings. *Can J Microbiol* **40**:993–999.

Zhaowu W, Kaiming B, Liping Y, Guifeng Y, Jinhua Z and Qili L (1993) Factors contributing to reinfection with *Schistosomiasis japonica* after treatment in the lake region of China. *Acta Trop* **54**:83–88.

Zhu Y-R, Chen J-G and Huang X-Y (1989) Hepatocellular carcinoma in Qidong County. In: Tang Z-Y, Wu M-C and Xia S-S (eds.) *Primary Liver Cancer*. China Academic Publishers, Beijing, pp. 204–222.

Zierler S, Feingold L, Danley RA and Craun G (1988a) Bladder cancer in Massachusetts related to chlorinated and chloraminated drinking water: a case-control study. *Arch Environ Health* **43**:195–200.

Zierler S, Theodore M, Cohen A and Rothman KJ (1988b) Chemical quality of maternal drinking water and congenital heart disease. *Int J Epidemiol* **17**:589–594.

Zmirou D, Ferley JP, Collin JF, Charrel M and Berlin J (1987) A follow-up study of gastro-intestinal diseases related to bacteriologically substandard drinking water. *Am J Public Health* **77**:582–584.

Zuckerman AJ and Harrison TJ (1995) Hepatitis viruses. In: Zuckerman AJ, Banatvala JE and Pattison JR (eds.) *Principles and Practice of Clinical Virology*, 3rd edn. John Wiley and Sons, London, pp 153–187.

Index